LIFE MORE ABUNDANT

THE SCIENCE OF ZHINENG QIGONG

PRINCIPLES AND PRACTICE

PRONOUNCED THE MOST EFFECTIVE HEALTH-ENCHANCING
QIGONG IN CHINA BY THE CHINESE SPORTS BUREAU

BASED ON THE ORIGINAL TEACHINGS
OF
MING PANG

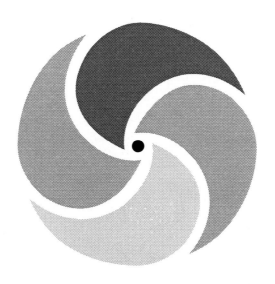

A GUIDE AND SOURCEBOOK FOR THE WEST

ENGLISH VERSION, NOTES AND COMMENTARY BY
XIAOGUANG JIN AND JOSEPH MARCELLO

LIFE MORE ABUNDANT

THE SCIENCE OF ZHINENG QIGONG

PRINCIPLES AND PRACTICE

BASED ON THE ORIGINAL TEACHINGS
OF
MING PANG

A GUIDE AND SOURCEBOOK FOR THE WEST

ENGLISH VERSION, NOTES AND COMMENTARY BY
XIAOGUANG JIN AND JOSEPH MARCELLO

1999

Editorial Assistant, Lynne Walker
Photographers, Guangbin Jiang and Yao Shen
Graphic Layout, Elizabeth Bonney
Photographer for Joseph Marcello's picture – Dominic Cavallaro

Xiaoguang Jin:
Jane_ZQS@yahoo.com
http://clubs.yahoo.com/clubs/zhinengqigongscienceinstitute

Joseph Marcello:
Marcello@shaysnet.com

ISBN 0-7414-0073-1

Published by:

Buy Books on the web.com
519 West Lancaster Avenue
Haverford, PA 19041-1413
Info@buybooksontheweb.com
www.buybooksontheweb.com
Toll-free (877) BUY BOOK
Local Phone (610) 520-2500

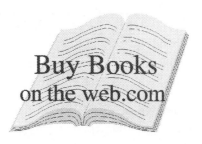

Printed in the United States of America

Printed on Recycled Paper

Published November-1999

Authors' Prefaces (1)

In China, for over the course of more than a decade, earth-shaking changes have been taking place in the realm of chigong (Chigong, Qigong, Chikung), and an unprecedented opportunity has arisen in its historical evolution, manifesting in the following ways:

1) A multitude of tens of millions of chigong practitioners has arisen. The traditional, once esoteric forms of chigong practiced by the sages and initiates have, in our day, become openly known and commonly practiced.

2) In its research upon the miraculous phenomena emerging from the practice of chigong, the achievements of modern science have provided incontrovertible evidence of the objective existence of chi.

3) The various benefits of chigong practice (the prevention and healing of illness, the attainment of longevity, the perfecting of mind and body, the development of higher intelligence, and other related benefits) have been rudimentarily, yet at the same time, comprehensively presented.

4) Chigong has developed from the stage of internal chi development (personal practice for the attainment of strength and health) to the stage of external chi development (exploiting the use of chi in one's personal practice and in the treating of others, as well as in other applications). It has evolved from the traditional stage of self-cultivation to the contemporary stage, wherein one benefits both oneself and others.

5) Both in their theories and their practice methods, almost all schools of practice have correspondingly reformed their traditional forms of chigong to meet the needs of the contemporary era.

Zhineng Qigong (The Cultivation of Intelligence-Energy) was born amidst the fervor of the great mass reform of traditional chigongs. Its emergence further promoted the development of chigong's potential. Zhineng Qigong has inherited the essential wisdom of those traditional chigongs - chigongs stemming from Confucianism, Buddhism, Taoism, Traditional Chinese Medicine, traditional martial arts, and folk religions. From ancient Chinese civilizations, as well as from the explorations of modern science, medicine and philosophy, it has also absorbed into itself the philosophical essence of the Concept of Entirety - The Oneness of Man and Nature.

In Zhineng Qigong, a thorough and integrated system of theory has been established and diverse levels of well-arranged practice methods, both easy to learn and to practice, have been created and compiled.

The Chi Field Technique (*Zuchang*) - a unique, broad-scale and highly effective teaching method - has been created, designed to establish and augment an intelligent energy field for the purpose of teaching and treating small and large groups of people. Moreover, the practices and principles of Zhineng Qigong have been synthesized with the development of the cultural and ideological realms of life, setting as their goal the liberation of the whole of mankind from poverty, illness and ignorance. This now enables chigong to take on a radically new image, as the paths of traditional chigongs are guided onto the broad highway of Zhineng Qigong Science.

In China at present, the development of Zhineng Qigong is spreading like raging wildfire. However, this is only the prelude to the emergence of a powerful and impressive science of Zhineng Qigong. In order to meet the present upsurge in the development of chigong science, and because chigong science is an empirical one based upon practice, it becomes necessary to develop thoroughgoing and widespread activities of mass practice. However, this alone is not enough, because chigong science is at the same time also a highly rational science; it possesses not only its own unique methodology and research methods, but also has its own unique methodological foundation. This is the essential difference distinguishing chigong science from other modern sciences. Because of this, chigong practitioners must raise the levels of both their comprehension of chigong theory and their personal accomplishment in chigong science. This will aid chigong in developing along the paths of a true science, as well as help to liberate the active mass practice of chigong from its confinement to a single method or skill, and guide that practice into the realm of chigong science.

This series of Zhineng Qigong textbooks has been written in order to meet the needs of fellow Zhineng Qigong practitioners of diverse levels; it follows the publication of *Popular Textbook of Zhineng Donggong Practice Methods* and *Brief Zhineng Qigongology* (a secondary textbook) and consists of the technical theories and fundamental applications of Zhineng Qigong science. There exists a total of nine volumes:

(1) *An Introduction to Zhineng Qigong Science.*
(2) *Fundamentals of Zhineng Qigong Science - The Hunyuan Entirety Theory.*
(3) *Essences of Zhineng Qigong Science.*
(4) *Practice Methodology of Zhineng Qigong Science.*

(5) *Technique of Zhineng Qigong Science - Superintelligence.*
(6) *A Summary of Traditional Qigongs.*
(7) *Qigong and Human Cultures.*
(8) *A Brief Introduction to Chinese Qigong History.*
(9) *Modern Scientific Research on Qigong.*

The subject matter of this series of textbooks is arranged in accord with the teaching requirements of students of Zhineng Qigong at the college level. *An Introduction to Zhineng Qigong Science* sets forth in general fashion the intentions and extensions of chigong, chigong science and Zhineng Qigong science. The unique characteristics of chigong science are also explored with reference to its research methods, methodology and methodological foundation, as well as to its relationship with modern science. The position and significance of chigong science in human civilization (especially in the realm of epistemology) are explored. This is a document of guiding principles and should be conscientiously studied and comprehended by every Zhineng Qigong researcher.

Essences of Zhineng Qigong Science embraces the quintessential principles of Zhineng Qigong. The profound mysteries of both Zhineng Qigong and traditional chigongs are analyzed with regard to such diverse areas as consciousness, cultivation, breath control and postural requirements, all of which have both inherited and further developed the essences handed down by traditional forms of chigong. In this text, not only is the general nature of a great many Chinese chigong sects - each having its unique strong points – explored, but revealed also are many formerly strictly guarded secrets of practice within these sects.

It must be especially pointed out that, in the chapter dealing with *The Exploitation of Consciousness*, the formation and the laws of the processes of consciousness, as well as its influences upon the activities of human life, have been deeply and completely explained. This part presents a totally new context in the field of chigong science. It declines the idealist and theist concepts of consciousness, and posits instead a dialectical materialist paradigm. Many subtle nuances pertaining to consciousness, which in the past were incapable of being properly described and expressed, and which could be grasped only through one's power of intuition, have been illuminated. This part then provides a text for readers to study, examples to follow, and methods to practice.

This is of immense impact and significance to the great majority of general practitioners presently practicing chigong, not only in the development of the ability to gather and transmit external chi to others, and in the acquisition of various supersensory perceptions and telekinesis, but also for undertaking advanced practice in the future.

In the above text, the two following points have been explored in detail, in accordance with ancient records and books, as well as the author's own personal experience in practice: understanding 1) the essential nature of various illusions experienced as a result of one's progress in chigong, and 2) the mysterious phenomena that may be experienced in distinguishing between the real and the unreal in one's chigong practice. This has not only broken with the existence of superstitious beliefs in chigong, but has also led the way to a higher practice discipline. This is an illusion-dispelling, barrier-breaking wisdom which must be diligently studied by every practitioner who wishes to explore the profundities of Zhineng Qigong.

The two textbooks - *An Introduction to Zhineng Qigong Science* and *Essences of Zhineng Qigong Science*, in fact, fall into the same category of general treatises of Zhineng Qigong Science (these can as well be regarded as the general treatises of Chigong Science). The general laws of chigong science, which are also the laws and conditions common to all sects of chigong, are presented; they are the essences of chigong and the common lifeline linking all types of chigong.

In the process of reviewing the various sects of chigong, if one understands this point, one may realize that there have been neither lofty chigongs nor lowly chigongs, but rather that every sect has emerged from the same source. With thoughts such as these guiding one's practice, one may make rapid progress, much like a hot knife slicing through butter.

In the textbook *Fundamentals of Zhineng Qigong Science - The Hunyuan Entirety Theory*, the Hunyuan Entirety Theory has, to a great extent, been explained. It consists of the following chapters: Hunyuan Theory, Entirety Theory, Human Hunyuan Chi, The Theory of Consciousness, The Theory of Morality, The Theory of Optimized Human Life and the Hunyuan Concept of Therapeutics.

The Hunyuan Entirety Theory is the theoretical basis upon which Zhineng Qigong science relies for its progress and development. It is also a world view and methodology according to which superintelligence and the objective world mutually act upon each other. It is the outcome of the combination of the ancient Chinese concepts of the entirety of life synthesized with the views of contemporary scientific thinking; it also represents the distillation of the chigong practice of the multitudes. Though there are many aspects within it that need further substantiation and perfecting, the Hunyuan Entirety Principle, by itself, has developed into a theoretical system of great integrity.

In the textbook *Practice Methodology of Zhineng Qigong Science*, the theory and methods of practice pertaining to the first three levels of Zhineng Qigong are introduced in detail, with both textual explanations and detailed illustrations. This book is both a good teacher and a helpful friend to practitioners of Zhineng Qigong.

In *Technique of Zhineng Qigong Science - Superintelligence*, the theory, practice methods and techniques for the implementation of the superintelligence of Zhineng Qigong science are introduced in detail. In the subject areas of chigong diagnosis (including super-vision, supersensory perception, remote-diagnosis) and chigong therapy (including external chi healing, remote-healing, and group-healing), the principles of diagnosis and healing are discussed in detail not only at a theoretical level; practice methods and practical secrets by which superintelligence can be quickly attained are also completely and unreservedly unveiled. Even if one has no teacher at one's side to give instruction, one can still quickly master the techniques so long as one practices conscientiously and in accordance with the methods introduced in this book.

In the textbook, *A Summary of Traditional Qigongs*, a number of traditional Great Vehicle chigongs are briefly and succinctly introduced. Most of these practice methods were handed down by the author's own teachers. Through the study of this book, not only can the reader grasp a general knowledge of the essence of traditional chigongs; she can also be clear about the factual origins of a number of traditional chigongs from which and upon whose foundations careful improvements and refinements in Zhineng Qigong science have been made.

A Brief Introduction to Chinese Qigong History introduces the history of Chinese chigongs - an evolution that has undergone a complete developmental spiral through "the negation of negation", from the simple to the complex and finally, from the complex to the simple.

In the remaining two books - *Qigong and Human Cultures* and *Modern Scientific Research on Qigong*, the little-known yet vital role the standing chigong has played in the past, presently plays, and shall play in the future, are comprehensively studied against the entire background of both ancient and modern civilizations.

It needs to be pointed out, with regard to a number of subtle and profound theoretical problems discussed in this series of textbooks, that although the author has tried to describe and explain them either in simple and accessible language, the sharing of examples from life, or in the use of existing scientific terminology, there are still many terms, phrases, and theories, that cannot be easily understood. This is because chigong science is a recently created science in the sense commonly understood by ordinary people; for most, there exists as yet neither the rational knowledge of chigong science nor the practical experience of chigong as empirical perceptual knowledge.

In fact, at the time of its own presentation, every innovative and epoch-making scientific theory failed to be comprehended and accepted by the reigning common sense of its time. Is this not so? For example, early in the beginning of this century, how many people understood Einstein's explanation of his theory of relativity? Now, not so very long afterwards, the theory of relativity has become an important concept in higher physics.

In 1946 in Brussels, when Blackett, a winner of the Nobel Prize in Physics, presented his paper on non-reversible phenomena in thermodynamics, not only was the new theory not comprehended - it was also vigorously opposed. A famous expert in thermodynamics even satirized Blackett in a questioning tone, "Isn't it a waste of time to study such things that vanish in a twinkle?" Nowadays - decades later, the concepts of non-reversibility, non-linearity and non-stability have not only become major issues attracting many interested people, but represent concepts that have also permeated or are in the process of permeating a number of different fields of science. Although this new science of chigong is not as unfamiliar to the Chinese as the above-mentioned once-new scientific theories were to their audiences, it still represents a totally new field in modern science. It is inevitable that people will initially feel at odds with it. But we believe that the correctness and soundness of its views and theories will be understood and accepted retrospectively, in hindsight of people's personal practice of chigong.

The last point to be made is that all of the theories and practice methods of Zhineng Qigong have been newly created. Although they have stood the test of the practice of millions of people, they still constitute a relatively recent undertaking, and one which needs further perfecting. So there must of necessity be some imperfections in this series of textbooks of Zhineng Qigong science as well.

The author has a heartfelt hope that other fellow practitioners in chigong circles can share their sincere comments and criticism, and that this may help chigong to play a greater role both in the enhancement of the mental, spiritual and physical health of human beings, as well as in the development of human civilization.

Ming Pang
May 1992

Authors' Prefaces (2)

1. Testimony

It was the cold winter of 1994, and I had just finished the last remaining metallurgical experiments for my doctoral dissertation. I had been recently diagnosed with serious neurasthenia and a wasting stomach inflammation. My stomach ached day and night, and even after resorting to sleeping pills, I went sleepless. I was extremely thin, weak and pale of face, and at a height of 5 feet, 7 inches, weighed just over 85 pounds. I could only take liquid meals. Worst of all, months earlier and prior to this diagnosis my husband had left Qin Huang Dao to do his post-doctoral research in Germany. It was my nine-year old son who prepared my meals for me when I was too weak to get up.

I was finally forced to give up writing my doctoral dissertation, and I turned first to Western medicine; it was ineffective, and the bad news from the doctors and nurses was that this disease was hard to cure completely and might develop into stomach cancer if the condition persisted too long. Two months later, I turned to Chinese medicine. It was more effective than Western medicine, but I was still too weak to resume work on my doctoral dissertation. Another two months passed; I was so anxious to obtain my doctoral degree that this terrible disease made me almost desperate.

Just at this critical period, a last hope entered my mind - chigong. There were four kinds of chigongs then being practiced on the campus of Yanshan University. Most of the practitioners were housewives, retired faculty and staff; there were also many graduate and undergraduate students among them. I had never believed in the healing effectiveness of chigong before that time; I just took it to be a tool for maintaining one's health - but not a healing art, to say nothing of a kind of science. And I didn't like the religious background of most of the chigongs, as I was educated to believe in no deities. Fortunately, one of my master's thesis classmates, Jiang Wenguang, now a post-doctoral researcher in Great Britain, recommended Zhineng Qigong to me in a three-hour conversation we had just after I had received the diagnosis for my condition. But even though he told me Zhineng Qigong had healed his serious kidney disease, I just laughed at him. I put away all the books he gave me and instead asked help from the doctors. I knew he was an officer of the Association of Zhineng

Qigong Science at Yanshan University, but I always thought he was a little bit not-quite-right-in-the-head.

One Friday afternoon, I noticed the posting of a free group healing activity given by the Association of Zhineng Qigong Science at Yanshan University.

Though I held strong prejudices against chigong, I couldn't resist the temptation to give it a try, being in such despair that, in my mental anguish, I thought of ending my life. That Saturday afternoon I found myself in a classroom with about fifty other participants, of whom I recognized only two or three as familiar, including Jiang. I felt shy and uneasy in what to me seemed so strange and peculiar a community. When Jiang began to establish a chi field, I still couldn't stop my mind from wandering away with doubts and curiosity. Then I heard a man's deep voice emerging from the tape player, giving directions for performing the exercises. I came to know later that this was the 45-minute tape of the Lift Chi Up and Pour Chi Down Method (*Peng Qi Guan Ding Fa*). Because I knew nothing about it at all, I couldn't help opening my eyes to see what the others were doing. Everyone was standing there, eyes closed, looking calm and reverent. I was assailed by a sense of guilt, and I immediately closed my eyes too.

Then I heard " Be humble and respectful . . . it is now the time to change your fate and to bring a bright future and destiny to yourself . . . ." I felt warm throughout my whole body, and a feeling of hope and gratitude arose from the depths of my heart. I was fascinated by that loving voice, and listened with rapt attention.

Suddenly, I saw a beam of red light within my head, and felt an unbearable pain in my stomach; I nearly fell down, and was helped up by a lady standing beside me. She was frightened by my pale, sweating face and called over two student practitioners. They immediately emitted chi into my stomach through both my head and my *Mingmen* point (though I didn't know what they were doing at the time). I began to feel better and sat there until the end of the whole 45-minute Lift Chi Up and Pour Chi Down exercise. Then all of the practitioners began to minister energy (*Fa-qi*) to those who wished to receive it. I was treated for the second time and I felt much better.

At the end of the healing session, I told my classmate my unusual experience during the gathering. He was delighted and told me that was caused by chi, and that chi had worked upon me! I had been too weak to stand the intense chi field, and thus had experienced a strong reaction. He assured that it was a good sign and that I would sleep very well that night.

He suggested that I should participate in their group practices every day in order to bring about a complete healing. I returned home full of hope and expectation. I did indeed have a deep sleep, and, since then, I've never doubted the existence and the effectiveness of chi. All my prejudices against chigong were gone. I threw myself into the group exercises, body and soul, practicing more than three hours every day, in the morning and evening, never once missing practice during my first two years.

It may be difficult to imagine all that my fellow Zhineng Qigong practitioners were doing at that time: 45 minutes of the Lift Chi Up and Pour Chi Down Method, 30 minutes - and sometimes one hour - of the Three Centers Merge Standing Form (*San Xin Bing Zhan Zhuang*), 90 minutes of The Body and Mind Form (*Xing Shen Zhuang*), 15 minutes of *Chen* Chi (one of the Eight Methods of Cultivating Chi), and dozens of wall squats (*Dun Qiang*).

At the beginning it was too hard for me to follow them; usually I would have to rest five minutes before I could do another five minutes of practice, but I never gave up. My stomachaches vanished almost unconsciously, and I could sleep well.

One month later, I resumed my work on my doctoral dissertation, and subsequently obtained my doctoral degree in December 1995. But I was not satisfied just to obtain my recovery; I wanted to know why it had happened. All of my spare time was then devoted to the study of Pang Laoshi's (Professor Ming Pang's) works, and I didn't miss an opportunity to participate in any available training programs. When I am unable to spend this much time in practicing the physical-movement forms, I continue to practice the mental and spiritual cultivation in my daily life and work.

2. Introduction

The Cultivation of Intelligence-Energy - Zhineng Qigong, founded by Professor Pang - (known by most North American practitioners as Chi-Lel™ *Qigong*), is one of the most popular new chigongs in China. Approximately ten million people practice it around the world every day. It has been officially certified by, and advocated by, the China Sports Bureau.

Over the past 10 years, more than 310,000 students (200,000 of whom were patients with various illnesses), have traveled to the Huaxia Zhineng Qigong Training Center, either to be healed or to be trained. The Center has achieved an overall healing effectiveness rate of 95% on more than 450 disease conditions. The applications of Zhineng Qigong science have also proven inspiring in many other fields.

No sooner had I arrived in the United States than I came to realize how little those in the West know about the broad-scale movement of chigong practice in China. There is an urgent need for authentic and accurate theoretical guidance among the Zhineng Qigong practitioners in the West.

I was surprised, after an investigation, to discover that there were no books introducing Professor Pang's works in English! Whereas Chinese practitioners regularly enjoy reading Professor Pang's books over and over again, English-speaking practitioners are restricted to taking notes from their teachers' oral instruction.

Although some practitioners have been practicing for a number of years, they still remain quite unclear about the principles underlying Zhineng Qigong science. A unique, totally new, highly advanced, complex and comprehensive science of life is thus mistaken for a simple self-healing skill.

As a Zhineng Qigong practitioner myself, I know quite well what Professor Pang's works mean to its practitioners. In the beginning, I never imagined that I might have undertaken a number of these translations and interpretations myself. I doubted that I could fulfill such a critical task in my second language - English, and again, with my relatively superficial understanding of Professor Pang's profound thoughts and insights. However, I received great support from a number of friends and practitioners, and finally found the faith to write down the first line.

Book II, The Science of Zhineng Qigong is a synthesis of the major theories and functional principles of Ming Pang's original text, freely rendered in contemporary Western language. A creative interpretation, faithful to the spirit and subtlety of Professor Pang's distilled thought has been chosen over a strictly literal translation. A subject-exposition style (different from the chapter-section style in the original Chinese textbook) has been adopted because of its convenience in quick referencing, freeing the author from the necessity of translating obscure ancient Chinese, excerpts of which Professor Pang includes in his works.

In the present English version, Professor Pang and the Center are first introduced to the reader. Following this, there is a detailed exposition of the basic concepts and definitions of chi and chigong, the unique features of chigong science and Zhineng Qigong science, and how best to practice Zhineng Qigong; following these there is an explanation of the relationship between chigong, Traditional Chinese Medicine, and special abilities. Finally the practice methods of the first level of practice (including practical extra disciplines) are presented, with accompanying illustrations.

Most of the present material was selected, translated and interpreted from two of Professor Pang's books - *An Introduction to Zhineng Qigong Science* and *Practice Methodology of Zhineng Qigong Science*; this has been augmented both by my own comprehension of Professor Pang's teachings, and insights drawn from my personal practice experience.

I would like to express my heartfelt gratitude to Ms. Lynne Walker for her proofreading, to Mr. Guangbin Jiang and Yao Shen for their photography, to Dr. Robert Hall Wagoner for hosting me at the Ohio State University, and to my friends and fellow practitioners, Shudong Liu, Tongyu Liu and many others in my Yahoo Zhineng Qigong Internet Club, who have offered their sincere support and enthusiastic encouragement.

My gratitude to Dr. Lin Jia and Ms. Yanfang Liu for their guidance in describing the acupuncture points.

This book is also for my husband, Dr. Yuli Liu, and my son, Kun Liu, who endured the pain of parting during my stay in the United States; for my father, Yongfu Jin, who clarified the ancient Chinese texts for me, and to my mother, Xiuzhen Wen, for her deep and everpresent love.

Finally, my inexpressible gratitude to Joseph Marcello, whose contributions to this work are irreplaceable and indispensable.

Although the material covered in this translation is only a very small part of the entire theoretical system of Zhineng Qigong science, I hope this guidebook will provide a relatively comprehensive introduction to this new science for English-speaking readers. The reader's comments and criticism are sincerely welcomed for the sake of future improvements in the present work.

Xiaoguang Jin
Columbus, Ohio
April 18, 1999

Authors' Prefaces (3)

*Life's end is not in a perfection that is final,
but in a completion that is endless.*

Sachindra Kumar Majumdar

The universe, and all within it, is a work in progress - including the world of mankind and its endless quest for understanding. With this in mind, the authors are keenly aware of the fact that the profundity of the treatise presented here - and the breadth of Professor Ming Pang's insight in general - almost certainly transcend their powers to faithfully render all of the subtleties and implications contained in a manner that does them the full justice they deserve.

That said, and while doubtless further refinements and clarifications remain to be made - both by ourselves or others committed to sharing this knowledge with mankind - we could no longer in good conscience countenance the painful and inequitable prospect of thousands – soon to be millions - of sincere, dedicated Western students any longer being deprived of the irreplaceable opportunity to study the writings and thoughts of Zhineng Qigong's founder, as he most certainly intended that they should.

To rely forever upon the wisdom of word-of-mouth - often received second- and third-hand - or upon knowledge derived solely through one's necessarily limited personal practice (or even that of one's friends and teachers) is both dangerous and needless, depriving one of the satisfaction of experience gained directly through personal initiative. This would be akin to living in a desert and forever being dependent upon certain more fortunately placed individuals who happen to have direct access to water. For such, the present volume presents a living well of great depth.

Thus, even with our present limitations of comprehension and experience, and with further insights yet to come, we have been impelled - both by our own personal hunger for knowledge as well as our inescapable sense of interconnectedness with our fellow human beings - to share these teachings, such as they are, with which all who wish to may at least begin the journey toward understanding - each for oneself, yet all together.

We willingly assume full responsibility for any omissions or misinterpretations found here, and we remain open to further enlightenment from any and every direction and source, consoled by the sincerity of our intent, the depth of our care, and the incalculable value of Ming Pang's wisdom.

It is crucial to bear in mind throughout the unfoldment of this rare document that it was conceived and written in a cultural climate long circumscribed by ideological strictures, and bound within a social framework largely unsympathetic to any but the most pragmatic and utilitarian aspects of art or science, and with a decided disinterest in spiritual truths.

It must be viewed to Ming Pang's credit not only that, amidst the volatile context of the Cultural Revolution, he succeeded in plumbing the profundities of man and nature, but that he succeeded so well, surviving, in the process, pressures which may have daunted a lesser spirit.

Thus, the Western reader may better understand the author's cultural proclivity for adopting a viewpoint which endeavors to interpret and resolve all phenomena, whether human, meta-human or cosmic, through recourse to unswervingly rationalistic conceptual structures.

In this light it may be easier to allow for the at times stringently pragmatic language with which the author attempts to convey highly subtle, if not manifestly transcendent dimensions of being.

The concluding irony in this historical intrigue is the ultimate salvation of chigong by the selfsame forces which initially threatened to erase it from Chinese culture, by virtue of their reliance upon its potent restorative and healing powers on virtually a daily basis. It is now well known that many of China's senior leaders were regularly treated by the ministrations of chigong masters, and were thus necessarily forced to spare chigong from exile - a living testimony, amidst a strategy of denial and suppression - of its seminal and life-giving potential for all mankind.

The path to awakening is never simple; I pay homage to my many teachers on the way: my mother, Angela Marcello, my brother Eugene Marcello, Sachindra Majumdar, Karlfried Graf von Durckheim, Vimala Thakar, Jiddu Krishnamurti, Roy Eugene Davis, Neville Goddard and Douglas Harding. With deep gratitude to Lynne Walker for her abiding faith, to Xiaoguang Jin for her great courage and trust, and to Ming Pang and Luke and Frank Chan for their profound commitment, I dedicate this work to those, like them, whose longing for Life cannot be quenched.

Joseph Marcello
Northfield, Massachusetts
April 21, 1999

Table of Contents

BOOK III - THE PRACTICE OF ZHINENG QIGONG

BOOK - IV LIVING WITH LIFE-ENERGY

The present volume consists of four distinct works, the centerpiece of which is *The Science of Zhineng Qigong*, a startling document by an individual of rare gifts who has given his life to the exploration of human life-energies - Professor Ming Pang.

Flanking this inspired exposition of revealed laws and principles, and fulfilling its promise, is *Life More Abundant*, a transcultural overview bridging the chasms of time, distance and custom, rooting those practices in Western tradition and illuminating them in their greater global context, and *The Practice of Zhineng Qigong: A Guide and Sourcebook for the West*, a manual of instruction for personal practice.

Following these, for the benefit of the serious student, is a volume of resources documenting a great number of ancient and contemporary life-energy enhancement modalities; while the traditional wisdoms are deeply respected, so too are the fruits of contemporary empirical research.

Finally, included are several rare and invaluable historical treatises on human health and vitality, offered by two Japanese masters, long unavailable in English. Taken all together, these gathered treasures may well offer mankind its best hope for the healing of the race.

BOOK I

LIFE MORE ABUNDANT

A GUIDE AND SOURCEBOOK FOR THE WEST

BY

JOSEPH MARCELLO

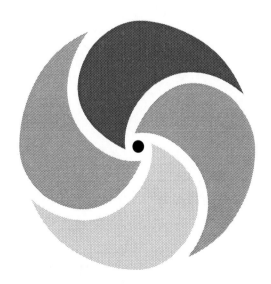

THE COSMIC CHALLENGE

The Power of Knowledge

Human life is like a shooting star amidst a timeless galaxy; brief, brilliant, and forever vanished. Its trajectory, however lofty, is seldom capable of fulfilling its arc of promise, its flame fading out too soon in the face of mortality and eternity.

The treasure of mankind has been its accumulation of dearly bought knowledge, and its supreme genius has been its invention of a system of sharing that knowledge with its individual members, by which the experience and insight of one can become the experience and insight of all.

Seen in this way, the journey of mankind is an ever loftier series of shooting stars, each born out of the promise of its predecessor, arcing ever more deeply into the recesses of the cosmos, each condensing within itself the luminescence of its forebears, and contributing its own.

In this way, there is hope for man in his endless quest into the mysteries of creation, and of his own being. He is no longer fated to merely repeat the weary evolution of his ancestors, and by extension, of the entire human race since the dawn of its emergence on earth.

Fortunately, neither all individuals nor all cultures were created with identical or even remotely similar desires, passions and life quests; a survey of global history reveals that different peoples and civilizations have mined and refined very unique and specific regions of natural, human and cosmic resources and potential. The legacy of China is truly profound.

THE INFINITE VOYAGE

Maps, Signposts and Wayshowers

The path to healing, though almost always a major life challenge, need not be a dark night of the soul - a stormy voyage upon uncharted seas without benefit of compass, moon or starlight.

While, if we are to become whole, the risks of the voyage must be made, and in the end made each alone, we would be wise to chart our course as the seafarers of old, by the maps of those who have gone before, and spent their lives upon these waters. They know the whereabouts of reefs and shoals, the lay of the shoreline, and the rhythms of tide and currents from long experience. Likewise, they know exactly why they cast an anchor or trim a mainsail, rig a rudder or heave into a storm wind.

How does this relate to the practice of Zhineng Qigong?

ENLIGHTENMENT OF BODY, MIND AND SPIRIT

The Totality of True Understanding

For those who are content to allow faith and trust to be their sole guiding forces, there need be no further inquiry; it is enough for them to obediently follow what they have been told and taught, leaving the rest to those they deem their betters, and to Providence - or chance.

But man is not only a being of feeling - even if that feeling be of faith; he is an indivisible entirety comprised of diverse and equally co-dynamic life principles - awareness, form, sensation, feeling, thought, memory and creativity - all of which are in ceaseless and synergistic intercourse with one another. However we may strive to fragment and isolate them, it is impossible to do so, for they are merely phases of one indivisible wave. Practice enlightens and fulfills theory, and to an equally important degree, theory illuminates and clarifies practice. To undertake the one without the other would be to attempt to walk with but one leg - and an awkward, unnatural and lopsided endeavor it would be. For beings of intelligence and cognition to forsake their powers of perception and discernment in favor of blind faith is only a disguised form of bondage - and not one enjoined by Ming Pang in his teaching, or for that matter, in his life. Rather are questioning and creative inquiry encouraged and addressed, for it is by and through this mutual exploration and response that human beings may best truly demonstrate their respect for one another, and that enlightenment may be shared in a dynamic and non-dogmatic way.

"Study to show thyself approved . . ." is a Biblical injunction equally applicable in any worthy field of study, Zhineng Qigong as well.

What this means is that, in such an entirety-being there is - and can be - no isolated or fragmentary experience of a thing, event, process or condition. Should a strong breeze suddenly chill the body, human consciousness will spontaneously and involuntarily probe into its source and reason; thus, sensation awakens cognition. Should a profoundly moving or troubling thought impinge upon one's awareness, instantly does the feeling nature respond in kind, and the metabolism; and so, cognition awakens feeling and sensation. Should a painful recollection arise from the deeper layers of the subconscious, immediately does the emotional nature reverberate, the mind simultaneously registers the disturbance with concern, and the body responds with tension; thus, memory awakens feeling, thought and sensation.

Despite our lack of complete awareness as often less-than-conscious beings, the truth is there are no mutually exclusive or isolated events in the human entirety field; it is indivisible and immanent, everywhere at once.

Thus, in practical terms, it is less than an ideal situation in which a person is limited to studying a thing or process in only one of its aspects, such as its practical or its theoretical aspect. By themselves, all individual aspects of a thing, process or system are fragmentary, even those which may provide obvious benefit, and with which we may be quite content.

This is no less true of the practice of Zhineng Qigong, which possesses a deep and seminal body of principles, theory, tradition, scientific documentation and practice wisdom. Professor Pang fully intended that these should constitute a living companion study to the practical instruction which has been handed down and generously shared with us. From the beginning, study, insight and the asking and exploration of innovative questions has been encouraged, with no restriction on the sharing of information, techniques, or relevant empirical data, no matter how provocative or revolutionary their implications.

FROM THE HUMAN TO THE SUPRAHUMAN

The Unfolding of the Cosmic Vision

In undertaking such a complete and multi-dimensional study, we can begin to realize the parallel evolution of all the facets of our being as a single, simultaneous whole. Now we too may know *why* we cast the anchor, or *why* we trim the mainsail, rig the rudder or heave into a storm wind. We know what we are doing, why we are doing it, where it came from and where it is leading us, and how we can illuminate and deepen our practice with the vision of the entirety of its vast underpinnings and expansive destiny.

Suddenly we may feel as if we have been given a marvelous pair of binoculars with which to gaze into the distant past, and a probing telescope with which to range ahead into the far-flung future, instantly transforming the moment-to-moment progress of our practice into a journey of truly breathtaking dimensions.

COMPASSION IN ACTION

The Liberation of the Mysteries

It has been erroneously assumed by some that concealment of such information, having long been the traditional approach with regard to many past practices, is the wisest choice. This was based upon caveats and protocols which have largely become obsolete and outmoded in our contemporary era of ever-expanding cultural global information-sharing. At their best, the ancient taboos on the revelation of such teachings were conceived out of a respect and a reverence for life, including the safety of those individuals seeking such knowledge; the purpose was the prevention of information concerning esoteric techniques involving the development and exploitation of various powers from falling into immature hands, with possibly injurious or even fatal consequences. Power was not to be wielded without wisdom and compassion, lest it become destructive.

At their worst, such hoarding of knowledge and harsh injunctions against its premature disclosure were motivated by human selfishness, suspicion, sectarian loyalties, and simple greed.

The time has long since come for the massive, needy body of humanity to come into possession of its inheritance - from all and any sources in which it may lie stored - in order to begin the journey back to wholeness. Esoteric provincialism and the cult of mystique have now come to the end of their fruitfulness, and are dying a lingering death.

Souls with a deep and genuine concern for humanity are arising, sifting the wheat from the chaff, and offering genuine spiritual nourishment to the people of the world. If defined by the fruits of his labors and nothing else - quite apart from any credentials or professed intentions - Professor Pang would have to be seriously counted among them, given the restoration and resurrection of lives experienced by the hundreds of thousands of suffering human beings who have had the good fortune to come into contact with him and his teaching.

In the past, he has been the first to encourage such free inquiry, and to fully address and explicate questions asked by the students and practitioners in their search for understanding. This is only reasonable, given that the development of human intelligence is among Ming Pang's most ardent endeavors. He well knows that without such active intelligence and understanding on the part of its practitioners, Zhineng Qigong will become prey to the dangers and temptations of mystery, myths, and illusions - the scourge of past qigong traditions.

In fact, in his attempts to clarify Zhineng Qigong theory for himself and others, he has availed himself liberally of the wisdom of modern Western science, derived parallel modes of thought as well as relevant frames of reference in which to couch his teachings.

THE DESTINY OF EAST AND WEST

The Twin-Spiraled Quest

While it would be unfortunate to harvest an orchard - or a wisdom - before its time, it would be an even greater misfortune to harvest it too late, or to fail to harvest it at all.

Much as the four millennia of wisdom of India has been harvested and put to fruitful practice in renewing and redeeming the lives of countless Westerners over the past half-century, so now is the harvest of China being threshed, milled and cast upon the waters of the West in forms too numerous to mention, and with equally great benefit, albeit it with some unavoidable trial and error.

To the West has been given the onus of the discovery and exploration of the world without - the cosmos - its functional laws and man's place within it, with an ultimate eye toward conscious creation of a new and higher order. To the East has been given the discovery and exploration of the world within, its respective functional laws, and of its place within man. While there are, inevitably, times and places where these exoteric and esoteric quests intersect and blend, they have, for the most part, existed in parallel, but estranged orbits since their primal parting.

Fortunately, these two traditions are not and need not be mutually exclusive or incompatible; they are, rather, complementary, forming two extensions of a single wave polarized in different directions and bound toward different destinations - the timeless wave of human consciousness in its quest to discover the truth of its world and itself, and to be free.

The distinct differences between East and West lie only in their respective convictions as to the direction in which the answer to this quest lies. The East has traditionally maintained that freedom is the result of inward knowing, while the West has been equally certain that outward understanding holds the ultimate conquest. Both have, by turns, succeeded admirably and failed miserably in their respective ways, depending on which

7

aspects of their respective life and cultures one chooses to view at any given time.

The esoteric fruits of Eastern explorers - while seldom matched by their Western counterparts - have largely been the harbored treasure of a privileged few, and until recently, inaccessible to the overwhelming majority of its peoples, who have continued to travail in relatively primitive conditions, and with correspondingly crude means. Thus, while the East may point to numerous examples of sages and adepts who have gone beyond the normal confines of mortal limitations, these amount to a minute fraction of the immense population of humanity, with its burgeoning burden of need and suffering, hunger and misery.

Conversely, the exoteric brilliance of the West - again, rarely equaled by any of its ancient or modern Eastern neighbors - has been its ability to create transpersonal structures and symbol-systems which enable the discoveries of one man here or there to become the legacy of all men everywhere; thus, while centuries of rhapsodic Hindu ragas have been invented and performed - often to mesmerizing effect - they have, in the absence of viable notational modalities, evaporated irretrievably into the mists of time, never to be heard since, whereas the transcendent polyphony of a Bach Brandenburg Concerto, once composed, is composed forever, and continues to grace the ears of earth for centuries yet to come - whether in Prague or Oslo, New York or Moscow - due to the universal reproduceability of the Western musical notation system. And so it is with medicine, architecture, agriculture, and a thousand other equally vital arts and sciences with which the West has endowed all the nations and cultures of the earth.

Now that these two waves of questing have come full circle, and as they begin to converge, it is the time for their inevitable reconciliation; neither succeeds fully on its own, however promising its merits, and neither can afford to exist without the fertilization and consummation provided by its estranged counterpart. Alone they are beguiling and fragmented; reunited they become seminal and complete.

THE GREAT REUNIFICATION OF BEING

The Marriage of Science and Spirit

The harvest of traditional Chinese energy wisdoms has now come under the structural aegis of contemporary science in a powerful and cogent way in the work and teaching of Ming Pang - a Grandmaster of traditional energy arts, or Qigong, as it is called in China.

Ming Pang has synthesized just such a hybrid. Culled and blended from a broad base of time-honored practices, shorn of all esoteric excesses and partisan peculiarities, Zhineng Qigong is the result of the wisdom of the ages as its path crosses the brightly lit fields of modern science, creating a practice eminently practical, a cultivation refreshingly lacking in cultism.

Daring to place itself under the searchlight of scientific scrutiny in the form of medical and para-medical technicians staffing its hospital at the Huaxia Zhineng Qigong Center in China, and treating an unceasing flow of patients numbering in the hundreds of thousands solely through the resources of chi, Zhineng Qigong has recently been pronounced the most effective health maintenance approach out of the most prominent traditional health practices by the China Sports Bureau.

Since energy is the common denominator of life and healing the world over, and as it has been since man's advent upon earth, it cannot be and never has been the sole possession of any one person, culture or nationality. Gifted individuals and age-old disciplines have evolved from all corners of the earth, from native American shamans and Indian gurus to African witch doctors and Chinese sages, all drawing upon the same reservoir of life. To see the unity in this diversity can be inspiring - at times even awe-inspiring: the phenomenon of humanity reaching out - and within - to reclaim that native force which is its birthright, and restoring wholeness to itself and its world.

Some have done it in humble ways, others in dramatic fashion. Some have been born with it, others have stumbled upon it on their journey. Some have been educated, others have not. Some have understood their gift, others have been mystified by it. Some have taught, others have remained silent.

But few, precious few if any, have been able to distill, standardize and share this power, and their wisdom concerning it, with the vast body of humankind.

It is here that Professor Pang's contribution attains perhaps its loftiest note, for in the depth and extent of his sharing, in the humility and power of his teaching, and in the rigorousness and efficacy of his approach, inclusive as it is of both science and tradition, his monumental work achieves a rare and remarkable universality.

THE UNITY OF ALL HEALING

The famous psychic seer Edgar Cayce, whose astoundingly accurate distance diagnoses and treatments for many illnesses are now successfully used by hundreds of mainstream physicians, gave the following invaluable insight:

> Know that all strength, all healing of every nature is the changing of the vibrations from within - the attuning of the Divine within the living tissue of a body to Creative Energies. This alone is healing. Whether it is accomplished by the use of drugs, the knife or whatnot, it is the attuning of the atomic structure of the living cellular force to its spiritual heritage, for all healing comes from the one source. (Reading 26961)

If this is so, then it becomes a simple matter to understand how all modalities and approaches - whether spiritual, secular, scientific or psychosomatic, in varying ways operate upon this one single dynamic - the heightening of the frequency of one's energy field. This may be effected through purer nutriments, physical exercise, breathing practices, emotional or psychological cleansing, electrical stimulation, chanting, fasting and prayer - to name just a few - but whatever the source or catalyst, the end result becomes the increased conductivity of the human system to the life-forces within, around and beyond it.

This enhanced conductivity enables a more unobstructed flow of force and substance by which the human psychophysical network maintains and renews itself, eliminating accumulations and blockages in the process, and maximizing its potential for optimal balance and function.

> Electricity or vibration is that same energy, same power, you call God . . . . that vibration that is creative is of that same energy as life itself. (Reading 2628-4)

In this light, we may view Zhineng Qigong as a practicum whose major purpose is the stimulation and renewal of the internal conductivity of the practitioner, in conjunction with the maximum receptivity of that practitioner to the vibrancy of the ambient life-field in which she exists.

And in this way we may easily and without internal conflicts resolve the seeming disparities of all the innumerable healing arts of mankind - Zhineng Qigong included - into one indivisible whole, preserving the integrity of each, yet maintaining an awareness of their ultimate unity.

ZHINENG QIGONG - THE CULTIVATION OF INTELLIGENT ENERGY

A Universal Offering

We - ordinary mortals for the most part - cannot be assured of finding just the perfect shaman; nor can we embark to the foothills of the Himalayas on a quest for the ultimate guru; we cannot be assured of the timely descent of the Holy Spirit - which falls and withdraws with alarming unpredictability, like a thief in the night - for the resolution of our needs; nor are we wise to depend upon the ever-burgeoning crop of premature psychics and soothsayers who are all too quick to attribute cosmic and 'karmic' dimensions to our personal sufferings - as if the source of creation had any need at all of its creatures' penitential agonies. And indeed, if there are lessons to be learned through such suffering, why should not such lessons be learned in a brief and telling moment - rather than a lifetime, allowing us then to heal, and to continue the adventure of life?

Respect and Compassion: Love in Action

It is obvious that a spirit of profound mutual support and cooperation embraces the shared environment of Zhineng Qigong practice. From one young Chinese woman, a Ph.D. research assistant, comes the following heartfelt description of life at the Center:

> I love the idea of sharing love and compassion with all the students. In the 24-day and 50-day healing classes, we treat the students as if they were our own fathers and mothers, sisters and brothers, sons and daughters. This loving chi, dominated by a clear healing intention, fills all of the Healing Center and results in amazing healing effects on the four to five thousand students. While in the Training Center, 16 training programs are available for the students of diverse levels.

11

We also share the love and brotherhood with the students taking the training programs. But, instead of healing, this loving chi is dominated by the clear intention to help the students to master various skills and abilities. Because students should first rid themselves of their illnesses at the Healing Center, they are then qualified to take training programs. Although the movements of every practice are the same, there are different requirements and strategies for those students wishing to be healed and those wishing to be trained, respectively.

While not a panacea, Zhineng Qigong does, at the very least, offer its participants the opportunity to address their destinies with their own hands, to set out upon a quest leading them in the direction of their own life-force, a quest which has been successfully executed by hundreds of thousands of prior travelers, and whose success they may eventually share. Without gurus, religious agendas or pecking orders, but rather with only the prosaic, perhaps slightly homely simplicity of the 'common man and woman', the 'salt of the earth', and those who have neither the background, training nor finances to be - or pretend to be - either exotic or subtle, exalted or arcane, the people of Zhineng Qigong simply hope, come, believe, follow, practice and, in great measure, receive. No one is excluded, all are encouraged, because all are part of the Greater Life.

What more can be asked of a teaching - or a practice?

A Total and Comprehensive Approach

This last pronouncement should extinguish the all too ready temptation on the part of energy-work eclectics to subsume Zhineng Qigong into a mindset that views it as yet 'just one more tool' in the ample arsenal of Qigong systems, with the misleading assumption that this too - in an age of patchwork, piecemeal disciplines - can be added to the stew.

However, such is not the case. Zhineng Qigong's impressive record - far and away superior to that of any presently examined method - could hardly be the random result of accident. Such dramatically effective outcomes, differing in quality and quantity from those of its peers, can only imply a mode of operation which differs distinctly and essentially from pre-existent methods of practice.

This, for some, is a difficult pill to swallow; they would prefer to carry on in the manner of adoring curators, collecting beloved additions to their ever-growing archives of esoteric - potentially life-saving - discoveries, deeming thereby that their lives have been further enriched; They may only dimly have begun to realize that, with the increasing ratio of treasures to time remaining, they may not have enough left to see the respective promise of these multiple treasures fulfilled in their life span.

It is a painful and intolerable thought to such inveterate esoteric hobbyists that perhaps these various practices may proceed along essentially and mutually incompatible lines; rather, the tendency of such well-meaning seekers is to hybridize and amalgamate, believing that they have further enriched their lot, and to move on to the next promising adventure.

This stubborn conviction arises from the perceived similarity between Zhineng Qigong and many of the chigongs of the past, such as those of Taoism, with their seemingly shared energy anatomies and modes of function. Nevertheless, if this were so, then the broad-scale effective results manifested by Zhineng Qigong would have been the results manifested by the prior methods - and they quite clearly are not.

While, in some instances, no overt damage may result from this eclectic approach, there is more than likely to be the less perceptible handicap of minimal or slow progress, or of poor results due to the neutralizing effect of crosscurrents or short-circuited energy. While Ming Pang is quite clear on the point that Zhineng Qigong works along essentially unique lines, and should not be assumed to function by the same model of operation as existent chigong practices, people will, as people always have, believe that which they wish to believe in order to do just as they wish to do.

However, Professor Pang is nothing if not respectful of others; rather than enjoining them to follow his way, he merely admonishes them that, should they find another practice effective, they continue to embrace it, and conversely, should they find this the case for Zhineng Qigong, then they should give it their sole allegiance.

On the less desirable side of the picture, an ongoing incompatibility of practices may generate mutually antagonistic energy strategies within one's organism, conflicting 'game plans' which neither enhance each other in their moment-to-moment sequence of deployment nor in their ultimate organic reverberations.

Thus, it is hoped that a word to the wise - if not always the humble - may be sufficient.

13

THE POWER OF SYNERGY -
THE INTELLIGENCE OF ENERGY

The Chi Field

It is true that special conditions are in effect in China which are not readily reproducible elsewhere, but this is no reason to discount the power of one's own endeavors wherever one may happen to be.

The phenomenon of the 'chi field' is perhaps the most potent of these. "Where two or more are gathered, there am I." While these are the words of Christ, this powerful saying might apply equally well to Zhineng Qigong; wherever a committed practice is consistently performed, particularly in concert with many others with whom one's intentions and actions are in harmonized resonance, a field of energy and intelligence (living information) is synergistically accumulated which far transcends the sum of its parts, and which manifests in at least two fundamental ways:

First, it exists as a reservoir of vibrant potential energy upon which the practitioners may draw, and which can be directed in any manner needed for the healing and 'wholing' of mankind.

Second, it exists as a self-sustained field of intelligent energy which, having complete and innate access to the organic information of all conditions and beings within that field, can spontaneously and dynamically manifest in a restorative, integrative healing manner without the express conscious direction of any particular individual associated with it, but rather by the synergy of the whole, just as, by force of gravity, floodwaters spontaneously seek to fill empty riverbeds. (In this second instance, it is not unlike the charismatic Christians' experience of the 'Holy Spirit', which, when achieving a critical intensity, moves and acts throughout the congregation in a highly spontaneous and dynamic manner, performing diverse healing and spiritually informational manifestations in different worshipers.)

While the magnitude and intensity of a chi field such as that generated by thousands of committed teachers and practitioners at the Huaxia center in China cannot be readily or easily duplicated elsewhere - relying as it does on the momentum of group intent sustained over a considerable time-span, this is not to say that it will not eventually be done, nor that a field of genuine presence and power cannot be formed wherever one happens to be.

HIGHER DIMENSIONS OF PRACTICE

The Total Exercise of One's Being, Body, Mind and Spirit

The true practice of any discipline, Zhineng Qigong included, cannot fail to impact all the layers of one's being. With this in mind, we should seek to approach our own practice with a quality of humility, wholehearted perseverance, and boundless faith.

The presence of nature is always a powerful starting place for such an endeavor, as is the company of those who share our spiritual intent. Simplicity, silence and humility allow the shedding of worldly cares and burdens, and a turning to the source. The practice of stillness and balance begin to align us with the axis of universal life, moving us beyond the limitations of anchorage in the personal realm, and through Imagination - spiritual perception - we begin to dissolve our ego boundaries, expanding our inner vision, sensation and beingness until we encompass the entirety of life.

Losing Oneself to Find Oneself

Slowly, softly, we practice. The world recedes into infinity. Tenderly, with floating hands, we probe the unknown, inviting its mystery within our own selves, like waiting children. Casting our impatience and our aggressiveness aside, we become like prayerful plants, extending our tendrils into the atmosphere to touch again, and be touched by, the power that gave - and still gives - us life.

Open, soft and surrendered, we feel all our quiescent vulnerabilities come alive within our physical, emotional and spiritual bodies, living reminders of all the shocks that flesh is heir to; yet we do not yield to the temptation to recoil, to close and to harden. This has been the way of humanity for too long, and to turn back now would be to return to imprisonment. Despite our trembling, we can only move forward, ever resurrendering and merging into dimensionless unity with that which lies within and beyond us.

Yet the emergence of these living and painful reminders of our past is no mere replay, nor evidence of our misbegotten practice, but an opening of the long-sealed Pandora's box of human woundings, and their offering up to the Greater Life which lies beyond.

The Merging of the Drop and the Ocean

In that Life lies, among other things, endless space, borderless dimension, which can and will easily accommodate and absorb that which so closely crowds, tortures and suffocates us within these little bodies and minds. It is precisely because we have knowingly or unknowingly chosen to harbor these conflicted energies, emotional shrapnel, scar tissues and congealed self-substances within this tiny mortal frame that it aches and heaves so fearfully and so desperately. We have never known, and no one has ever taught us, how to release ourselves and our contents to the primal self and content of the universe, and to invite and receive that One and its content within our own being.

Many have taught or preached of this bond, this life-connection, between what has variously been called the creator and the created, the manifest and the unmanifest, God and man, Universal Being and personal existence - but few have had the fortune to effectively transmit a sense of, and a feel for, its actuality to those they so ardently wished to help.

While an inspiring conception of such a relationship is a wonderful seed, it needs the soil of wisdom and the water of practice to insure its emergence into a sprout, a tendril, a leaf, a tree and finally a fruit - and a fruit with many new seeds for others.

Here is where Zhineng Qigong offers its deepest gift. Taking mankind where it is, in the realm of cognitive, religious, cultural and personal beliefs and concepts, it yet offers a palpable and practiceable method of re-establishing and enhancing its field of living energy, and in so doing insures that, organically, if subtly, those beliefs and concepts will dissolve, reform and deepen in accordance with the influx of new and vital energy and information moving within the mind, body and spirit.

CULTURAL HONESTY - THE PATH TO AUTHENTICITY AND POWER

To Thine Own Self Be True

However, while experience shapes belief, belief may also powerfully shape and filter experience. One culture, experiencing this influx of life force, may choose to interpret it in a purely scientific way, another, schooled in scriptural lore, will choose to proclaim it a purely metaphysical

16

phenomenon; those whose cultural conditioning has prohibited demonstrative emotional expression - as perhaps various Asian cultures - will, without knowing it, automatically interpret the phenomenon to be a non-emotional, entirely pragmatic process, while those whose programming has included deep immersion in the emotive realms of life, such as music and the arts, or those of the Romantic cultures, will spontaneously experience the most personal and intimate of encounters.

Many a dedicated Western explorer has foundered upon the shores of time-honored eastern disciplines due not to any shortcomings of knowledge, perseverance or technique, but rather due to a stoical but misguided belief that she could or should successfully adopt an essentially alien aesthetic without integrating its essence into her being by a process of intuitive insight and interpretation which allows for the dynamics involved (which are, to be sure, universal) to be absorbed and assimilated in the ontological aesthetic of her native soil.

No one truly can - or should - attempt to work against the overwhelming momentum of her cultural matrix by endeavoring to emulate either the personal, social or spiritual trappings of artificially adopted archetypes - at least no one for whom authenticity, creative power, and growing access to one's deeper self are vital.

While such cross-cultural infusions are undeniably enriching, of great beauty and penetrating wisdom, and serve to balance the often inhuman excesses of the crudest aspects of Western culture, (and the same may be said of the noblest aspects of Western culture with regard to its purification of the darkest aspects of the eastern world) - such psychospiritual 'grafting' almost always produces the severest negative reverberations at the deeper levels of one's being.

Though these are often slow in manifesting, manifest they will, and with a vengeance. In the words of C.G. Jung:

> An ancient adept has said, 'If the wrong man uses the right means, the right means work in the wrong way.' This Chinese saying, unfortunately all too true, stands in sharp contrast to our belief in the 'right' method irrespective of the man who applies it. *In reality, in such matters everything depends on the man and little or nothing on the method. For the method is merely the path, the direction taken by a man. The way he acts is the true expression of his nature. If it ceases to be this, then the method is nothing more than an affectation, something artificially added, rootless and sapless, serving only the illegiti-*

17

mate goal of self-deception. It becomes a means of fooling one-self and of evading what may perhaps be the implacable law of one's being. (Author's italics, J.M.) This is far removed from the earth-born quality and sincerity of Chinese thought. On the contrary, it is a denial of one's own being, self-betrayal to strange and unclean gods, a cowardly trick for the purpose of usurping psychic superiority, everything in fact which is profoundly to the meaning of the Chinese 'method'. For *(in the latter case)* these insights result from a way of life that is complete, genuine, and true in the fullest sense; they are insights coming from that ancient, cultural life of China which has grown consistently and coherently from the deepest instincts, and which, for us, is forever remote and impossible to imitate. .

However this does not mean that we cannot be fertilized, enriched and transformed by such insights and their related practices nor, ultimately, that we, perhaps in a way yet unknown, may not carry them to an even greater pinnacle of perfection and power by cross-fertilizing them with the seeds of our own considerable, complex and growing body of learning from the fields of science, spirituality and transpersonal psychology.

Yet the explorer, the seeker, the one so fertilized and catalyzed, must ever breathe the air of her homeland and express herself in the language of her native heart - even in the process of taking into herself the fruits of foreign cultural orchards, or, to the degree she fails to do this, pay the irretrievable price of her own self-betrayal.

While these may be natural, necessary and right for those living within such traditions, brocaded garments, tea ceremonies, severe formal observances, shaven heads and chronically stoical demeanors, when self-consciously adopted by others, may point to a deeper underlying cultural insecurity and immaturity, not too unlike children beguiled into a game of cross-cultural 'pretend' - in which the spontaneity of true life is all but extinguished, and by which the much cherished fruit withers on the vine. In such carefully enacted cultural emulations there is no redeeming upsurge of life from the deep, with all its spontaneous power and originality, because the living rhythms of the native cultural soil by which one has been nourished have been rejected, tied off at the root, and abandoned.

There can be no argument that the Western world needs its own psychic, spiritual and practical equivalents of these practices and traditions, and the genuine fruits that they offer - but if they are to have any hope of spontaneously thriving within our lives they must be undertaken and integrated in a culturally authentic manner.

Obviously it is possible, with seemingly total fidelity, to adopt foreign disciplines, philosophies and cosmologies into one's being, but the total 'success' of such a thorough graft is only prelude to the completeness of its eventual failure to truly nourish us in a way that does not turn our lives into effigy.

Let the buyer - the seeker - then *truly* beware. Let her learn deeply, accurately and thoroughly all that there is given to know, and let her, in a spirit of humility, neither adulterate nor re-prioritize that which she has learned. But, above all, let her exercise the intuitive capacity to extract the essence of what she has learned from its time-bound and culture-encrusted containers so that she is left with a practice - and not a prison.

It is in this spirit that we have chosen to describe the present work as *A Guide and Sourcebook for the West*. While there exist some words which have, due to the uniqueness of their meaning, become viable English terms - such as *chi* - there are many others that need not and should not be carried over, lest we add a head to the one we have already.

Likewise, and more importantly, we would do well to have an awareness of the distinct cultural patterns through which Zhineng Qigong has arrived upon our shores, and which need form no subtle or overt part of our adoption of the practice itself.

THE NEW WORLD

North America: The Polycultural Paradox

Deriving as it does largely from the eastern and western European, African and Latin cultures, as well as its own indigenous tribal cultures, the persona of the North American continent is blended from powerful expressive colors, despite the more internalized natures of some of its Nordic inhabitants; bold and extroverted, with, for better and worse, strong individuality and creativity, forging their paths amidst a pluralistic society such as the other nations of the world could never have dreamed. Young, pragmatic, impetuous, idealistic, at times brash and blundering and then again, brilliant and generous, American culture continues to defy all confining molds.

In every way the antithesis of the stepchild of the New World, China has evolved by slow growth, earth-bound toil, long patience in the presence of hardship, an abiding gentility of spirit amidst a virtual cultural homogeneity, with an almost uncanny conformity of the individual to the group-life which subsumes any individual autonomy or behavioral anomaly. Humble, hardy, self-effacing and possessed of profound respect for life and for the authority of the social system, the Chinese culture is slow to share, much less scatter, the precious content of its humbly nurtured heart, lest it disquiet the hearts of others by its excess.

It consistently amazes Westerners to see just how content - and even happy - Chinese peoples can be in finding their lives embraced, governed and fulfilled by an almost childlike group obedience to club, committee, society and state. Yet those caught up in Western culture may also find themselves wistfully wishing for such ready fellowship and peer acceptance.

Conversely, the Chinese may gaze upon their Western counterparts and wonder at the wanton excesses which the cult of individualism has wrought upon the shallow-rooted society of the West, with its endangerment of person, family, social good and planet. Yet those under the yoke of Eastern cultural sanctions may privately hunger to feel the exhilaration of such rarely experienced personal freedom and creativity.

Without weighing the relative merits of these imponderables, it is enough to know that these essential and profound differences cut at the quick of the shared humanity of East and West, and vital to honor them in both ourselves and others.

Coming Home

What this means in practical terms is that in order to be successful in one's practice of Zhineng Qigong, one need neither be, act, think, eat, live nor relate as if somehow one were in even the remotest way Chinese - because in fact, the essence and functioning of chi - or intelligent energy - is neither Chinese nor of any other national pedigree - but a universal, transcultural fact.

So let us not sacrifice our natural ways, our personal uniqueness, our native language and our pioneer spirit as Westerners by succumbing to the all too easy temptation to make the fateful spiritual trade, for there is nothing to gain and much to lose thereby.

20

PURITY, PASSION AND PERSEVERANCE

Native Liabilities and True Commitment

Having said that, there are some uniquely Western pitfalls to overcome, if one is to avoid compromising the great potential inherent in the practice of Zhineng Qigong. The first is adulteration. It is with good reason that Professor Pang has admonished against combining Zhineng Qigong with the practice of other chigongs.

A second area of strategic importance is the issue of perseverance. It has been said, not entirely without truth, by those Chinese practitioners who have had both experience at the Huaxia center and in the United States, that Westerners cannot stand hardship. Heard the wrong way, this statement might seem to give reason for offense; after all, America was created out of hardship, has fought her wars encountering severe hardships, and continues today to address the newly emergent hardships of the world in countless ways. Have her people suddenly become weak-willed and spineless? What can the statement mean?

Through heavy reliance upon technology, a great number of contemporary Westerners have become accustomed to expecting instantaneous results in many areas of their lives, from quick fixes in medicine to instant gratification in areas as diverse as entertainment and relationship. The idea of slow, organic growth through time and self-initiative, cycled through the seasons of nature, has largely been replaced by an instantaneous- quantum-leap world view; this is but the illegitimate stepchild of the sound bite mentality promulgated by the popular media and the computer culture.

Beneath these blatant, all too visible layers of American society there exists a deep substratum of immensely seminal human beings working just beyond the confines of media-driven cultural conventions; original and independent, energetic and resourceful, awake to the subtleties of life, aware of the need for sustained focus and self-effort, and committed to living by the highest human values, they provide and sustain the core of practices, disciplines and lifestyles which fertilize not only their own lives, but - through the American's uncanny gift of synthesizing pluralistic streams of human knowledge - the life and new birth of the entire world.

Going Beyond Limitations

Many Chinese witnesses have shared the most moving testimonies of the commitment, courage and dogged persistence with which the simplest of people – peasants, housewives, students or grandmothers - have undertaken their practice of Zhineng Qigong. Some ailing, some in critical condition, some on the verge of death, some unable to support their bodies in an upright position, practicing on their backs or tethered upright to posts or trees, persevering day and night against seemingly insuperable odds - lifelong chronic conditions, personal fears, fatal diagnoses and unspoken temptations to suicide; - yet all of them working, practicing, willing themselves onward through pain and weakness, and through all of the tortures of the damned which assail the minds of those for whom hope has been abandoned.

A moving account of one Western practitioner now teaching in the Midwest provides but a brief glimpse of this tenacity for life:

A few days later, we were participating as a group in the Three Centers Merge Standing method with perhaps two hundred or more students. I was in the stance listening to the sounds surrounding me, aware of the teachers quietly walking through the crowd correcting postures. I tried to ignore the agonizing pain in my body until I felt I could no longer continue. Then I began noticing sounds around me. A woman beside me was spitting and coughing up something, and had been for some time. A lady somewhere behind me was quietly vomiting. Yet they were not complaining, and continued. Why? They believed . . .

Shortly after an intense group session, an attractive Chinese woman approached me. Although I speak no Chinese, I was able to understand that she wanted to speak with my teacher, Luke Chan. I caught Luke's attention. As his gaze shifted from me to this woman there appeared to be no immediate recognition - until she began speaking to him. His eyes lit up; he threw his arms around her and asked to sit down and share her story. She explained that she came to the Center in 1993, paralyzed from the chest down. For the last ten years, her husband had gently rolled her body over every two hours to prevent bedsores. Incapable of caring for any of her personal needs, she was basically a vegetable. After five months at the Center, there was no change in her condition; in fact, she had become worse. Nevertheless, her husband continued to practice La Chi and administer Fa Chi to her daily. Luke asked her what had motivated her to continue. She remembered Pang Lao-Shi saying, "You never know when you may have spontaneous healing." She simply kept believing! Eventually she began to have slight feelings and movements in her fingertips. All the students in her dormitory gathered around her, giving her encouragement and congratulations. Shortly thereafter she was able to move her whole hand and then her arm, little by little regaining control of her body. Through perseverance, belief and daily practice, she gradually improved. Soon she was able to sit up and have her husband push her in a wheel chair to actively participate in the group sessions.

In 1995, Luke had videotaped a little girl, about five or six years old, demonstrating the wall stance. He continued to videotape this child as she walked to her grandmother, who was slumped in a wheelchair, and began lovingly administering Fa Chi. This feeble-looking grandmother is today the woman mentioned above. She can now stand upright, proudly beside her husband, and walks with the use of a cane. And, as her husband pointed out, not only is she walking, but all of her internal organs, which were previously dysfunctional, are now healthy. They both smiled proudly!

These vignettes provide us an important glimpse of just what a profound depth of faith and tenacity are possible for ordinary human beings who, more than anything, wish to retrieve their lives from the prison of illness, the limbo of hopelessness, or even the jaws of death. The humble heroism of such individuals offers an inspiration to all, the more so because they, for being so ordinary and human, might well be ourselves. And the moment we undertake the path that they have trodden, we become them.

Truly, the intensity of one's practice will be in direct proportion to the depth of one's sensed need, provided that faith lights the way. Even a desperate need will not result in a strong practice if faith is lacking. Faith illuminates the path ahead, and practice provides the momentum to walk it.

ZHINENG QIGONG IN THE NEW WORLD

Chi-Lel™ Qigong

Under the name of Chi-Lel™, and with the blessing of Professor Pang, Zhineng Qigong has begun to take firm root in American soil, due to the pioneering work of Luke Chan and his brother Frank, two individuals who have been creating a cross-continental network of practitioners through their ongoing one-, three- and six-day workshops and seminars. Dedicated, like Johnny Appleseed, to implanting the American landscape with seeds which will bear much wonderful fruit, these two committed teachers have, with integrity, humor and humanity, nurtured American Zhineng Qigong through its infancy, and are now guiding it into its first years of harvest.

Galvanized almost solely by Luke Chan's bold, moving translation of documented healing testimonies from the Huaxia Center, *101 Miracles of Natural Healing*, Zhineng Qigong, under the trade name of Chi-Lel™, succeeded in capturing the imagination of many American students and inspiring them with the faith to undertake practice.

Starting without benefit of a national awareness of chigong, such as exists in China, and having had to educate many of those who came in such subtle matters as *chi*, while at the same time bolstering their sometimes flagging efforts with encouraging words and ideas, Luke and Frank Chan have succeeded in an often alien territory, due largely to their passion for sharing the gift of Zhineng Qigong with others, as well as the genuine hunger of Western people for such knowledge.

Luke's approach to this task is refreshingly honest and direct:

> . . . After finishing my manuscript, I gave it to my editor for review and later received a call.
>
> "I like your stories, but. . . ," my editor hesitated.
>
> "Yes?"
>
> "They are *truly* incredible."
>
> "You don't believe them, do you?"
>
> "Of course I do, but it's the average American I'm thinking about. They might be turned off by these miracles. You want to sell books, don't you?"
>
> "Well, what's your advice?"

"You might want to tone them down."

As our conversation ended I felt unsure. Should I alter these interviews to make them seem more reasonable?

Then I recalled the emotion of a cancer patient who had been waiting three years to die because there wasn't any cure for his bladder cancer, and who finally, with the help of Chi-Lel™ was given a fighting chance to recover and live. And I thought of a woman who, when being told by doctors that she was just too old for any treatment, refused to give up and fought her deadly disease with Chi-Lel™ and finally survived to tell her story. Then there was the lady who had secretly practiced Chi-Lel™ at home for two years because she was afraid of being ridiculed for believing in miracles, and who, when she finally went to a group practice, was embraced and "welcomed home." How could I deny these stories of human triumph over suffering?

To change these accounts to suit average beliefs would be a denial of encouragement and hope to those who truly need it. So the stories in this book remain exactly as they were told to me. Furthermore, I will endeavor to compile a sequel - of miracles involving Americans who've had the courage to try and triumph with the help of Chi-Lel™.

Attempting in various ways to stem the Western student's penchant for theorizing and speculation, Luke and Frank have consistently concentrated on imparting the fundamentals of practice in a very personable, pragmatic manner. Their working strategy is simple: Do the practice correctly and faithfully, experience the benefits, and you will understand. But forever understanding and never practicing is only a recipe for frustration and failure.

In this light, one understands their decision to steer clear of the more esoteric aspects of practice, such as dramatic, difficult or controversial techniques and ideas which might threaten to distract new students from the task at hand - establishing a firm foundation of basic practice. It is an amusing and enlightening experience to watch Luke re-route an overly intellectual questioner's complicated queries, pointing his nose instead in the direction of simple, sustained practice - the avenue to all answers.

Their Chi-Lel™ workshops introduce participants to such core practices as Gathering Chi, Three Centers Merge Standing, Lift Chi Up and Pour Chi Down, Wall Squatting and the Level Two Body and Mind Form. The preparation is careful and the practice is closely monitored, so that each student comes into possession of a clear understanding of the forms, postures and movements, as well as a sense of the inner subtleties of relaxation, balance, body-tone and visualization techniques involved. A strong atmosphere of support, synergy and interconnectedness is created in the culminating activity of these workshops and seminars - the creation of chi field, followed by a group healing session in which all participate, well or ill, young and old, beginner and initiate. Thus has Professor Pang's vision begun to become a global reality.

Likewise, through their umbrella organization, Benefactor Press, they have made available both audiotapes and videotapes comprising an invaluable series of instructional materials covering all aspects of their teaching; these are to be highly recommended for both the novice and the initiate. Having the virtue of visual continuity and clarity, the videotapes offer immense benefit to those students who have yet to receive personal instruction, or those who wish to refine and perfect their technique through repeated exposure to Luke Chan's clearly articulated demonstration of the practices. In addition to these handsomely produced instructional videos, there is also available a series of audiotapes which feature Luke Chan's guided instruction in English, simultaneously layered over a recording of Professor Pang's resonant voice leading the same practice in Chinese. It is not possible to describe the electric effect of Ming Pang's potent voice in empowering one's own private practice; at times it sounds like the living expression of an ancient tree, or the deep vibration of an ocean wave, penetrating one's being. The sense of connection with Professor Pang becomes immediate and palpable, and one senses a renewed strength and faith.

In addition, Luke and Frank Chan are to be admired for their creation of a series of networking systems which bond together the Chi-Lel™ community and provide information, enlightenment and encouragement; 1) a quarterly newsletter, *Chi-Lel™, Qigong News*, which features articles by and about Americans who have been practicing Chi-Lel™ and experiencing recovery from illness and healing of many different disease conditions - and 2) an internet web site, complete with testimonials, workshop calendars and an online forum where students and practitioners share encouragement and information. Singlehandedly, these two guides have brought Zhineng Qigong into the front lines of the American healing scene, where it deserves to be, and have enhanced it with modern communication technologies.

The following is but a sampling of excerpts from the most recent of their many newsletters:

Good News From Santa Fe (GW):

It is time for another wonderful six-day retreat. I learned so much at the Sedona Retreat.

Sante Fe is really responding to Chi-Lel™, like mad. There are more than 150 at this point and at least five to ten new people come a day! We are practicing at a local fitness center that donated the space, since I am doing this free as a community service. My vision is that by summer every neighborhood park will have a group doing Chi-Lel™ there! It would be a lot like China, yes? We are already getting many testimonials. I am encouraging people to use the web site forum to spread the news. Here are some for you:

1. Jay: severe diabetes with sugar level at 400 when he started Chi-Lel™. Now, 35 days later, his blood sugar level is down to 150! He comes to the group daily and also is doing La Chi and Chi Massage and 30 wall squats a day.

2. Nina: with environmental illness, one of the first to start at my house, is now, four months later, no longer experiencing sensitivities to chemicals, smoke and fragrances. She is losing weight without changing her eating habits and she is happier than she has ever been.

3. Robin: dealing with bladder and kidney problems for seven years. Now the pain is gone and she can feel in her abdomen and she is roller-blading! She does wall squats and La Chi and Lift Chi Up and Pour Chi Down with the group.

4. Nicole came the first day depressed and suicidal. After we did the Lift Chi Up and Three Centers Combo tape, she said she felt a lot of pain in her nose and then heard a crack and her septum adjusted itself! She hasn't been able to breathe through her nose for 30 years! She also is no longer depressed and is joyful daily.

We did the Full Moon with 35 people last night! We send you love, chi and joy.

Hao-La!

As an inspiration of the depth of human endeavor possible, Luke Chan includes a cover article documenting the history - and updating the present status - of one Teacher Zhang: "As I read a recent letter from Teacher Zhang, I was filled with awe and respect. Her faith in Chi-Lel™ has rekindled my spirit to spread this wonderful art to the world. I hope you too, will find her letter uplifting. To give you some background, here is an excerpt of what Teacher Zhang told me in 1995." (Miracle #66 of *101 Miracles of Natural Healing*):

I stared at Teacher Zhang's youthful face in disbelief as she told me that she was sixty years old. Furthermore, she asserted that she had recovered from more than twenty illnesses. Seeing my amazement, Teacher Zhang showed me a faded photograph of herself taken almost thirty years ago. The picture showed her dark brown eyes resting in a hollow skull, staring into the camera. Her neatly combed hair and pretty dress couldn't cover the emptiness and suffering of a sick person.

"During the Cultural Revolution, my husband was branded as a 'poison weed' and our lives were turned upside down. Under such tremendous stress, I started to develop severe headaches, ringing in my ears, a running nose, and toothaches; I also had difficulty swallowing food. As time went on, my illnesses became more and more severe. I had kidney infections, and ulcers, spleen problems, arthritis, paralysis on the left side of my body, and an irregular heart rate."

"Were you very weak as a child?"

"No, I was a healthy child. Indeed, in school I was the envy of the other girls as I was an excellent sportswoman and a good singer. But in just a few years my illnesses turned me into an old woman who couldn't sing or walk. Wearing winter clothes year-round, I endured pain every day and I moved as if I were walking on a layer of water. Indeed my life was poisoned, and I was slowly choking to death."

"It must have been a very difficult time for you."

"Yes, it was and it became harder. Just as I thought I had seen the worst, my lungs contracted tuberculosis. Where before people hadn't cared about my illnesses because they were busy in their revolutionary activities, now I was despised and isolated because of my contagious disease. I stayed in the hospital for two and a half years.

"Then the good news came that the Gang of Four had fallen into disgrace and my family was resurrected as being innocent.

I was joyful as my mental pressure was released. However, my physical illnesses continued to plague me for another ten years."

"So when did you learn Chi-Lel™?"

"It was not until 1989 that I was introduced to Chi-Lel™ and I have loved it ever since my first week of practicing it."

"What do you mean?"

"After the first week of practicing my stomachache disappeared. With that encouragement, I began to take seriously by practicing the movements every day for long hours. It took me two years to conquer all my illnesses. Ultimately, four years ago, I became a teacher in the Center."

*　　*　　*

Dear Luke,

As you requested in your last letter, I am sharing with you my daily routine in the Center as a teacher.

I get up at 4:00 a.m. and practice Wall Squatting or Bend Body Arch Back (level two) until 5:30 a.m. before everyone gets up. Then I join the teachers' group practice from 5:40 a.m. to 7:00 a.m. We alternately practice different levels of Chi-Lel™.

After having breakfast, I lead our class to practice and F a Chi to our students for three and a half hours. (Teacher Zhang teaches a class of students facing the challenge of deafness.)

From 12:30 p.m. to 2:30 p.m. I have a two-hour nap time - these are the most treasured hours of the day! Then I will continue to teach class until 6 p.m.

After dinner, I practice with the same teachers' group from 7:20 to 8:30 p.m. For another hour, I will visit our students at their dorm to make sure everyone is okay. After all the students and other teachers go to bed at 10 p.m., I will practice Wall Squatting or Bend Body Arch Back for another hour and a half.

So I practice about 16 hours a day with only six hours sleep. I love it. The more I practice, the more energy I get. I'm 65 years old and I feel younger and younger. I don't need any medicine or needles. Every year I have one or two chi-reactions and I overcome them with more practice. Each time after the chi-reaction, my practice has reached another level.

Please tell my story to your Chi-Lel™ friends. I am a living proof that Chi-Lel™ works. I had suffered with more than twenty illnesses for decades but now I am free. I know I can live to more than a hundred. I believe Chi-Lel™ will bring health and happiness to the whole humankind.

Luke Chan concludes: "Teacher Zhang, we, too, believe Chi-Lel™ will bring much joy to the world. Thank you for being a guiding light. We love you."

Without the groundbreaking efforts and continuing support provided by Luke and Frank Chan, Benefactor Press, and a fast-growing core of instructors and practitioners throughout the United States and Canada, the reality of Chi-Lel™ - North American Zhineng Qigong - would still be only a dream.

Further reading:

Chan, Luke, *101 Miracles of Natural Healing*, Benefactor Press,
    Cincinnati, Ohio, 1996.
The Chi-Lel ™ Qigong News, Quarterly Journal, Benefactor Press,
    Cincinnati, Ohio.
Jahnke, Roger, *The Healer Within*, Harper San Francisco, 1997.

LIFE ENERGY AND THE VITAL CENTER OF MAN

In light of Zhineng Qigong's insistence on chi - intelligent life-energy - as the source and substance of all existing things, and also in light of the centralization of this life-substance within the human form in the *dantian* or lower belly - it is enlightening to find profound corroboration in the lifework of a contemporary Western master of the art of healing.

A famous American healer, William Gray, a man whose services were highly sought after by prestigious members of congress, the military and the Washington elite, and whose gifts and wisdom were the subject of a prolonged study by the physician Dena L. Smith, was the subject of two books by Ruth Montgomery.

Reliable witnesses, including doctors and nurses, have seen this man stop heart attacks, heal crippled arthritics, dissipate large tumors, arrest glaucoma, and rebuild a disintegrated jawbone, simply by placing his hand on what he terms the 'magnetic field' - that is, the lower abdomen or pelvic area.

With this declaration, Gray provides a stunning Western parallel to, and confirmation of, the energy traditions of the East.

Mr. Gray's otherwise excellent appearance was marred by a great protruding stomach, which I had assumed to be fat; but when I commented on the pump-like movement of the pulse in his forearm, he stood up and asked me to push my fist into his stomach. I couldn't even make a dent. To my surprise, it was as solid as bone. Mr. Gray answered my unspoken question by explaining that this was his over-developed magnetic field, from which he transmitted energy to those he healed.

Endowed from birth with unusual powers of healing and psychic perception, Gray spoke simply but eloquently of his perceptions:

"This is where you live," he says, as he lays the palm of his hand on that area. "In here is an intricate system, grouping together the main trunk nerves and their branches and relay systems which extend throughout the body. The lungs draw in the energy, but the magnetic field must draw the energy from the lungs in order to radiate it through the body. Everything is centered in the belly.

"The solar rays give us life, but the position of the planets at the time of birth makes us the individuals that we are. Characteristics and personality occur at conception; individuality occurs at birth. Your individuality is governed by your fixed sign. This establishes your magnetic field, which consists of three different frequencies derived from the Power of Powers. You are thereafter influenced by the vibrations of all the planets of this universe. We are no stronger than our magnetic field. Shortness of breath, irritability, and illness are among the signs that insufficient energy is being distributed. When the depletion of the magnetic field continues, the nerves are partially starved for their fuel or energy, creating spasms or nerve tension through the body. This depletion, unless corrected, can develop into serious ailments . . ."

Mr. Gray says that in the lower abdomen is the master brain, an intricate system forming the magnetic field . . . He says that some of the symptoms of insufficient energy distribution are shortness of breath, nervousness, confusion, restlessness, irritability, bloat, pain, and a feeling of heaviness. Their

31

intensity depends on the degree of depletion of the magnetic field, which is caused by fear, anger, hatred, shock, or improper or deficient nerve fueling.

"A child is born with a strong or a weak nervous system," he says, "which is determined at conception and is the result of his parents' energies. If the mother and father are of mated frequencies and are well and strong at the time the child is conceived, that child ordinarily has an easy birth and a strong, healthy nervous system. If the child is the result of mismated energy currents, and the future parents are nervous, discontented, or unhealthy, the baby usually has a weak nervous system, and may also have a difficult delivery. Because of this, he is the victim of low energy and nerve depletion for most of his life. But even when a child inherits a weak magnetic field, that tension can be released shortly after birth by someone with the properly blended energy who is able to convey this energy to the infant's magnetic field *so that the infant is freed from bondage and open to the universe, and is thereby able to draw his normal capacity of energy from the atmosphere.* (Author's italics J.M.)

As to the source of his great reservoir of healing energy, author Ruth Montgomery writes:

> . . . the boy frequently accompanied the doctor on his horse-and-buggy rounds, helping him to diagnose and treat sick patients. In school he was a lack-luster student. Instead of attending classes, he would slip off into the woods to make friends with bears and deer, or sit quietly beside the river, 'tuning in'.
>
> "Tuning in on what?" I prompted.
>
> "On the ring," he replied. At my look of puzzlement, he declared that a protective ring of energy encircles each planet and stores within it all knowledge since the beginning of time. He said all thoughts and inventions are "taken off the ring" and anyone who will listen properly can pick up whatever information he needs.
>
> "For as long as I can remember I have been receiving a continuous flow of information coming over the air from The Universal Ring of Wisdom, explaining the Ancient Wisdoms of life.

. . Receiving this information was always as constant and natural to me as breathing . . ."

How close this comes to Professor Ming Pang's description of the primordial information/energy field which engulfs planet earth, and upon which we begin to draw in our practice of Zhineng Qigong.

Gray continues:

"The theory of energy as the life-force and body activity is as old as the ages, and there are many well versed in the Ancient Wisdom to whom most of this is known. The world we live in is composed of gases and energy. All substance - plant, animal and human life - results from the unlimited combination of energy frequencies acting on these gases. Every plant, animal and human has its own individual energy frequency to establish and maintain life, growth, and development. At birth, the first breath of life is our direct supply, our lifeline with the Universal Power . . . Life itself! At any time that this energy flow is cut off from the magnetic field, the energy which originally sets this field becomes a part of the Power it came from. So long as this energy is established and flows through without obstruction, we are in tune with the Universal supply of energy."

THE THREE LIFE-CENTERS OF MAN

Heaven, Earth and Humanity

While many subtleties and subdivisions might be given, the primary vortexes of the human life force and its activity are embraced in the three essential energy centers: The Earth Center, the Human (or Personal or Heart) Center and the Heaven Center.

The Earth Center embraces the primordial, pre-human realm of natural forces and activities which embodies the origins and root-system of man's life on earth. It governs the instinctual, pre-rational and evolutionary levels of cosmic life, including the primal life of mankind.

The Heaven Center embraces the immanent, transcendent and meta-human dimensions of life, which comprise the ultimate potentialities of mankind, extending to realms beyond the terrestrial; it governs the superphysical, visionary and trans-evolutionary levels of life, embracing the cosmic totality, both manifest and unmanifest.

The Human or Personal Center embraces the marriage of the converging forces from the Earth Center and the Heaven Center, wherein a unique dynamic balance of time and eternity, place and infinity, and embodiment and transcendence is achieved, resulting in the antagonistic yet complementary life-polarity unique to human beings.

While the core and essence of the lives of the great majority of human beings is lived through the Personal or Heart Center and is heavily filtered through the various initial layers of the Heaven Center, such as the intellect, the social matrix, cultural and race conditioning, and psychospiritual archetypes, to a great extent that personal and cognitive life unconsciously draws upon the primal, pre-personal power of the Earth Center, from which it emerges like a lotus from the lake bottom, and from which it continuously - and often unknowingly - draws its sustenance.

Thus, it is in the finely balanced synergy between these three centers that the truly fruitful life is actualized.

While the initial practice of Zhineng Qigong does not dwell on the extended implications of transformations upon and within these three 'elixir-fields', and while it does not require even a rudimentary understanding of the effects of practice upon these three energy centers, it is, in fact, designed to directly impact each of them in turn.

Such movements as the push-pulls at shoulder level are involved with the circulation of life-force through the mid-body center, while, in their initial phase, those of pouring chi down clearly involve the upper center; the emphasis of yet other movements is upon drawing the flow of chi through the lower center. Ultimately the flow of movements and chi is felt to be integral and uninterrupted, proceeding throughout the entire body.

IMAGINATION - THE SECRET OF PRACTICE

If one were to distill the profundity of Ming Pang's insights and teachings on Zhineng Qigong into their purest essence, it might well be this:

The dynamic spiritualization of matter, and conversely, the dynamic materialization of spirit, are achieved through the conscious dilation of the human energy field unto the circumambient cosmic force-field within which it exists, re-establishing the heightened interchange of primordial unconditioned energy with conditioned human energy.

34

This comes eerily close to a palpable expression of Einstein's revelation of the reversibility of matter and energy.

Beyond the necessity for learning correct technique and following this up with consistent and correct practice in a spirit of sustained faith, there remains what may be considered in some senses that most vital element if one is to be successful in achieving the dual transmutation of spirit and substance in her practice of Zhineng Qigong: the faculty of Creative Imagination.

While it may be Einstein whose scientific thinking comes closest to the essence of Zhineng Qigong's transubstantiation of matter and energy (substance and spirit), it was also Einstein who stressed the necessity of transcending that very same process of scientific thinking.

How then, to go beyond this impasse?

The sage of science offered the answer - and not he alone - but innumerable sages and initiates from spiritual traditions of every origin:

Imagination is more important than knowledge.

- Albert Einstein

What he meant by this is that 'reality', at least insofar as it is ordinarily known, is more often than not, not a reflection of the universe's ultimate truth, but rather a statement only of mankind's present ability - or more precisely, inability - to perceive it. Anchored in the consensus of reality as generated and sustained by the group-mind of his time and culture, as well as by the limitations of his senses, man rarely succeeds in transcending the web of social and scientific fictions defining his existence on earth. For most, rather, this consensus is the 'way things are', and easily mistaken for reality.

By 'imagination' is not meant the vague and fantasied imagery of reverie, dream or rumination, but rather the clear and focused interior perception of a super-subtle sensory awareness that penetrates the veils of material manifestation, without yet violating them.

A wise man once said, "Imagination which is based upon reality is no imagination." This is to say, if an imaginal process is founded upon an underlying reality - such as a home builder trusting that he will find water where a skilled dowser has instructed him to excavate – and if water is indeed eventually forthcoming, then we may conclude that, while proceeding purely by faith and imagination, such efforts are actually rooted in deeper realities.

On a subtler level, this implies that imaginal exercise upon non-visible realities, such as internal or external energy centers and fields of force - far from being futile fancy - may yield very palpable fruits.

Thus, while imagination may be the passtime of fools, it may equally well become the workshop of reality. As such, it can play a vital and indispensable part in leading one to the shores of direct experience in one's inner quest. Man's habitual adoption of points of view and self-concepts which define and ultimately limit his life and potentialities has become such an unconscious process that he actually believes in the realities of the ideas - or imaginations - by which he imprisons himself.

Perhaps the deepest and most damaging of these assumptions is his utter assurance and conviction that he exists distinctly apart from the rest of creation, an autonomous and independent entity. This, though, is nothing more than a highly convincing illusion generated by his gift - or curse - of creative self-awareness, by which, if only in thought, he may conceive himself to be segregate, extracted from his larger body - the universe; as a result he is often compelled to exert an illusory control over the fathomless immensity from which he unknowingly draws his very life.

Due to this now pandemic habit of instinctually conceiving itself to be isolated from the body of creation - separate, cut-off, and opposed, humankind has for centuries been paying the costliest of prices - its aliveness, well-being and its spiritual health. Despite its ability to survive and endure such psychic and physical self-deprivation, it is questionable whether a life poised upon such a severe rupture in the fabric of creation can truly be called living. For many, it has spelled alienation, disease and even death - whether psychic or physical. Throughout the millennia, the formation and development of what man is pleased to call his 'self' has depended upon an antagonistic positioning of this little 'I' against the great 'I' of Being, until it has assumed the status of an incontrovertible reality. However, common sense - let alone true insight - would dictate that nothing can or does exist independently of its ground, its background and its immediate or extended interrelationships with its world - nor can or does its world exist independently of it. Further, this co-relationship is not merely the juxtaposition of mutually alien entities, but rather the ceaseless interplay of spatio-temporal phases of one totality in spontaneous communion and communication with itself at different levels. The human level, in overly exercising its powers of free will and cognitive consciousness, has come to focus excessively on the purely subjective side of this reality, losing touch with the true nature and dimension of the totality underlying and embracing its very being.

The human spirit now finds itself bound on one side by its imprisonment in the restrictive realm of body consciousness - replete with all the pleasures and agonies of sense life - and, in the psychospiritual dimension, confinement in national, tribal and personal identities which have divided it from its fellow creatures, its spiritual heritage as an heir of the universe, and its very self.

By the exercise of Creative Imagination - supersensory perception - the primal division between spirit and substance may be seen through and dissolved, the ancient wound healed, and mankind and the universe may be restored to wholeness.

PENETRATING THE VEIL OF MATTER

Sensation - The Phantom Foe

What our consciousness concludes about an experience is far more crucial than what is actually experienced, for by that conclusion - for good or for ill - and not the experience itself, hangs our very destiny.

A far greater number of human beings have failed in their struggle not so much from the reality of true defeat, (if in fact there be such a thing), but rather from private convictions of fatalistic proportions. The severest battles are fought - and won or lost - within the borders of the mind and the boundaries of the human will - the one force which can never be usurped by, overridden by, or deferred to, another.

However deep or shallow our sufferings, it is not so much the measurable weight of their burden that either prepares us for or prevents us from their ultimate conquest - but rather solely our inner convictions about them. We all know of individuals who have almost literally lifted themselves out of seeming hopelessness by dint of their own refusal to give up, redeeming themselves from situations which many another would have long since proclaimed hopeless. And conversely we have all come across people with relatively light burdens who, empty of faith, have glanced at the climb ahead and visibly trembled, turning wearily back to re-enter - and lock - their narrow prison-cells, utterly convinced of the cosmic immutability of their fate.

Within the parameters of this crucial difference lies the whole span of human life and death, success and failure, rebirth and self-entombment. Why does one woman shake her head wearily and surrender, while another lifts her eyes toward the horizon, vowing never to turn back? What subtle inner movement plunges one into the abyss, and the other toward the heights?

For want of a term, we may choose to call it the 'conclusivity of feeling' or the 'terminality of sensation'. What this attempts to describe is that almost indescribable internal sensing - uniquely different in each individual - which somehow conclusively and irreversibly confirms the finality of a given outcome in that individual's consciousness. It implies a point of inner threshold beyond which the subject either can not or will not conceive of herself as ever capable of proceeding. The question of whether or not this conviction may have reasonable or even overwhelming corroborating evidence is irrelevant with regard to the subjective attitude of such a person, because, upon closer inspection, it is not so much the prevailing evidence which contributes to the fatalistic conviction as it is the psychospiritual readiness to accept such a possibility.

Now, what creates such a readiness of acceptance for fatalistic outcomes in the lives of human beings? In very great part, if we take care to observe closely and carefully, we will see, both in ourselves and others, that the principle, process or syndrome which fully contains the power of beguiling us and capturing our awareness to such a dangerous and dizzying extent is founded upon the primacy of sensation - physiological, neurological or psychological experience as translated by the intellect and interpreted by the ego, functioning within the confines of a limited vision of human potential.

Since life first manifested in physical form, sensation has been the benchmark by which creatures - non-human and human, have calibrated their state of being, registered and responded to their environment, and related to their own psychophysical existences. Sensation has been the constant pre-technological computer read-out through which mankind has charted the warp and woof of its life on earth. It has been the common denominator of such diverse experiences as pleasure and pain, hunger and fulfillment, anxiety and ease, birth and death. Sensation - the unceasing data-flow of moment-to-moment existence, is, for the overwhelming majority of earth's population, the god of man's secret worship, the unvoiced reality he privately swears by. What the flesh says, what the body confirms, what the feelings reverberate - and finally, what the mind concludes - all these attain instant and unquestioned actuality in the consciousness of their beholder.

And what is wrong with this arrangement, then? Where would we be without it? To a great extent, mankind's survival depends upon the respect of and response to sensation - heat, cold, light, danger, and so on.

Only this: that a life bound and determined by sensation is a life which is bound and determined; that an existence for which sensation is lord and master is an existence which can never transcend the slavery of sensation; that sensation, however essential and needful for the balanced responses of life on earth, represents only an incomplete piece of the picture of man's totality, his entirety and fullness; that those - whether in Zhineng Qigong, in spiritual spheres or in the worldly walks - who dare to go beyond the limitations of sensation are those who, by that very definition, find themselves going beyond the limitations of sensation. This is not unlike the famed madness of the Wright brothers, who, unwilling to concede the obvious truth that nothing heavier than air could ever soar aloft, ultimately made of their madness a new type of genius which transcended the very limitations of the obvious.

What does this mean in practical terms? And what might it imply for us?

Each of us, either consciously or unconsciously so calibrates and judges his or her life in much the same manner at each point along the journey. It is vital - even while a prisoner - to realize that we are self-imprisoned, or if free, self-liberated. We may not in one courageous leap be willing to reverse the habits of a lifetime and to step beyond the bars of our cell bars which have never really been in place, but only remarkably well imagined; but at least we will begin to see where the secret of freedom lies - and in whose hands the judge's gavel has always been held.

When we are suffering, sensation naturally takes dominion over our awareness by its very bothersome, insistent or oppressive nature - and becomes the motive for our subsequent behaviors and life choices, including our spiritual practices. And while sensation bears some relation to the actual condition generating it, that relationship is not always directly proportionate nor even at times remotely congruent. The fact is, sensation is no arbiter of the ultimate or even temporary reality of a condition or situation. It is a creature of the nervous system as it interacts with the consciousness and becomes interpreted and filtered through the memory and the belief system of the individual personality. It is much like a hall of mirrors in a fun house; somewhere, in either remote space or time, there is or has been a source image - which now comes to be reverberated and refracted, proliferated and reconfigured in ways which bear little fidelity to its original and essential nature, but which nonetheless succeed in monopolizing the individual's field of awareness, including her thought and feeling and imaginal life. Thus, it comes to have a much greater power than it might otherwise have had, due to the magnification and self-corroborating phantom reality of its own making and sustaining.

In the face of this silent, persuasive phantom life, one may be sorely tempted to believe that nothing is succeeding, that little is happening, and that past conditions and causes are, if anything, as stubborn as ever; and with this comes the weakening of the personal will and the temptation to give up. One judges oneself and one's life by false standards - false because they are incomplete - and is incarcerated by one's own self-sentencing.

In fact, it is paradoxically the case that, the stronger and more pressing the sensations of various perceived conditions or imbalances become, the closer one may be to unraveling the illusion of the paper tiger of sensation. When one's life becomes open and permeable to healing energy, and the various layers of the subtle bodies are unveiled, a phenomenon is experienced in which one senses more clearly than ever the root cause of the condition or illness, as if one had just freshly experienced it - and this may be rapidly followed by the total dissolution of the entire symptom-complex, along with its attendant sensations. The inner bodies, being composed of progressively finer layers of energy, are the substance upon which the sensations have been so seemingly indelibly imprinted; until they have been accessed, penetrated and cleansed, they continue to convey re-stimulated phantom sensations consistent with the primal pattern of the wound or insult to the system.

HEALING OF THE INNER PERSON

The Effect of Zhineng Qigong on the Mind and Spirit

Until now, Western students have received relatively little or no information or instruction about how Zhineng Qigong practice impacts the mind, emotions and spirit. One reason for this is simply the much more dramatic and visible nature of physical healing, which causes the focus of attention to be limited solely to these areas. As yet there has been no opportunity for non-Chinese-speaking students to avail themselves of Professor Pang's writings on these subjects, due to the absence of translations.

Even so, one encounters virtually no open discussion of such matters even amongst the Chinese Zhineng Qigong practitioners due to the reserve and introversion so common to the national cultural temperament. It might well be considered a major indiscretion and moral failing to even hint at having such problems or issues, much less to openly share such delicate and long-veiled matters. In part this stems from the historical sublimation of psychic and emotional aspects in Chinese culture, leading to an internalization of this entire realm of life. The acknowledgment of the psychological and emotional dimensions of life - as such - has never been a tenet of Chinese culture; rather it has sought to explain and transform these dynamics either into physiological-energy phenomena on the one hand, or abstract metaphorical and spiritual principles on the other.

This in large part explains the virtual absence of psychologists, psychoanalysts, psychiatrists and other healers and explorers of the mind in Chinese society.

This, however, is no reason for Westerners to pretend that, after a lifetime of immersion in the psychological and emotional levels of life, they are not deeply imbued with, driven and shaped by them, and they are wise to include and address them in a dynamic way in their practice of Zhineng Qigong, and to do this without fear of concern that, because no such parallels seem to exist in the Eastern practice, they are somehow doing something wrong. Thus, if powerful or provocative emotions or insightful thoughts arise, these may (and should) be honored and taken as opportunities for inner transformation, without allowing them to compromise the integrity of one's practice.

This is all the more relevant when one ponders the fact that, with the cultivation and accumulation of more abundant internal chi or life-force, one may be inviting further suffering if one's views and attitudes toward life and the world have not undergone corresponding improvement. In fact, in China the emphasis is squarely placed upon parallel spiritual development along with chi-development, and many Chinese practitioners have been seen to benefit psychologically and spiritually by virtue of their practice of Zhineng Qigong, even after years of previous mental and emotional suffering.

THE LONG JOURNEY HOME

The First Step is the Last

The pilgrimage into self-healing and self-knowledge, like life itself, presents itself as a successive series of foothills – or perhaps mountains - each unfolding before our gaze as the seemingly final challenge to be surmounted - only to reveal, once we have scaled its summit, a further peak looming upon the horizon. Fortunately, the choice is not ours to make; just as we cannot take two breaths at once, nor live two moments together, so, no matter how great the distance or the endeavor to be made, we are always facing only a single challenge at any and every given moment of our lives - the one that lies before us.

Much as we might like, we cannot make all the steps at once, arriving suddenly (and perhaps prematurely) at the end of the adventure - a solution that would deprive us of incalculable opportunities for growth, human bonding, self-giving and serving, as well as of insights too numerous to mention; nor can we stand still, refusing to make a step, or pretending that there is no step which needs to be made - at least not without great danger of taking up residence in the 'City of the Living Dead'; for our spirits, in essence, are nothing if not creative.

Rather, we need to accept the moment-to-moment sacredness of ordinary life - the only life that we have been given to live, and to embrace its soft, slow, patient rhythm of growth; we need to trust the tiny, transient and seemingly inconsequential molecules of existence which comprise our daily walk as the means by which Being has chosen to manifest itself in time and space. In so doing, the unbearable loneliness of human existence opens out upon the headwaters of the immutable aloneness of universal consciousness; and while the joys and torments of the human realms are never to be avoided or escaped, they yet find their resolution in the embrace of a greater dimensionality which restores all that was deemed lost from the purely human point of view.

In a very real sense, then, getting there *is* being there; the journey *is* the destination; becoming *is* Being. The Universal Life reveals Itself as our very own moment-to-moment existence.

> *It is not in the stars to hold our destiny,*
> *but in ourselves.*

-William Shakespeare

BOOK II

THE
THEORY AND PRINCIPLES
OF
ZHINENG QIGONG

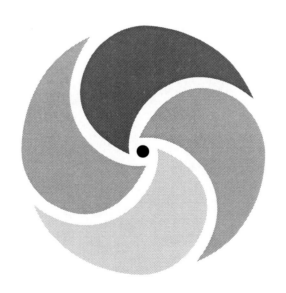

A fruit of the five-thousand-year-old Chinese culture, and a uniquely new, highly advanced life science - Zhineng Qigong has won the hearts of millions of people. Numerous miracles of healing, virtually unbelievable experimental results, and extraordinary powers have been the rewards of those who practice it. Zhineng Qigong represents a revolutionary leap in the exploration of the mysteries of human life.

A. GENERAL

1. Professor Ming Pang (*Pang Lao Shi*)

(The following section (A) is based upon information collected from various sources other than the writings of Ming Pang - X. J.)

Professor Ming Pang, the founder of Zhineng Qigong science, is known as *Pang Lao Shi* by his students. He has achieved great attainment in Traditional Chinese Medicine, diverse forms of chigong, various martial arts, and modern and ancient philosophy; and, while not a physician, he is well versed in Western medicine.

From early childhood, Professor Pang began his training in various types of traditional chigongs. His teachers, numbering nineteen grandmasters in all, came from backgrounds in Buddhism, Taoism, Confucianism, Traditional Chinese Medicine, martial arts, various folk chigong practices, and many other disciplines.

In 1980, Professor Pang announced the birth of Zhineng Qigong. Since then, millions of people have joined the growing mass movement of Zhineng Qigong practice.

Professor Pang has authored a number of seminal works on Zhineng Qigong science: nine textbooks for two-year full-time college level students, as well as other elementary and secondary textbooks. He is also the editor-in-chief of several chigong journals in China.

Professor Pang is the President of the Zhineng Qigong Branch Society of China Qigong Science Association. He is also the President of the Center of Qigong Intelligence Science. His other titles include: President of the Huaxia Zhineng Qigong Training and Recovering Center, Chairman of the board of the Zhineng Shen Food & Drink Corp. Ltd., and President of the Huaxia Zhineng Qigong Science Institute.

2. Professor Pang's works

Professor Pang has authored more than a dozen books. Those published are as follows:

    a. Elementary level:
      1) *Popular Textbook on Zhineng Donggong.*

2) *An Exploration into the Profundities of Qigong.*
b. Secondary Level:
   Brief Zhineng Qigongology.
c. Advanced level (Series of textbooks for two-year full-time college level students):
   1) *An Introduction to Zhineng Qigong Science.*
   2) *Fundamentals of Zhineng Qigong Science - The Hunyuan Entirety Theory.*
   3) *Essences of Zhineng Qigong Science.*
   4) *Practice Methodology of Zhineng Qigong Science.*
   5) *Superintelligence. - The Technique of Zhineng Qigong Science*
   6) *A Summary of Traditional Qigongs.*
   7) *Qigong and Human Cultures.*
   8) *A Brief Introduction to Chinese Qigong History.*
   9) *Modern Scientific Research on Qigong.*

3. The Center

The Center refers to the Huaxia Zhineng Qigong Training Center, Wenquanpu, Funing County, Qin Huang Dao, (Post code - 066326), Hebei, the People's Republic of China.

It consists of:
   a. Department of Instructors' Training.
   b. Department of Teachers' Training.
   c. Correspondence Department.
   d. Recovering Department No. 1.
   e. Recovering Department No. 2.
   f. Recovering Department No. 3.
   g. Huaxia Zhineng Qigong Science Institute.
   h. Editorial Office of the Journal of Zhineng Qigong Science.
   i. Clinic.
   j. Office of General Affairs.

The Center (formerly called Zhineng Qigong Training College) was founded in November 1988 in Shijiazhuang. It was approved by the Education Committee of Hebei Province in 1991 and was renamed as Hebei Huaxia Zhineng Qigong Training Center. In 1992, the founding of the Hebei Huaxia Zhineng Qigong Institute was approved by the Science and Technology Committee of Hebei Province. In May 1995, the Hebei Huaxia

Zhineng Qigong Recovering Center was approved by the Public Health Office of Hebei Province and founded at Fengren County.

At the present time, the Center has developed into an integrated training-recuperating-research community entity, with a faculty and staff of more than 600, and an average enrollment of 4,000 students per month from March to December of each year. In July and August the enrollment can reach up to 5,000-6,000.

During the past ten years, 310,000 students have been trained at the Center, among them, 3,377 professors and scientists and 1,769 foreign students from twenty countries and districts around the world. The Center is an organization dedicated to the principle of serving humanity with high-quality training, high-quality healing, high-quality service and low fees.

The Recovering Departments, the Editorial Department, the Clinic, and the Correspondence Department are now located at Huaxia Zhineng Qigong Recovering Center, No. 7 P.O. Box, Zicaowu, Fengren County, Hebei Province (Post code - 064000), the People's Republic of China.

Because of the rapid development of Zhineng Qigong, the two sites are always overcrowded with newly arriving students. A new center - The Center of Qigong Intelligence Science (known as Zhineng Qigong Town) - went into construction at Shunyi County, Beijing, in March 1996.

It is designed to hold 20,000 teachers and students, with schools of all levels, from an elementary school to a college, on site. The first stage of construction has already been completed. It opened on April 6, 1999. Sections of the Department of Teachers' Training and the Department of Instructors' Training have now moved to this new center.

When the overall construction is completed, all of the various departments will be moved into this new home. That day will be a great day of celebration for the ten million practitioners of Zhineng Qigong.

4. Training programs available at the Center

The following are full-time programs available at the Center:
  a. Twenty-four day recovering program.
  b. Fifty-day recovering program.
  c. Ten-day tuition-free training program for scientists and professors.
  d. Twenty-four-day Body and Mind Form (*Xing Shen Zhuang*) training program for instructors.
  e. Twenty-four-day Five One Form (*Wu Yuan Zhuang*) training program for instructors.

47

f. Twenty-four-day superintelligence (special abilities) training program for instructors.

g. Twenty-four-day half-tuition summer vacation training program for teachers and students from elementary schools, high schools, colleges and universities.

h. Thirty-day half-tuition advanced summer vacation training program for teachers and students from elementary schools, high schools, colleges and universities.

i. Fifty-day superintelligence training program for coaches.

j. Fifty-day advanced training program for support-coaches.

k. Fifty-day advanced training program for instructors.

l. Three-month training program for coaches.

m. Three-month secondary training program for medical coaches. (It is legal for these officially certified coaches to provide Zhineng Qigong treatment, known as Zhineng Qigong Therapy, in hospitals in China.)

n. Two-year college level training program for Zhineng Qigong teachers.

o. Two-year college level correspondence program for Zhineng Qigong teachers.

p. Other correspondence programs for instructors of different levels.

5. Zhineng Qigong practitioners around the world

According to incomplete statistics, about ten million people all over the world, the great majority of whom are in China, practice Zhineng Qigong every day. Most practitioners practice it twice a day, both in the morning and evening.

In China, every county and city has its own Zhineng Qigong Society, and there are also a number of overseas Zhineng Qigong organizations and groups in many countries and districts. Such places include Hong Kong, Tai Wan, Japan, Singapore, Malaysia, Indonesia, Thailand, New Zealand, France, Switzerland, Great Britain, Russia, Spain, Holland, Norway and the United States.

6. The rate of healing effectiveness at the Center

To the present, the most remarkable benefit of Zhineng Qigong practice has been its ability to prevent and heal disease. Not only have those suffering from common or frequently occurring diseases been successfully healed, but in addition, many patients diagnosed with and dying from difficult and complex illnesses have also recovered their health through the practice of Zhineng Qigong.

During the past ten years, 200,000 students with many kinds of illnesses have been treated at the Center, some of them being among the few rare cases of such conditions encountered anywhere in the world, while other such conditions were not yet even accorded names by medical authorities. An overall healing rate of effectiveness of 95% has been achieved at the Center.

According to incomplete statistics, the 450 disease conditions (embracing 210 categories of disease), included all types of cancers (including cancer of the liver), ascites caused by the cirrhosis of the liver, long-term paralysis (including paraplegia), and deaf-mutism (including congenital deaf-mutism and conditions caused by drugs). There were also detachment of the retina, thighbone necrosis, leukemia, congenital brain hypoplasia, atrophy and inflammation of the stomach, diabetes, hyperthyroidism and hypothyroidism. Other difficult-to-heal diseases included displacement of the uterus, pulmonary emphysema, heart disease, long-term high blood pressure, arrhythmia, asthma, psoriasis, lupus erythematosus, early stage cataract, neurologic tinnitus, neurologic itch, tuberculosis of the bones, and protruding lumbar vertebra, all of which responded successfully to treatment.

Between September and October in 1997, the cure rate of high blood pressure at the No. 2 Recuperating Department was 75.86% (22 healed out of 29 patients); 66.67% for coronary heart disease (12 healed out of 18); 50% for diabetes (18 healed out of 36); 63.64% for all types of stones (14 healed out of 22); and 22.72% for cancers (5 healed out of 22). Between August and September in 1998, at the No. 1 Recuperating Department, the cure rate for deafness was 29.4% (12 healed out of 34.)

In December 1996, 142 cancer-warriors attended the Meeting of Zhineng Qigong Cancer-Warriors at the Center. Among them, 138 have remained healthy over an eight year span, and four have remained healthy over a five year span. As of October 1998, fifty types of cancer have been healed at the Center.

Zhineng Qigong practice is a very effective drug-rehabilitation discipline. Between February and September in 1993, and in July 1996, Zhineng Qigong Drug-cessation experiments in Lanzhou successfully helped 1,800 people free themselves of dependence on drugs. Between October and December in 1997, and May and October of 1998, teachers from the Center helped another 1,700 people free themselves of drug dependency at drug-cessation clinics in Lanzhou. Between March and November in 1997, six drug-users went to the Recuperating Center. They all had a history of taking drugs between eight to nine years, and had experienced many other drug-cessation treatments. After one or two months of Zhineng Qigong practice and treatment at the Recuperating Center, all six students have completely ceased using drugs.

7. The Hunyuan community - a new medical model

Zhineng Qigong practitioners have been exploring a new type of medical model - that of the Hunyuan Community. This model employs Zhineng Qigong as its principal means of treatment, absorbing the essences of the models based upon biomedicine, social medicine, and psychological medicine, organically unifying the special functions of the mind and chi and carrying out healing activities within a chigong community; this promotes and guarantees the physical and mental health of the members of the community with a high level of quality and efficiency.

Emphasis is placed not only upon healing, but also upon wellness, prevention of illness, optimization of life, self-development and self-perfection, and the ultimate harmony with nature and society. In the medical model of the Hunyuan Community, the power of the chi field is emphasized and the building of a chi field is carried out through the whole of the recuperative process.

Special attention is paid to the controlling role played by the consciousness. Maintaining a healthy, positive and optimistic psychological state is the essential content of the recuperative activities. 'Healing-talk' (chatting or dialogue between a teacher and students) is a unique recuperative modality of the medical model implemented at the Hunyuan Community.

This model turns the process of recuperative activities into a process of social activities. All activities at the Hunyuan Community, such as the practice of the forms, study of the theories, chi field healing activities, scientific research, activities of living, communication and recreational activities, have become vehicles of the recuperative process. The individual behaviors of the community members have been transformed into collective recuperating activities.

8. The Huaxia Zhineng Qigong Science Institute

The Huaxia Zhineng Qigong Science Institute, in cooperation with other universities and institutes, has performed a number of experiments on the application of Zhineng Qigong science since 1989. The strategy of focus was shifted from mass practice of Zhineng Qigong to mass scientific research activities. Six Zhineng Qigong Symposiums were held at the Center, amassing 4,224 research papers exploring Zhineng Qigong enhancements various fields such as agriculture, industry, forestry, animal husbandry, fishery, medical treatment, education, sports, and the arts. Twenty-four state-level scientific institutions, 61 province-level research institutions, and 90 colleges and universities have been involved in these research projects. A number of well-known professors and scientists personally participated in the research projects.

Some of its achievements are both astonishing and inspiring. For example, chi-treated crops can yield up to 10-30% more than non-treated ones. A cancer cell stopped splitting within 50 minutes under the control of a chigong teacher. Chi-treated batteries could be more quickly and more effectively charged.

9. The Journal of Zhineng Qigong Science

This monthly Chinese Journal of Zhineng Qigong Science released its first issue in 1992. It contains many columns:
    a. Professor Pang's latest speeches.
    b. Theories and methods of Zhineng Qigong science.
    c. Experiences of the practitioners.
    d. Cases of recovery.
    e. Questions and answers.
    f. Reports and papers on scientific experiments.
    g. Correspondence information.
    h. Recent Zhineng Qigong developments in China and overseas.
    i. News from the Center.
The Journal has become an indispensable tie linking Professor Pang and the Center with the ten million practitioners of Zhineng Qigong.

10. The clinic at the Center

The main purpose of the clinic is not the treatment of patients but rather the undertaking of physical examinations, and the verification of the effectiveness of the treatment. All patients take standard examinations both upon their enrollment and before their departure. The clinic has accumulated voluminous data covering hundreds of thousands of cases.

11. Full Moon and New Moon practices (*Zishi Gongs*)

In China, there are two national Zhineng Qigong Nights (*Zishi Gongs*) every month, the night of the full moon and the night of the new moon (the fifteenth and the last nights of the month by the Chinese lunar calendar). Wherever Professor Pang is, he regularly leads the national practice twice a month, and the ten million fellow practitioners concurrently join the tremendous chi field both in order to benefit others and also to be benefited themselves. Miracles also take place on such nights.

The time of practice is approximately 10:30 - 12:00 p.m. (Beijing Time). According to the theory of Zhineng Qigong science, time and space are viewed as an entirety. If one cannot practice simultaneously with the Chinese practitioners due to one's work (nights in China are mornings of the same day in North America), one may put it off until evening. As long as one consciously connects oneself with the millions of fellow practitioners in one's consciousness, the results will still be good.

B. CHIGONG SCIENCE AND ZHINENG QIGONG SCIENCE

1. The importance of clarifying the implications of chigong (qigong)

Since the 1980's, the mass practice of chigong has been surging in eastern countries and rippling out to other parts of the globe. Its great vitality and seemingly miraculous effects are impacting all fields of modern science.

The benefits of chigong practice in the areas of the prevention of illness, improvement and enhancement of health, and the attainment of longevity have been recognized and accepted by numerous people. The mistaken notions of chigong as merely being a blind feudal belief system or a form of sorcery have gradually been dispelled.

However, commonly held views and understanding of chigong are of every description: some regard it as a therapy - a branch of Chinese medicine or medical science; some view it as a part of sports or sports therapy; others think that it is an evolution of the martial arts. Although each of these understandings is reasonable in some way, they are all incomplete.

In these present times, when chigong will eventually come to flourish all over the world, such fragmentary understandings will definitely obstruct the scientific research into chigong and bring about setbacks for both chigong students and practitioners. It is vitally necessary to explore and define the correct and complete implications inherent in chigong, and to place it within the rightful context it deserves.

Chigong is the rare treasure of the cultural heritage of China. It is subtle and profound, and its nourishing waters emerge out of a long history and from far-distant sources. In order to rightly explore the profundities of chigong, it is essential to start our exploration with both its depth and its breadth.

On one hand, with regard to its depth, the relationship between chigong and the human life processes must be studied and endowed with all the rigorous standards inherent in modern scientific research. On the other hand, the history of the origin and development of chigong, as well as its relationship to ancient Chinese cultures, should be examined against the entire background of the history of these cultures. (This is discussed in another book - *A Brief Introduction to Chinese Qigong History*.)

With regard to its breadth, chigong relates to many schools of thought. It is true that, down through history, the three major religions, Confucianism, Buddhism, Taoism and the other nine schools of thought attached great importance to chigong. The Confucianists looked upon it as the fundamental method by which to cultivate oneself and to pursue one's studies (the performance of scholarly research). The Taoists regarded it as the secret through which to realize "immortality". The Buddhists thought of it as the way to become a Buddha, or the founder of a new sect. Medical doctors looked upon it as a supremely ingenious method for the prevention of illness and the prolongation of life, as well as a way of diagnosing and treating illness.

Because the aims, practice methods, benefits and applications of chigong in these sects vary from each other, the terms for chigong also differ. For example, Chinese medical doctors called it Absorbing Vitality (*She Sheng*), Preserving Life (*Yang Sheng*), Guiding and Directing Chi (*Dao Yin*), and Moving Chi (*Xing Qi*). The Taoists called it Breathing in and Out (*Tu Na*), Internal Vital Chi (*Nei Dan*), Nine Cycles to Return to

Vital Chi (*Jiu Zhuan Huan Dan*), Metaphysical Practice, Heavenly Microcosmic Circulation (*Zhou Tian Ban Yun*), Preserving Life and Keeping True Vitality (*Bao Xing Quan Zhen*), and The Practice of Tranquillity. The Confucian scholars called it Self-Cultivation, Keeping the Heart Upright, Keeping the Mind Honest, Holding the Spirit in the Mean, Preserving the Spirit and Cultivating the Mind, Preserving the Nocturnal Chi, and Tranquil Sitting. The Buddhists called it Stopping and Observing (*Zhi Guan*), Zazen Meditation (*Can Chan*), Dhyana Meditation (*Chan Ding*), and Yoga. There are other such names, too numerous to mention individually. In order to help the reader grasp a relatively comprehensive understanding of chigong and its related issues and implications, the various types of chigong and their respective benefits will be introduced in a general manner in the first section of this part.

2. Chi (*Qi*)

Chi (*Qi*) is the most profound and fundamental concept in both ancient chigongs and Traditional Chinese Medicine. With regard to chi, it is easy to refer to the breath and to that which we breathe; thus some have translated chigong as "Breathing Exercise", which is not truly accurate. Although breath control occupies a vital position in many schools of chigong, the chi referred to in chigong is entirely different from simply that which we breathe.

In the theoretical view of classic Chinese cultures and traditional chigongs, the concept of chi embraces at least the following three implications:

    a. The Life-force (Chi) in the world of nature (external or exogenous universal force, the original Primordial Life-force, or the most basic source matter in the universe).

Chi is the finest, most elemental and most rarefied source-substance constituting both the universe and all things within it. Chi is formless and invisible. Ordinary people can neither see it nor feel it, yet it nonetheless exists and fills the entire universe. "*It is too vast to arrive beyond, yet too fine to penetrate into.*"

It was originally termed chi (*qi*) or Oneness (*yuan*), or undivided chi (*yuan qi*), Tao chi, Taiji or Great Oneness. The ancient Chinese believed that this invisible and formless chi was the source of all visible and physical phenomena.

In other words, all varied, complex and ceaselessly changing phenomena are the manifestations of dynamically converted chi. The birth,

54

growth, decline, and dissolution of every existent thing is the result of the infinite transmutations of chi, and man is no exception. Wang Chong (an ancient sage) said, *"Water condenses into ice, chi condenses into man."*

In Zhineng Qigong science, this energy-substance is referred to as the original Hunyuan chi (the Primordial Life-force, the most basic source matter). It is very fine, homogeneous and even. It fills the entire universe and permeates all things. It is a unity and cannot be divided. It exists with neither beginning nor end. It nourishes all things in the universe and especially benefits those who are open and selfless, nature-loving, warm-hearted and indifferent to either fame or gain.

b. Life-force within the human body (internal physical chi).

This is a special and invisible substance which maintains the normal functioning of the human life processes. Chi is the very basis of the human life processes. Zhang Jingyue (an ancient sage in the Ming Dynasty) said, *"The life of man relies completely upon this chi."* In traditional Chinese medical theory, it can be variously classified as true chi (*zhen qi*), vital chi (*yuan qi*), chi flowing in the main and collateral chi channels (*jingluo qi*), chi within the internal organs (*zangfu qi*), prenatal, inborn or innate chi (*xiantian qi*), postnatal chi (*houtian qi*), and so on, according to its distribution throughout and functioning within the human body.

In Zhineng Qigong science, the highest level of primordial energy (Hunyuan chi) in the universe, is called unity-of-consciousness chi or human brain Hunyuan chi (the chi of unified human consciousness). Some of its characteristics are similar to those of original Hunyuan chi, but it is much more complex in its composition.

In addition, the chi of unified human consciousness is volitional, that is to say, it has subjective initiative, and it can cause both original Hunyuan chi and other levels of Hunyuan chi to change and transmute themselves in various ways. One of the goals of Zhineng Qigong practice is to heighten the ability to gather and condense, and to disperse and to dissolve all levels of Hunyuan chi.

c. The interaction and transmutation between natural chi and human chi.

According to the theories of chigong, the process of human life is the process of unceasing interaction and transmutation between human chi and universal chi. If one can successfully absorb the universal chi in order to nourish the body and mind, one will appear sound and healthy; if this is not the case, then one is either in a state of illness or the process of dying. This is so because man is a part of the universal chi.

The aim of chigong practice is to strengthen this process so that man can live a better life. It can be inferred from this then that the chi in chigong refers both to the chi of the natural world and the chi of the human body.

As a specific philosophically defined category, the notion of chi is usually affirmed and defined as one of "simple materialism". It is also willingly accepted as a vague but key element at work within the human life process.

However, does chi objectively exist? Is it a substance? People may feel that presenting positive replies to these questions is neither a reliable nor credible endeavor.

Usually, the notion of chi is equally looked upon existing in the same category of such principles as the Five Elements, *Yin* and *Yang* in ancient Chinese culture, or the "Four Great Elements" (earth, water, fire, wind) in classic Indian philosophy.

These principles are regarded as the result of a simplistic process of abstraction of the objective world on the part of ancient cultures limited by incomplete knowledge, rather than as elements having real and independent existence. This is because no homologue or corresponding conceptual structure for chi can be found within the framework of modern science.

However, in reality this is not the case. Since 1978, in China, a series of experiments has been in the process of being carried out verifying the physical and biological effects of chigong external chi.

These experiments have proved that external chi not only acted upon various instruments and specimens (both organic and non-organic), but that it also caused changes in them. These visible changes were observed, but were incapable of being explained by modern scientific theories.

As we know, in the universe, only the interaction between various manifestations of a substance can cause changes in its dynamic state. Because of this, in view of genuine materialism, the existing experiments on the physical and biological effects of the external chi of chigong, while they have not been able to reveal the mystery of just what chi is, can yet convincingly prove the objective existence of chi, and also prove that chi is a kind of superfine matter. This concept is of vital importance to the present development of chigong science.

Generally speaking, the chi of chigong stems from the Chi Theory of classic Chinese philosophy. A complete and correct knowledge can be obtained only by studying chigong against the background and over the entire historical span of classic Chinese cultures.

Modern scientific experiments have proved that chi does exist, and that it is a new, subtle and primal form of matter, but this new form of matter has not yet been objectively brought to light by modern science. These two ideas are the cornerstones of Zhineng Qigong science and of all chigongs.

3. Gong

In Chinese, the word 'gong' has several meanings related to chigong:
   a. Skills, achievements and merits (both spiritual and physical abilities or capabilities) obtained through chigong practice.
   b. Time and effort spent on chigong (skill-cultivation).
   c. Practice methods of specific chigongs and forms.
   d. Practice plans or schedules.
   e. Actual practice of chigong.

4. The origin of the term 'Chigong' (Qigong)

Although, as a specific body of learning, chigong has existed in China for thousands of years, the term 'chigong' (qigong) first appeared in the book *Smart Swordsman* (*Ling Jian Zi*) by Xu Xun during the Jin Dynasty. It referred to that cultivation in which internal changes were caused by chi-related practices (such as moving chi, and applying chi) as well as the cultivation of one's moral nature (embodying virtuous actions), in order to achieve a measure of skill. From this, it can be easily inferred that, although the implications of chigong practice included the cultivation of chi and the moral nature, 'chigong' was not the term employed for this dual practice.

From then on, the term chigong came to assume a religious connotation, and did not exercise any great influence in any sect until the advent of the Ming and Qing dynasties, during which period religions gradually tended to collapse. The martial arts were closely interwoven with chigong, eventually forming martial arts chigongs.

In the book, *Tendon-Transforming Scripture* (*Yi Jin Jing*), a classic work on the Shaolin martial arts which greatly influenced the later martial arts chigongs, the principle of chi was repeatedly emphasized. Great stress was placed upon the application of chigong in the shadow boxing arts of the Wudang sect of Taoism. The former excels at 'hard' forms of chigong, such as the skills of the Iron Shirt discipline and the Golden Bell Armor (*Jin Zhong Zhao*), in which the chi-shielded practitioner functions just as if he were covered by a huge golden bell, impervious to injury by guns or blades. The former discipline stresses the internal transmutation of spirit, mind and life-force.

At the end of the Qing Dynasty, in the book, *Secrets of Shaolin Shadow Boxing Arts*, there appeared a chapter entitled, "Expounding on the Subtleties of Chigong", in which it was clearly pointed out that, *"The doctrine of chigong includes two aspects: one is the nourishing of chi and the other is the cultivation (practice) of chi."* It also presented clear and detailed practice methods. The term 'chigong' gradually increased in influence.

In 1931, Wang Zhulin published *Detailed Explanations on Mind Qigong*. directly employing the term 'qigong'. In 1934, Dong Hong authored a book *Qigong Therapy - Special Therapy for Lung Diseases*. In 1938, Fang Gongbo published another book - *Records of Successful Cases of Qigong Therapy*, and also founded the Gongbo Qigong Hospital. It is remarkable to note that chigong was actively applied in medical treatment at that time

It was in the 1950's that the term 'chigong' began to be widely used and became popular. In 1953, Liu Guizhen codified his own experiences of both chigong practice and clinical treatment into a series of practice methods. With approval and support by the Health Office of the Province of Hebei, he termed his method Chigong Therapy. He founded the Tangshan Clinics for Recuperation in Tangshan, and a Chigong Sanatorium at Beidaihe, in Qin Huang Dao. He also authored two books - *The Practice of Chigong Therapy* and *The Practice of Internal Nourishing*.

The chigong therapy advocated by Liu Guizhen was not a single method, but included The Practice of Internal Nourishing, Strength Discipline, Fitness Practice and Walking Practice. According to Mr. Liu Guizhen, the implications of the term 'chigong' were "The sum of tranquil-sitting, controlled breathing, the directing and guiding of chi, as well as internal cultivation."

Between the end of the 1970's and the beginning of the 1980's, unprecedented changes occurred in the advancement of chigong. Chigong was not only applied to the healing of illness, but also upon a broader and greater scale; a number of scientific experiments were also carried out, especially experiments involving external chi healing.

The term 'chigong' became not only a synonym for methods of practice geared toward preserving life, healing illness and keeping healthy and fit; it was also regarded as a special body of learning accepted through common practice. Following and largely due to the foundation of the China Qigong Association and the China Qigong Science Association, chigong has with increasing frequency been lifted onto the throne of science - it has become chigong science. The implications embraced by the term 'chigong' have become quite different from those that have previously existed.

5. The definition of 'chigong'

Chigong is a practice based in and on the Entirety Concept of Life. During the process of this practice, the mind is introverted through one's own initiative (psychospiritual adjustment, postural requirements and breath control comprising the extensions of its internalized activities), the life process of man is re-formed, perfected and enhanced, and the natural instincts are transformed into conscious intelligence.

This definition of chigong (which is set forth by the author) points out its theoretical basis, clearly states its special practice methods and contents, and delineates its aims of practice. It embraces the totality of the distinctive features of chigong:

a. Chigong is a practice based upon the theoretical framework of the Entirety Concept of Life. It includes the following aspects:

1). The universe is an entirety that contains numerous levels of substance. These diverse levels of substance embody each other, are in a ceaseless process of mutual transmutation, and together constitute the substratum of all things in the universe.

2). The human body is an entirety. Traditional chigong and Traditional Chinese Medicine hold that man is a unified spirit-body entirety, of which the spirit is the director, the internal organs the central substance, with the chi, blood, main and collateral chi channels (*jingluo*) the interlinking network integrating these. In Zhineng Qigong, man is regarded as a unified body-chi-spirit Hunyuan entirety.

3). The oneness of man and nature (*tian*). This refers to the existence of man and nature as a dynamic unified entirety.

This entirety concept of the oneness of man and nature not only underlies the common theoretical basis of all forms of chigong, but also constitutes the essence of ancient Chinese civilization. Western scientists have also begun to study this theory.

In view of their highest potential development, the theories of all chigong sects must be refined and elevated to this level. This is only a matter of time. It is true that it was the ancients who, through chigong practice, created the entirety concept of the man/nature unity. This concept is still in the process of continuous evolution.

This principle, together with the practice of chigong, has been uninterruptedly undergoing repeated cycles of ever-deepening development. If we trace back into the historical origins of chigong prior to the establishment of this theory, we find that the practice was only a kind of blind process, a primitive form of chigong which cannot be compared with modern chigong practice.

        b. Chigong is characterized by its unique method - the special practice of interiorizing consciousness. This method of Inner Perception embraces the following two implications:

First, the activities of consciousness of ordinary persons are usually extroverted toward external things that are largely irrelevant to his or her own life processes, while the activities of consciousness of a chigong practitioner are interiorized in order to merge with his or her own life processes.

Second, the activities of consciousness of ordinary persons are usually scattered outward, moving from this to that, from the one to the many, while the activities of consciousness of a chigong practitioner are centralized within, upon a single object which is of sole concern, proceeding from the many to the one.

This point is the soul of the definition of chigong. It is a standard by which to evaluate whether a fitness method is or is not truly chigong. For example, the methods of establishing health found in pharmacology, medicine or sports cannot be called chigong because by these methods the mind is not interiorized, enhanced and rendered healthy.

        c. It is clearly pointed out that the aim of chigong practice is the re-forming, perfecting, and enhancement of one's abilities in relation to one's own life process.

It embraces the diverse areas of maintaining health, developing intelligence, heightening one's feeling nature, tapping one's potentials, and freeing oneself from the confinement of instincts in order to stride into the dimension of freedom and conscious intelligence.

        d. It is pointed out that chigong is a practice process in which practice methods are applied for the purpose of keeping oneself spiritually and physically healthy, and for further enhancing one's abilities in relation to one's own life process.

If one knows the theories and methods of chigong but does not practice oneself, one can only be regarded as a person of learning in chigong (placing one in the realm of chigongology), but one cannot be regarded as a chigong master.

60

The chigong referred to here is a practice process of self-molding and self-refinement in accord with the theories and methods of chigongology.

This definition is the outcome of a comprehensive investigation and examination of the history and the present state of chigong, as well as the future of chigong science. Does it apply generally to all sects of chigong? Indeed it does, because all schools of chigong, even at their diverse respective stages, place their emphasis upon mental or spiritual cultivation. This definition also applies to popular relaxation methods, sitting meditation, and many forms of yoga found in other countries.

This definition thus stresses the exploitation of interiorized consciousness, but without specifically mentioning chi; this not only avoids the unique limitations of definitions of chi found in traditional forms of chigong, but it also grasps the essence of those schools in which chi is emphasized, and where there is a pronounced focus upon the practice of the transmutation of chi. This is because thought (idea) is the commander of chi; wherever a thought (idea) reaches, there chi also arrives. Thus the emphasis upon consciousness does not in any way exclude the principle of chi, but rather incorporates the principle of chi within itself.

In the view of the Hunyuan Entirety Theory of Zhineng Qigong, the activities of consciousness are the core motive contents and processes of the Hunyuan chi of the human brain, and though these are described as the unity of consciousness, they are also the special formative manifestations of Hunyuan chi.

6. The differences between physical exercise and chigong practice

The fundamental difference between physical exercise and chigong practice lies in the way the mind is used. In all sports (isolated muscle-building exercises are an exception), one directs one's mind outward toward the objects of the game - the balls, the equipment and so forth, instead of interiorizing the mind in the direction of one's own physical body and stream of consciousness.

If one's consciousness is not integrated with one's own life activities, then one cannot take advantage of the unique role of the medium of consciousness in implementing the enhancement of one's vitality.

The results of chigong practice and physical exercises are also different. The specific differences lie in the following aspects:

a. Contents of exercise.

Chigong practice consists of spiritual cultivation, moral cultivation, breath control and physical movements, whereas, in the practice of sports, only physical movement is involved.

b. Physical movements.

In chigong practice, the movements of the body serve the direction of the mind and the chi. The practitioner enjoys the subtlety and comfort of his practice in a relaxed body and with a peaceful and tranquil mind. While engaged in sports, the activity of the mind serves the movements of the body while the actions of the muscles and tendons execute various skills.

c. The process of the mind directing the body.

In chigong practice, the mind is interiorized with the purpose of giving various conscious directions controlling the body, while in sports, the mind is put in command of the body through the reflexive actions of the physical activities.

d. Metabolic changes.

In chigong practice, the life processes are maintained in more optimal balance, thereby renewing one's life energy and enhancing human vitality. In sports, the stimulation of one's vitality is derived through increasing the production and expenditure of bio-energy.

In addition, through chigong practice, latent human sensitivities can be heightened and the "sixth sense" may be developed, such as the ability to see through objects, remote-vision, remote-hearing, remote-sensing and other supersensory abilities. However, in sports, endurance only is strengthened, and no special abilities are tapped.

7. Types of chigongs

There are thousands of different chigongs.

(Note: more than 2,400 sects are registered in official record, of which, only 11 have obtained permission to be publicly disseminated in China up to the present time, with Zhineng Qigong ranking first among them. - X. J.)

There are many ways to classify these chigongs:

a. Based upon the contents of practice.
   1) Mind practice forms (*xing gongs*). The main purpose of these chigongs is the cultivation of the mind.
   2) Life practice forms (*ming gongs*). The main purpose of these chigongs is the maintenance of strength and health.

3) Mind-life practice forms (*xing-ming gongs*). The main purpose of these practice forms is both the cultivation of the mind and the maintenance of strength and health.

Zhineng Qigong, with its unique set of practice forms, is a new type of mind-life cultivation created on the following bases:

b. Based upon the postures.
   1) Standing practice forms.
   2) Sitting practice forms.
   3) Lying practice forms (forms practiced while recumbent).
   4) Walking practice forms.

c. Based upon physical movements.
   1) Static (still) practice forms (*jing gongs*) (with fixed posture and no physical movements).
   2) Dynamic practice forms (*dong gongs*) (with physical movements).
   3) Dynamic-static practice forms (*dong-jing gongs*) (fixed postures alternating with physical movements).

d. Based upon the functions of chi.
   1) Hard chigongs. The internal chi is concentrated upon a specific part of the body in order to demonstrate unusual resistance to external harm such as the traditional practices of "Hand Breaks Metal and Stone", "Belly Against Steel Fork", "Throat Against Long Rifle", "Head Against Hammer", and "Unburned in Fire".
   2) Soft chigongs. In these chigongs, chi is used to prevent and heal illness and to maintain fitness and health.

e. Based upon their respective sources.
   1) Medical chigongs. The aim of these chigongs is the eradication of illness, the prolongation of life, and the exploration of the mysteries of life. They are the foundation and essence of Traditional Chinese Medicine.
   2) Taoist chigongs.
   3) Buddhist chigongs.
   4) Confucian chigongs.
   5) Martial arts chigongs.

f. Based upon their respective benefits.
   1) Healing chigongs. The prevention and healing of illness is the primary benefit of all chigongs. This effect is obviously greater in healing chigongs.

2) Fitness chigongs (designed mainly to maintain the practitioner's strength and health).

3) Intelligence chigongs. The main purpose of these chigongs is the improvement of ordinary intelligence (including both physical capabilities as well as wisdom-potential), and the further stimulation and development of superintelligence. Intelligence Chigong - Zhineng Qigong - has become the abbreviated special term for Zhineng Qigong science.

Broadly speaking, all chigongs can be classified into two types: closed-style chigongs and open-style chigongs. Zhineng Qigong is a new open-style chigong.

8. The common key elements of all chigongs

a. Spiritual (mental) cultivation. Properly employing the mind to attain perfect command of one's volition in certain special ways, in order to heighten one's ability to "consciously direct the body".

b. Moral cultivation. This is the general implementation of the above point in one's daily life; it is also the condition of conscious practice.

c. Breath control. This refers not merely to the biological process of breathing, but rather to an interactive process closely connected with one's consciousness.

d. Postural requirements. Both moving practice forms (forms using sequential movements), and still or static practice forms (forms using fixed positions), require specific postures for their execution. These postures are closely associated with the cultivation of conscious awareness.

(Note: The above-mentioned four points comprise virtually all the fundamental essences of chigong. These are expounded in detail in *Essences of Zhineng Qigong Science. - X.J.*)

9. The historical stages of Chinese chigong

Statements about both the laws of the activities of human life, as well as traces of the existence of chigong, can be found in the early-recorded history of Chinese civilization. For example, the most ancient and monumental work on Chinese philosophy - *Laws of Changes (I Ching)* - expounds the general laws of the evolution of all things in the universe, including human life, from a philosophical viewpoint. It not only lays down a theoretical basis for ancient chigong theory and practice, but also discusses a number of specific practice principles and methods. This suggests that, in the period of time predating recorded history, chigong had already come to be widely practiced.

The exact period of chigong's emergence is unverifiable. According to existing records, even in the period of remote antiquity during which primitive communities flourished, mankind had already mastered the practice of chigong. Its later development can be classified into three periods:

a. The period of simple chigongs (from remote antiquity to the Qin Dynasty)

This period was comprised of two ages:

1) The age of pre-history: Chigong existed in its potential and formative stage. There are no reliable documents or records by which to verify this hypothesis.

2) The age of Spring and Autumn and the age of Warring States: This was the golden age of the simple form of chigong. At that time, sages arose in great numbers and hundreds of schools of thought contended with each other.

Almost all of the theories of the various schools of thought concentrated upon man and human life. Each established its own system of theory by taking the social problems of the period as its prime subjects of study. However, in this pursuit, the prerequisite for the acquisition of correct knowledge was the researcher's own accomplishment in spiritual and physical cultivation, implemented through the processes of accurate observation and correct reasoning.

Therefore, the various sages of diverse schools of thought possessed their own methods of moral and physical cultivation - chigongs which were in accord with their own theoretical systems. Among these schools, the practices of the Taoist, Confucian, medical, fitness and immortality sects made the greatest contributions to the development of chigong.

There were two outstanding specific features in the chigongs of this age: first, chigong was comprised not only of skill but also of learning (scholarship or knowledge). Second, although chigong was more or less involved with various religions, it had little to do with religious theology, and it still retained its own original character. Thus, this period was called the period of simple chigongs.

b. The period of religious chigongs (from the beginning of the Han Dynasty (circa 220 A.D.) to the end of the Qing Dynasty (1912).

There were also two stages in this period:

1) From the beginning of Han Dynasty to the Sui and Tang Dynasty (ending circa 906 A.D.)

As feudal society was established and consolidated, the Confucian school of thought became elevated to a status of universal respect; at the same time, in its relationship to the monarchical power, it fell to the status of an indentured servant. Chigong was similarly affected, being gradually driven out of the halls of learning and, in the popular view, relegated to the realm of witchcraft and folklore.

Conversely, as Buddhism was introduced into China, became domesticated and flourished, and as Taoism was developed and established, chigong gradually evolved from a method of self-cultivation into a religious practice.

The noteworthy features of chigong at this stage included its transformation from being merely a body of learning into once again being a set of skills, while its practice methods became specific and practical. Second, chigong came to be exploited by religious sects.

2) From the beginning of the Song Dynasty (circa 906 A.D.) to the end of the Qing Dynasty (ending circa 1912 A.D.)

Feudal society passed its golden age and gradually began to collapse. Cultural confinement became increasingly more severe. Thinking became rigid and, eventually, ossified. Chigong fell completely under the aegis of religion and assumed a subservient status to religious theology.

The noteworthy developments of chigong during this period consisted first in the fact that, simultaneous with its becoming subsumed by various religions, its practice methods were becoming more specific and practical. Second, the practice principles and methods of numerous diverse sects such as Taoist, Buddhist, Confucian and medical practices mingled with and became indistinguishable from one another. Third, as time went by, numerous sects arose and fought for supremacy with increasing ferocity. Fourth, the emergence of martial arts forms of chigong laid the foundations for the undermining of the many religious chigongs.

3) The period of modern chigongs (from the beginning of the Republic of China to the present)

As the feudal dynasties collapsed completely, and under the further onslaught of modern science, chigong broke out of the prison of religion. On its primary levels, chigong has been widely applied in the field of medicine and has come to be accepted by a growing number of people as an effective traditional healing method.

Since the late 1970's, scientific experiments have proved that chi is a substance, and that the state of energy-cultivation (chigong state) is an inherent, newly discovered state, and one of higher stability than that encountered amidst the activities of ordinary human life. The light of science began to disperse the religious shrouds which had been enveloping chigong. The development of chigong had entered a uniquely new era.

10. Contemporary needs and requirements for the practice of chigong

With regard to the practice methods of chigong, what are the needs and requirements of our own time? The answer can be summed up in these words: Chigong must offer us a practice which is simple and clear, rational and reasonable, easy to learn, safe and highly effective.

Simplicity and clarity refer to the need for the theories and practice methods of chigong be simple and clear; there are no particular requirements or restrictions for practice environments; the forms can be practiced easily and conveniently and do not require a great deal of time.

Rationality and reasonability refer to the need for chigong's theories and practice methods to coincide with the principles of classic chigongology and also, as far as possible, to embody the essence of modern scientific thought, while at the same time rejecting the encumbrance of unenlightened historical beliefs.

The phrase 'easy to learn' refers not only to the need for the practices to be capable of being easily mastered, but also means that there are laws and rules having wide applicability by which to abide. Such a practice meets not only the needs of the old, the weak and the sick, but also the young, the strong and the healthy; it must be of benefit not only to those whose work largely involves physical activity and labor, but also to those whose endeavors are chiefly in the domain of the mind.

Safety refers to the need for the practice to insure its adherents freedom from the possibility of experiencing abnormal symptoms, and high effectiveness refers to the need for such a practice to achieve beneficial results quickly, and within a short time period.

Based upon an understanding of these requirements, in recent years, new explorations into the ancient chigong have been undertaken by a number of individuals of high ideals and integrity. Our present form of Zhineng Qigong is a reflection of these new explorations.

It is capable of addressing the needs of diverse kinds of practitioners at correspondingly diverse levels. Zhineng Qigong is such a new kind of chigong, and fulfills all of the above-mentioned requirements.

11. The benefits of chigong practice

    a. The prevention and healing of illness.
    b. The enhancement of health.
    c. The prolongation of life.
    d. The development of intelligence.

12. The reason for the healing effect of chigong practice.

According to the theories of Traditional Chinese Medicine and chigong, all diseases are caused either by the shortage of blood and chi or by the abnormal circulation or movement of blood and chi. In such cases, various life processes become unbalanced.

Through chigong practice, on the one hand, the blood and chi can become plentiful, and on the other hand, the smooth and unimpeded circulation of blood and chi can be promoted.

In this way, it may be said: "One never falls ill when one's blood and chi function (or circulate) well," and "When plentiful healthy chi dwells within, unhealthy influences cannot interfere."

The mechanism by which this occurs is generally identical with that of acupuncture and moxibustion, as well as massage therapy, in Chinese medicine. The difference lies only in the specific methods of practice.

Some may wonder how a pathogen, such as a bacterium in the patient's body, is dispelled. Traditional Chinese Medicine and chigong formulated the foundations for the functioning of chi: when healthy chi is plentiful and circulating well, all unhealthy elements will die or disappear. Bacteria are no exception. Is this true? Most certainly! Many Zhineng Qigong practitioners can provide such ironclad evidence.

Repeated modern scientific experiments have also proved that immunity is greatly improved after chigong practice; the number of white blood cells and their pathogen-engulfing abilities and parameters are all considerably increased.

In addition, the chi sent forth from a practitioner can also kill germs and viruses. If this out-sent chi works outside the body, the same chi will surely work inside the body as well, where the mind, the chi and the internal anatomy are interconnected in a much more intimate way.

The healing effect is the initial benefit after one commences one's chigong practice, and it is also the most elementary one. It can be regarded as the ongoing reward while one is passing through the life-long journey of chigong practice; it is also the foundation by which to transmute oneself through the sustained practice of chigong.

Strictly speaking, the purpose of chigong practice is not to directly heal or to cure illness, but to readjust the life processes as a whole. Stabilizing, mutually interactive transformations, wherein things return to normal, always occur after the practice of chigong: high blood pressure becomes lower, while pressure that is too low becomes higher; the obese lose weight while the thin gain weight. All functions become normalized.

There is one thing that should be pointed out; this is, that although the healing range of chigong is truly broad, and its effectiveness is genuinely amazing, it is not omnipotent.

It should be clear that, as with any other existing science, it is not absolutely applicable for every situation or condition, but rather has its own range of effectiveness. It is wrong to believe that chigong heals no real illnesses, and it is also inappropriate to deify chigong.

13. Enhancement of health through chigong practice

Practicing chigong can balance yin and yang, adjust and promote the circulation of chi and blood, clear and open the main and collateral chi channels, and cultivate the true chi, so that the quality of human life can be improved and enhanced.

Through the practice of chigong, the weak become strong, the sick become healthy, and the old become young again. Millions of practitioners have obtained these benefits, and many modern medical experiments have also proved this.

a. Effect on the nervous system.

Chigong practice can repair and adjust the nervous system so that it can function more optimally. During the practice of chigong, alpha waves appear in the practitioner's EEG (electroencephalogram), while the waveamplitude increases and there is a concentration of waves in the region of the forehead (differing from their concentration at the back of the head during closed-eye meditation).

The left and right hemispheres of the brain appear to be synchronized, which indicates that the functioning of the brain is better balanced. At the same time, through the control of the autonomic nerves, chigong can adjust the nervous system and can improve and enhance the ability to move, to sense, and to think.

b. Effect on the cardiovascular system.

Chigong practice can cause the heart to function more efficiently, improve the macro- and micro-circulation of the blood, and have an anti-aging effect upon the nervous system.

c. Effect on the respiratory system.

During chigong practice, oxygen consumption and CO_2 production are both reduced, the respiratory rate is reduced, and the functioning of the lungs is greatly enhanced.

d. Effect on the digestive system.

Chigong practice can increase the secretion of saliva and digestive juices in both the stomach and the intestines, as well as promote the peristaltic motion of the intestines. In this way, the digestive functioning of these organs can be strengthened.

e. Effect on the internal system.

Through chigong practice, the brain's pituitary body and all the organs of the internal system can be appropriately adjusted. For example, the metabolic level of adrenaline declines, the growth hormone diminishes, and the concentration of cholesterol in the blood may be reduced.

Not only have medical experiments demonstrated the above-mentioned excellent effects of chigong practice, but so also have the experiences of millions of practitioners. Worldwide, practitioners of Zhineng Qigong have experienced its manifest health-enhancement benefits, including the prevention and healing of illness.

Moreover, the figure-enhancing effect of chigong practice is great. For example, on a normal diet, one person lost 22.5 kilograms within three months, another person lost more than three kilograms in one day, and an underweight person gained eleven kilograms within three months, achieving a normal weight. Several adults between the ages of 34 and 37 grew three to four centimeters taller.

There have also been further dramatic health benefits, such as the emergence of new teeth and the growth of new hair in the aged, as well as the disappearance of spots and freckles, and other similar results.

14. Attainment of longevity through chigong practice

The experiences of many chigong practitioners have also confirmed the above statement. At the Center, there are many teachers in their seventies and even eighties who are still happily working as hard as younger teachers do. Their sharp minds and agile bodies are greatly admired by the students.

Many experiments have also proved that the secretion of sex hormones can be adjusted through chigong practice. Beijing Qigong Association studied 600 aged persons, 300 in a chigong group and 300 in a non-chigong group. Seven parameters related to intelligence were then tested. The comparison showed that the aging process of the persons in the chigong group was obviously slower than that of those in the non-chigong group; there were also a small number of people who showed no signs of aging.

Why? According to modern biology, the normal life span of a living thing is five to seven times its growing period. The growing period of man is 25 years, thus the normal life span for man is 125 to 175 years.

Because most people violate the natural, vitality is harmed or damaged, and the normal life span cannot be realized. Through chigong practice, the practitioner may learn how to come into accord with the laws of life, and how to enhance vitality; thus the goal of being healthy and living long can be attained.

15. Development of intelligence through chigong practice

a. Cognitive ability is heightened.

Not only can the practice of chigong build up health in the practitioner, it can also stimulate the emergence of infinite wisdom and power. This is because "being calm and tranquil" is a basic requirement for the practice of chigong. An "inwardly calm and tranquil state" is the third state, differing from both sleeping and waking states. It is a state in which not only is rest provided, but also in which fatigue is relieved.

More importantly, it is an effective way of optimizing the life processes, and especially of keeping the functioning of the brain in better balance, so that the working efficiency of the brain cells can be greatly improved.

In ordinary people, only a small percentage of the fourteen billion brain cells is used, while the great majority remain idle. If the brain cells can be kept in better balance, obstructed channels can be opened and the potentials of the brain can be developed.

According to traditional Chinese medical theory, true chi is the source and impetus of both physical and mental activities. The state of calmness and tranquillity experienced during chigong practice is the best condition in which to increase internal true chi and promote its circulation. Plentiful true chi provides the reliable source material for the cognitive processes; it also renders the cerebral organs sharper and more sensitive.

A number of experiments carried out at various elementary schools, secondary schools and colleges in China have proved that the examination results of student practitioners improve considerably after three to six months of Zhineng Qigong practice.

b. Inspiration emerges more easily.

Inspiration is a special mode of functioning of the cognitive process; there is nothing mysterious about it. The emergence of inspiration requires the following conditions:

1) Both theoretical and practical knowledge are necessary in order for the possibility of inspiration to occur.

These are the prerequisites which must be in place for the receiving of inspiration. It is impossible for a musician to receive an inspiration in physics, or for an artist to have an inspiration in chemistry.

2) An even distribution of all acquired data in the memory "database" is essential.

If one part of the brain is in a state of excessive stimulation, the emergence of inspiration can be restricted due to the fact that the activity of the stimulated part can obliterate or disrupt the accurate reflection of the nature of the subject or object perceived. Only with the removal of this obstruction of access to information within one's field of awareness can the reformatting of vital data naturally occur, permitting the nature of the subject or object perceived to be clearly reflected.

3) The presence of, or relationship to, an external stimulus is an indispensable precursor to the process of inspiration.

This may be either the initial motivation or induction for the inspiration or the last datum needed. The primary conception for inspiration usually appears in a symbolic, representational or illusional manner. In this light, the nature and mechanism of lucid dreams is explained in the author's book, *Essences of Zhineng Qigong Science*.

Through the practice of chigong, first, all of the functions of the brain can be improved and sharpened; further, the brain cells may be kept in a chigong (or energy-sensitive) state - a state in which they are maintained in optimum order. All the preceding provide the necessary conditions for the emergence of inspiration. As long as a practitioner is diligent and hard-working, he or she may be rewarded by creative inspiration at any time and anywhere.

3) The temperament and moral nature are developed.

An unstable mood, especially one such as impatience, impetuosity and anger, is caused by a shortage of internal chi; the mind and spirit are not being sufficiently nourished by true chi.

Through the practice of chigong, as more true chi is produced and re-plenishes the brain, and as the mind is successfully nourished by this chi, its functions are enhanced and stabilized; inward peace and tranquillity are acquired, and anger and worry disappear.

In addition, the smooth, unimpeded circulation of the chi throughout the body can result in an open nature and a full vigor, which provide the physiological conditions for helping others in need. In the theory of Zhineng Qigong science, the close relationship between chigong practice and moral cultivation is thoroughly explained.

For example, maintaining a spirit of open-mindedness and warmheart-edness is quite important in maintaining and increasing the internal neu-tral chi. After the practice of Zhineng Qigong, many practitioners have im-proved their relationships with both their family members and their col-leagues. Their levels of self-cultivation have been greatly improved.

4) Potentials are developed.

No one knows how many potentials are stored within the human body, but one point is certain: the ordinary functions found therein comprise only a part of the whole; there are many human potentials that have never been tapped.

Some people possess certain special abilities in varying degrees; this is a fact which has been proved by scientific experiments. These include, for example, diverse abilities variously described as "reading with the ears", "seeing through the human body", "remote-vision", "remote-hearing", "remote mental-control", "mind-sensing", and telekinesis. These abilities are actually the inborn potential abilities of all human beings. The problem is that ordinary people do not know or have not learned how to use them.

Through chigong practice, these abilities can be awakened and mas-tered by ordinary people. Different practice methods facilitate the devel-opment of different abilities.

Chi-Transmission Therapy (transmitting chi and giving positive af-firmations to the sick in order to bring about healing) can be mastered through a 24-day Zhineng Qigong training. Many students can dissolve benign tumors in seconds. After a three-month Zhineng Qigong training, many students can do "chi-diagnosis" and "mind-sensing" (including "re-mote-diagnosis" and "treatment").

In the larger view, the potentials of mankind are very great. If, through one's own initiative, the mind can be correctly used, many potentials can be developed through special training.

16. The significance of chigong development

Although it is based upon a complete theoretical system for improving the mental, spiritual and physical health of mankind, chigong is not only an exercise method; it is also an ancient and recently reborn science related to the mysteries of human life. The development of chigong is of great immediate significance as well as profound historical significance in light of the current needs of humanity.

a. Chigong can provide health care and develop intelligence.

The practice of chigong can benefit both the young and the old: it is beneficial in helping children to develop their intelligence, in aiding teenagers to grow healthily, to adults in the prevention of aging, and to the elderly for the prolonging of life. It is the optimal choice for the wisest investment of human intelligence.

b. The level of skill in the practice of self-cultivation can be heightened.

The importance of the molding of temperament as well as the cultivation of the moral nature is discussed in light of the requirements of chigong practice. Thus, practitioners are capable of consciously improving their levels of self-cultivation. This is of great significance in promoting moral education and in creating the renewal of society and a better world.

c. Chigong is closely related to Traditional Chinese Medicine.

When the secrets of chigong are fully revealed, the mysteries of the fundamental Chinese medical theories - the Theory of the Main and Collateral Chi Channels (*Jingluo* Theory) and the Theory of Chi and Its Transmutation (*Qihua* Theory) - will be quite easily brought to light. This will further substantiate and refine the theories of Traditional Chinese Medicine, as well as improve the accuracy of diagnosis and therapy.

d. Chigong is an important part of ancient Chinese civilization.

Many of the achievements of ancient Chinese cultures had numerous and intimate linkages with chigong practice. Through chigong research, the esoteric details of ancient Chinese civilization can be further unveiled so that its cultural heritage - which is as well the treasure of the whole of mankind - can be more freely and fully carried forward.

e. Chigong is very advantageous to economic development.

Not only can the practice of chigong heal common and frequently occurring illnesses; it may also reverse serious and complicated diseases. Health care costs and medical expenses can be greatly reduced.

The development of methods of applying chigongology to the outer world is also very promising. For example, chi technology can improve agricultural production. Current experiments have not only resulted in gratifying preliminary results with regard to a great number of crops, but also with regard to experiments of a more immediately applicable nature, such as large scale production-enhancing experiments. Chigong technology is also highly effective in implementing industrial production. As Zhineng Qigong becomes more widespread, and the Technique of the Chi Field is applied on a wider basis, greater success will be achieved in all walks of life.

f. Modern scientific research on chigong will advance the development of modern science.

Research on chigong theories and the various special abilities possessed by chigong practitioners can advance not only the rapid development of bionic engineering, but also the whole-scale and coordinated development of modern science; this in turn will aid the advancement of the entire spectrum of the diverse sciences. In the future, achievements in chigong science research may possibly result in great breakthroughs in the natural sciences

g. The development of chigong will open up an entirely new dimension in the knowledge of mankind.

In the universe, all forms of matter exist in different modes, or dynamic states, which can be classified into three types: the functional processes of inorganic matter, the functional processes of organic matter, and the functional processes of consciousness. All three of these activities are integrally embodied in the human body. In the material universe, modern science has opened a gateway into the realm of inorganic matter - as huge as the macrocosm of the Milky Way, and as fine as the microcosm of the quantum level; yet science is incapable of further developing its exploration into the mysteries of the science of life itself.

The potentials tapped through the practice of chigong can help us experience and observe all kinds of information related to the life processes. As chigong develops, the mysteries of human life will eventually be unveiled, and a new field of knowledge will be revealed.

Many scientists have predicted that the twenty-first century will be the epoch of the science of life-mysteries. Chigong has opened up a new way of understanding the laws of human life processes. Whoever masters chigong may hold a lead in the life science of the new century.

Until now, all civilizations have been established upon the foundations of external energies. After man learned to use fire, he gradually learned to use hydraulic energy, atmospheric wind and electrical energy as well as atomic, solar and other forms of energy. In the process of both researching and actively applying these energies, the different branches of modern science as we now know them have been established, and these have created better conditions for man's existence in the natural world.

Chigong sets its sights upon the development of the internal energies of human beings, and their human potentials. Various demonstrations of chigong and special abilities manifested through its practice have proved that tremendous energy lies dormant and undeveloped within the human body - energy that can be mobilized and utilized. If mankind can use this energy in an unrestricted way, greater freedom and initiative can be achieved in the realm of the natural world, and this will result in a civilization of correspondingly higher quality.

17. Chigongology

Chigongology is a body of knowledge embracing the specific practice methods, principles and fundamental theories of chigong. In chigongology, chigong itself is the object of research, and this is based upon a specified methodology and view of life and the world. It studies the principles and methods of raising the human life functions to higher levels of integrity, and through such practice of chigong, it also studies the ways and means of attaining superintelligence.

18. Chigong science

Chigong science is a science founded upon the basis of the Entirety Concept - perceiving things as a whole. It employs superintelligence, including various innate special abilities attained through chigong practice as means by which to uncover the laws of human life within the unity of man, society and nature. This new science also applies these laws in the service of mankind, helping humanity to make the great leap from the dimension of life governed by necessity into the realm of freedom.

19. The unique features of chigong science

The ultimate aim of all scientific development is the attainment of liberty, freedom and happiness for mankind. The research of chigong science is focused upon man himself, and man himself is the central subject of study.

Chigong science is a unique science which had its emergence in the 1980's. The object of its research is man himself. It differs not only from the social sciences, which study only the social laws and attributes of man, but also from the natural sciences, which study only the natural laws and attributes of man (including human microstructures and functions).

What chigong science studies is the unity of form, energy and consciousness, the unity of man, nature and society, and the complete body of laws inherent in the life processes of this unity. Its research methods, methodology, and methodological basis differ from those of existing branches of modern science. These distinguishing features are as follows:

- a. Chigong science possesses its own unique system of theory.
- b. Chigong science possesses its own unique research means - the method of Inner Perception.
- c. Chigong science possesses its own unique objects and ranges of research.
- d. Chigong science possesses its own unique research aim.

20. The unique system of theory of chigong science

This system of theory is different from the theoretical systems of modern science, which form the basis of modern methodology and epistemology for all branches of modern science.

If we take Zhineng Qigong as an example, its system of theory consists of:

- a. Fundamental theories, such as the Hunyuan Entirety Theory and the Hunyuan Chi Theory.
- b. Specialized theories, such as those introduced in *An Introduction to Zhineng Qigong Science*, *Essences of Zhineng Qigong Science*, and *Practice Methodology of Zhineng Qigong Science*.
- c. Theories on application technology, such as the Theory of Superintelligence, Zhineng Qigong Diagnosis and Therapeutics, and application theories of Zhineng Qigong science in other fields.

Over the course of the last nineteen years, the experiences of millions of practitioners have proved that these theories are reasonable, reliable and valid. As more such experiences continue to be accumulated, the entire related system of theory will also continue to expand in both its scope and its depth.

21. The unique research method of chigong science

Chigong science employs its own unique research method, which has been termed the Inner Perception (*Neiqiu*) Method, while the counterpart utilized in modern science is the External Observation (*Waiqiu*) Method (the process of practical application, induction, deduction, and the tracing from effects back to causes), and other such related methods.

Nei means internal, inner, while its opposite - *wai* means external, outer. *Qiu* means to seek the answer to, the solution to, or the truth of something. Inner Perception and External Observation refer mainly to the respective cognitive functions or the diverse modes of reasoning.

A complete system of methodology (chigongology) has been created based upon both ancient and modern experiences of chigong practice. This is the quintessential intrinsic feature of chigong science, and also the heart of the whole of chigong science. If there existed no such unique system of methodology, there would have been no chigong science.

The definition of the Inner Perception Method given by the author in Zhineng Qigong science, is as follows: the Inner Perception Method is *the* fundamental method of Zhineng Qigong science. It is the method by which to facilitate the development of superintelligence (including the inborn or innate special abilities) in a) understanding, enhancing and renewing the personal life processes of human beings, b) understanding and improving the interrelationship between man and nature, and c) understanding and transforming the attributes of the natural world.

The specific nature of the superintelligence discussed here (special abilities of both a spiritual and physical nature) differs from that of the ordinary intelligence of ordinary people. It is developed and acquired through the practice of chigong.

The concrete methods involved include information-receiving methods (Interior-Vision, Remote-Vision, Remote-Hearing, Mind-Sensing and other methods), and information-transmitting methods (Chi-Transmitting Method, Mind-Sight Method, Idea-Transmitting Method, and others).

Although, as a scientific research method, the Inner Perception Method was put forward by the author relatively recently, the idea of self-perfection through inward perception was the creation of the ancient Chinese. The Inner Perception Method has been formulated upon the basis of the practice of inner perception found in traditional chigongs.

22. The unique objects and ranges of research in chigong science

The objects and ranges of research in chigong science are the human life processes, as well as the other levels and processes of the natural realm. In the study of the human life processes, chigong science explores not only the characteristics of different functional states (such as waking, sleeping, illness and lucid dreaming) and super-states (such as energy-sensitive states and states in which there is the functioning of extraordinary abilities). It also studies the laws of transformation between different states; this latter endeavor is the more important. For example, the visible life processes, the invisible chi processes, the functions of consciousness itself and the natural laws related to human life all constitute subjects of study.

The applications of superintelligence in different fields are further studied in order to establish sub-theories of chigong science; for example, Chigong Therapeutics, Chigong Music, Chigong Arts, Chigong Sports, Chigong Physics, Chigong Chemistry, Chigong Astronomy, Chigong Geology, Chigong Agriculture, Chigong Biology, Chigong Engineering, and other specific subject areas.

23. The unique aim of chigong science research

Simply speaking, the aim of the scientific research on chigong is to understand and to master both the laws of the human life processes and their correlation with nature, and to use this knowledge to improve one's own well-being.

The elementary aim in the first stage of chigong science is the prevention and healing of illness, the prolonging of life and the perfecting of body and mind. At a higher level, the ultimate aim of chigong science is, step by step, to enhance and renew the life processes, to develop human potentials, and to succeed in helping humanity in making the great leap from the life dimension of necessity to that of freedom.

In fact, genuine chigong scientific research - especially the applications of such research - can only truly begin after the ability of superintelligence has been tapped or developed. The process of healing and health-enhancement is but the very preparatory stage of Zhineng Qigong; this is true for most chigongs and most chigong practitioners.

All the above-mentioned features indicate that chigong science possesses all of the conditions necessary to constitute an independent science. It is a recently born science, parallel to but independent of other contemporary sciences, and it can not and should not be contained by other branches of modern science. It has brought the dawn of the revelation of the mysteries of both human life and the life of the universe. It is a product of our time - the proud son of the union of chigong and science and it will bring forth - and flourish amidst a new scientific era.

24. The implications of Inner Perception in traditional chigongs

As we know, through the practice of chigong, quantum leaps may take place at different levels within the human body. Chigong can not only prevent and heal illness - it can also develop one's intelligence potential, as has been stated above.

When one's inner sensory ability (including higher-sensory perception) becomes sharp enough, one can actively perceive the various life processes within the human body.

These life activities include the functioning and individual processes of the internal organs and tissues, the flowing, gathering, dispersing, opening and closing movements of the internal chi, and also the activities of various networks of chi channels. In traditional chigongology, all these inwardly perceived life activities were termed 'internal geography'; the perceiving process itself was called interior vision (inward-seeing) and the means of acquiring such knowledge was called inner exploration or inner perception.

It needs to be pointed out that, during the simple era of chigong, before the classic chigongs of the Qin and Han dynasties, the implications of inner exploration and their various specific techniques were generally applied to the directing and enhancing of one's healthy chi, one's wisdom, and one's own abilities.

However, the ancients called this "*turning within oneself for the solution*" or "*returning to oneself*", rather than formally terming it inward exploration or inner perception. For example, Mencius said, "*The ancients first turned to their own minds for help, and only thereafter, others.*" Confucius said, "*Gentlemen seek solutions from their own brains.*"

From the above quotes, it can be inferred that the process of "*turning within oneself*" is actually undertaken in order to enhance one's accomplishments and abilities (including one's moral cultivation) in one's practice of chigong.

Further, the ancients also realized that superintelligence could be developed through such inner exploration.

Although, to some extent, the ancients understood the functions and mechanism of the technique of inner perception, they did not widely practice it. This is because the application of superintelligence would consume high-level energy; even though those same ancients, who advocated more pragmatic forms of cultivation, characterized such *"tire-the-brain, drain-the-spirit"* techniques by such descriptions as *"the magnificence of self-cultivation,"* they also admonished, *"but the most foolish thing to do"* (Han Feizi - an ancient sage).

In later dynasties chigong gradually became religious in nature - the practitioners pursuing such goals as becoming super-beings or Buddhas; such chi-damaging and spirit-consuming superintelligence practices were strictly forbidden. The axiom *"know how to do but do not do"* resulted from this mandate.

It can be inferred from the above summary that, in traditional chigongs and in the self-cultivation of the ancients, inner perception was only a guiding principle, the aim of which was the procuring of healthy chi and the enhancement of various abilities. Thus, it fell into the category of chigong practice.

In chigong science, the purpose of the Inner Perception Method is the acquisition of superintelligence through inward perception, this was followed by the active and conscious application of this superintelligence with regard to both understanding and reforming one's own life and the life of the universe. Thus it has entered not only the field of scientific methodology but also the realm of philosophical methodology. The Inner Perception Method of chigong science embodies its own unique implications.

25. The implications of perceiving inwardly in the process of the Inner Perception Method

a. The process of inner perception during common chigong practice.

For ordinary people, superintelligence can only be obtained by inwardly perceiving one's own activities of consciousness. First, one must turn one's mind within in order to raise the level of one's life processes to a state in which superintelligence may become functional. This is a process of practice which embraces clearer aims and requirements than those so generally embodied in the ancient axiom *"turn within oneself"*.

Only through the practice of such inward perception can one's sensitivity and clarity of consciousness be enhanced, can obstructions to awareness be dispelled, and can sensory abilities and the potency of their respective results be enhanced. Moreover, only when these abilities reach a certain level can the Inner Perception technique be successfully applied to the objective realm.

      b. The process of perceiving inwardly in the application of the Inner Perception technique.

In applying the Inner Perception technique, initially, one must focus one's consciousness inwardly, achieving the super-functional state described above; then one is in a position to receive or transmit information. While in a super-functional state, one's attention is focused upon the activity of the processing of data within the field of awareness. The more successful the inward focus of one's mind, the better the results will be.

Only when the focus of consciousness is turned within in order to achieve a state of superintelligence can it successfully act upon external things. This is a process of practice through which the practitioner greatly expands upon the fruits referred to in the ancient strategy - *"the insight within extends without"*.

26. The distinctive features of the Inner Perception Method

      a. The distinctive features of the method of inner perception in the understanding of matter.

The cognition of a thing achieved by the Inner Perception Method has the feature of entirety:

      1) Through means of superintelligence rather than means of the ordinary sensory organs, information about the characteristics of a thing in all its aspects is received directly, simultaneously and multi-dimensionally. Thus, an objective cognition of a thing can be obtained without logical thought or analysis.

      2) The totality (or entirety) of space. Knowledge of a thing can be obtained without its being limited by spatial limitations. The ability of diagnosing at a distance is one such example.

      3) The totality (or entirety) time. The knowledge of a thing can be obtained without reference to its limitations in time; there is no differentiation between the past, present and the future; these three temporal states emerge simultaneously. Precognition is one such example.

      4) The totality (or entirety) of time and space. The knowledge of a thing can be obtained without reference to time and space. In any given thing, the unity of time and space forms a real existence. This is a common characteristic distinct from the

solidity of a thing, and constitutes a feature which is possessed by everything in nature.

When one can experience, observe or perceive this special unity, one is able to exploit the ability of penetrating into matter as one pleases. (For example, one can remove an object from a sealed container without breaking or opening it.)

It should be pointed out that the process of understanding the entirety of a thing, as stated above, is a step-by-step process proceeding from the easy to the difficult and from the elementary to the advanced. It is also proportionally related to the level of power that the subject or practitioner has attained. Moreover, the cognitive process itself also represents a unity comprised of observing and thinking; the latter constitutes a very important principle in the sphere of epistemology.

b. The characteristics of inner perception in acting upon matter.

Not by means of any human organs (such as functional organs) can the subject directly apply superintelligence to act upon an object without touching it. For example, when a chigong practitioner sends chi into a human body, or into various laboratory instruments or specimens, changes may take place in them. In chigong circles, one also finds those who possess the ability to move objects with the mind, as well as similar related abilities.

27. The difference between The Inner Perception Method and introspection in psychology

Although, in psychology, the object of introspection is itself also the subject of cognition, and the major focus of the observation and analysis involved are the psychological processes of the self, this observation and analysis still belong to the objective realm. The peak experiences which have been described by various researchers (which are similar to the internal states of peace and tranquillity in chigong) have appeared spontaneously rather than deliberately.

As generally understood, introspection is a process involving a kind of internalized thinking. This thinking method differs from the turning within of one's awareness found in the practice of chigong. Moreover, psychological introspection involves ordinary thinking rather than super-thinking.

The Inner Perception Method of chigong science is an entire process, moving from the inward focusing of one's consciousness to the uplifting of one's own functional state to that of a higher level. Thereupon, while one is in an advanced state of life-functioning, one proceeds to heighten one's conscious awareness of the internal life processes. Finally, there occurs a further leap to an even higher-level state of life-function.

In this approach, the essential point is the bringing about the leap of one's life-functions to a higher level. Without such progressively higher functional leaps, it cannot rightly be called or confused with the Inner Perception Method which we have discussed here.

28. The logic and applicability of the Inner Perception Method for research into life activities

In the realm of cognition, the common doctrine holds that the measuring tool must be more accurate than the object measured. Moreover, the level of functioning of the subject must be higher and more complex than that of the object.

It is because of this doctrine that man has explored both the macro universe and the micro quantum world, and it is likewise due to this axiom that man cannot cognize his own life processes. The reason for this is that the life-functions of the whole of the human realm are intimately connected with the higher-level functional activities of consciousness.

This is due to the fact that man is an organic unity consisting of body, chi, and spirit (substance, energy and consciousness). It is impossible to use spirit, which is based in and upon the body and chi (matter and energy), to "measure" the activities of the body and the chi controlled by the consciousness.

The Method of Inner Perception is employed while one is in a super-functional state attained through the practice of chigong. In this state, on the one hand, the cognizing functions (including cognition through synthesis of consciousness) are more accurate; on the other hand, the activities of consciousness also function at a higher level than those of ordinary people. Thus it is possible to comprehend the subtleties of the human life processes.

Such super-functional states, termed chigong-states of functioning, (described in shortened form as 'chigong-states'), do appear in some experienced practitioners. Many experiments have proved the existence of such states; moreover, it has also been proved that the super-functioning of chigong masters is also related to the above-mentioned chigong-states.

29. Noteworthy achievements through the application of the Inner Perception Method

There have been many noteworthy achievements in the application of the Inner Perception Method.

a. The Theory of the Main and Collateral Chi Channels, as well as the Theory of Chi and Its Transmutation were established upon foundations laid by the active application of the Inner Perception Method.

Both the Theory of the Main and Collateral Chi Channels and the Theory of Chi and Its Transmutation constitute the theoretical essences of Traditional Chinese Medicine and ancient chigongs. They have both successfully stood the test of practice in both Chinese medicine and chigong for thousands of years.

These theories have also been proved in a preliminary way by modern scientific experimentation: by means of these we now know that chi has an objective existence, and that the main and collateral chi channels are internal balancing systems differing from the nervous and circulatory systems, the subtleties of which are still unknown to modern science.

Even the highly developed modern sciences are not capable of uncovering the subtleties of chi and its networks; how then did the ancient Chinese know of the invisible and ethereal existence of these entities? The only answer is: through the practice of chigong and by means of techniques of inner perception. Much evidence of this can be found in ancient Chinese medical records and books.

b. Modern experimental results.

At present, a growing number of people have joined the mass movement of chigong practice. Many phenomena related to chi channels and chi transmutations have appeared in various practitioners. Moreover, it has been demonstrated that, under some stimulation, a number of sensitive people are also able to experience the existence of the main and collateral chi channels.

Several special photographic experiments have demonstrated that the distribution of biological light in the human body coincides with that of chigong light, that the energy pathways in the human body coincide with the distribution and flow of chi along its channels, and that the vital points along those energy paths coincide with the classical acupuncture points.

Although modern science cannot explain what form of matter chi and the chi channels are comprised of, and how these phenomena occur, it has at least proved their existence.

30. The possibility and practicality of the majority of people using and mastering the Inner Perception Method

Special abilities exist not only within the special few, they are also dormant in ordinary people. They are the latent potentialities of the whole of the human race.

Experiments have shown that the special abilities dormant in ordinary people can be tapped by special training. In the Huaxia Zhineng Qigong Training Center, after a three-month full-time Zhineng Qigong training, approximately forty percent of the students are able to attain the ability of diagnosing through the use of the mind alone, and five and ten percent of the students can achieve the capacity to perceive sensorily at remote distances. It is both possible and practical to use the superintelligence acquired through the practice of chigong to understand both man and nature.

31. The principles of the Inner Perception Method

a. Superintelligence is an indispensable prerequisite.

The faculty of superintelligence is indispensable in the processes of both understanding and transforming the world. Herein, superintelligence may be understood to mean inborn special abilities; but more importantly it refers to that higher intelligence which is acquired by special training - chiefly chigong training.

The practitioner's level of superintelligence directly decides the range, depth and accuracy of her cognition of the world. It also controls the degree and the reliability of her effectiveness in beneficially transforming the world. In chigong science, the dependence upon superintelligence is quite similar to the dependence of modern sciences upon instruments, equipment and the skill of those performing the research.

The Inner Perception Method possesses the disadvantages of its somewhat mysterious status and of its reliance upon highly intuitive thought processes; these can be overcome only by the widespread dissemination of the knowledge of chigong and by the active participation of a progressively greater number of people.

b. The process of application of the Inner Perception Method is a process of perfecting or optimizing one's own life processes.

In chigong science, the process of applying the Inner Perception Method is also a process of chigong practice in which the practitioner's level of function can be enhanced, and by which her life processes can also be optimized. The most important task of chigong science is to study the entirety of the process of health-enhancement, and its laws. This research process is also one of gradual self-perfecting, progressing from lower to higher levels.

For the researcher-practitioner, the progressive application of the Inner Perception Method, in accordance with the Hunyuan Entirety Theory and corresponding practice methods of Zhineng Qigong, actually constitutes a process of self-perfecting. Zhineng Qigong places its emphasis of practice upon both internal chi and external Hunyuan chi; the external Hunyuan chi of nature is absorbed into the body in order to enhance one's life functions. Great attention is paid to improving one's ability to bring external Hunyuan chi into full play.

      c. The application of the Inner Perception Method must be based upon knowledge obtained through the External Observation Method.

Knowledge obtained through outer observation refers to knowledge gained by the respective approaches of modern science and philosophy, as well as other generally existing knowledge obtained by means of ordinary intelligence.

In the process of exploring the object of cognition through super-intelligence, conscious instructions are given through the faculties of ordinary intelligence. If one's ordinary knowledge is neither broad nor deep enough, it will be impossible to issue the proper conscious instructions to the faculty of superintelligence in order to explore the object in question.

The processes of distinguishing and judging by means of one's own frame of reference are based upon ordinary knowledge, and are necessary in analyzing the information acquired through superintelligence. Ordinary intelligence is also needed in order to guide superintelligence in acting upon the object of its inquiry. The evaluation of the results of the application of superintelligence requires not only repeated experimentation through the practice of the Inner Perception Method, but also, within specific parameters and to a sufficient degree, corroborating proof yielded by the External Observation Method.

In the most complete view of chigong, the Inner Perception Method is not purely a process of inward perception because it also embraces within itself the External Observation Method. Moreover, in studying human life and the life of the natural world, the tremendous data obtained by the Inner Perception Method also needs to be processed - by analysis, induction, synthesis, deduction and other methods of logical inference - all of which constitute the fundamental or basic operative principle of the External Observation Method - data processing. Without these, it is impossible to obtain correct and complete knowledge of the many complex and multi-faceted processes of life.

32. The methodological foundation of chigong science

Methodology is the general principle by which people are educated in ways in which to understand the universe; this is closely related to the particular cognition of the nature of the universe (or world view) at work. Generally speaking, methodology and world view are intimately related to each other and are always coupled.

A certain methodology will result in a specific corresponding world view; a specific world view also mandates a related methodology. In a sense, they are in a mutually indivisible and interdependent relationship.

The methodological foundation of chigong science is the Hunyuan Entirety Theory. It comprises the unity of ontology, methodology and epistemology; it is the basis upon which Zhineng Qigong science relies - and it can also provide a necessary frame of reference for chigong science.

The Hunyuan Entirety Theory consists of the following components: the Hunyuan Theory, The Entirety Theory, The Theory of Consciousness, The Theory of Morality, and the Human Hunyuan Chi. In the following text, only the first two parts are briefly introduced.

33. The Hunyuan Theory

The common pursuit of mankind seems to be the ceaseless exploration into the origin of the universe. This is true at virtually all times and in all countries.

An ancient Greek philosopher held that every substance in the universe was formed by discreet and indivisible particles - atoms; this is the well-known Atom Theory.

In contrast to this theory, the Chinese sages summed up the basic nature of the universe as invisible, continuous and indivisible existence. Lao Tzu (*Laozi*) termed this most basic existence the *Tao*. Some called it Vital Chi (*Yuan Qi*), while others called it *Yin/Yang*.

In fact, *Tao*, Vital Chi and *Yin/Yang* can be summed up in one word - chi. This chi is neither air nor gas, but a special and superfine source-substance. In classic chigongology, this is described as the "all-things-from-one" theory of chi.

In the view of this theory, all visible physical things are transmuted into manifestation from invisible and formless chi - "*Being comes from non-being (entity-comes-from-non-entity)*". Visible substance can also be transmuted back into "nil" (or no-thing-ness). (This "nil" is not emptiness but rather that condition of non-visible being which exists prior to and in contrast to the visible world - and refers to chi.) Repeated cycles of "being-into-nil" and "nil-into-being" transformations constitute the evolution of all things in the universe.

Upon the basis of the achievements in cosmology inherited from the ancient sages, the author has set forth the Hunyuan Theory in a synthesis embracing modern science and philosophy, as well as his own practical experiences in Zhineng Qigong science.

In Chinese, *hun* means to blend and transmute, to mix and to form, and *yuan* means a unity or oneness. Simply speaking, the meaning of Hunyuan is the blending and transmutation of pre-existing substances or entities into a new unity, or oneness.

However, in Zhineng Qigong science, Hunyuan is a special phrase embodying many implications. Hunyuan Theory is comprised of three parts: the Hunyuan Concept of Matter, the Hunyuan Concept of Change, and the Hunyuan Concept of Time-space.

34. The Hunyuan Concept of Matter

a. In the universe, nothing exists as an isolated form, but rather all things exist as wholes - Hunyuan entireties, blended and formed by two or more key material elements.
b. In the universe, all things exist in either of two states: the state of Hunyuan chi or the state of physical manifestation.
c. With regard to all physical manifestation, the Hunyuan chi of things exists not only within them, but also around them.
d. Both Hunyuan chi and physical substances have diverse levels of manifestation.

35. Matter existing in the state of Hunyuan chi

Matter existing in this state is formless, superfine and invisible, and has no physical manifestation. Although it is formless and invisible, and represents a condition in which the body and the chi co-exist in an undetectable, mutually indistinguishable state, it is a result of the transmutation of the chi, the physical body, and its own essence through a mutual process of inter-blending.

36. Matter existing in the state of physical manifestation

Matter existing in this state (physical manifestation) is visible and has the characteristics of three-dimensional existence. The gathering, accumulation and concentration of Hunyuan chi culminate in the formation of substance; conversely, a substance can also be dispersed and dissolved back into the condition of Hunyuan chi.

Invisible super-physical (or subtle) Hunyuan chi can be regarded as a specialized form of Hunyuan chi, while visible substance can be considered a generalized form of Hunyuan chi; one can be transmuted into the other, and vice versa. The universe is such a Hunyuan entirety, wherein these two states of matter act upon each other, dynamically changing and evolving from one state into the other.

37. The existence of Hunyuan chi within and around all things

Visible substance is the gathered or condensed form of its inherent Hunyuan chi, while the Hunyuan chi surrounding it is its attenuated, dispersed form of existence. The greater the density and volume of a substance, the thicker and broader the Hunyuan chi around it becomes. Any change in the character and structure of a substance will also cause relative changes in the Hunyuan chi around it, and vice versa.

Every substance is the unity of its own physical and superphysical existences, which is called its Hunyuan entirety in Zhineng Qigong science. Different Hunyuan entireties can either act upon each other - to be blended and transmuted into new Hunyuan entireties of a higher level, or they can be dispersed and dissolved into Hunyuan entireties of a lower level.

People with superintelligence can experience and be aware of this character of unity within the Hunyuan entirety, but modern science is incapable of detecting it.

This is because, when modern science tries to understand one characteristic of a thing, it takes as its prerequisite the exclusion of the totality of its characteristics. That is to say, it is not capable of simultaneously studying the characteristics of a thing in all its diverse aspects.

For example, this is the reason modern science can reveal the characteristics of a thing in physics and chemistry, but cannot reveal the specific nature of the life processes which are embodied in the central formation of a Hunyuan entirety.

38. The diverse levels comprising Hunyuan chi and physical substances

Because substance is evolved from Hunyuan chi, the most primordial and original state of subtle matter is the original state of Hunyuan chi, which can be called original Hunyuan chi. It is a superfine, homogeneous and unique substance with no differentiation in its nature, which fills the whole universe and permeates all things.

It is a unity, and incapable of being divided. It can evolve and transmute itself into different states of superphysical (and subphysical) Hunyuan chi, and can further gather and accumulate into all kinds of three-dimensional manifestations (substances).

In the process of gathering and accumulating Hunyuan chi, when the entirety of the body, the chi and the nature embodied within it becomes condensed to the point of reaching a 'critical density', a physical substance is formed with the visible manifestations of form, energy and mass.

At the same time, its Hunyuan chi is also coherently distributed from the interior to the exterior of the substance, completely surrounding it. Together, both the central physical form and the surrounding Hunyuan chi constitute a Hunyuan entirety.

All known substances in modern sciences, from basic atomic particles to planets, to animals and to mankind, are the manifest transmutations of different states of Hunyuan chi.

In Zhineng Qigong science, the highest level of Hunyuan chi in the universe is termed chi of unified human consciousness. It constitutes the formation and functional processes of Hunyuan chi of the human brain.

Several of the characteristics of the chi of the unity of consciousness are similar to those of original Hunyuan chi, but there is a difference in their respective levels. The former chi is much more complex in its composition.

In addition, the chi of unified consciousness is volitional, that is to say, it has initiative. This form of chi can cause both the original Hunyuan chi and other levels of Hunyuan chi to transmute in various ways. One of the goals of Zhineng Qigong practice is to heighten the ability to gather and condense, disperse and dissolve all levels of Hunyuan chi.

Since 1997, the scientific research of Zhineng Qigong has developed in depth, and the research into the verification of the basic theories of Zhineng Qigong has been enhanced. A number of experiments have been conducted with the purpose of verifying the fact that Hunyuan chi can be successfully transformed into light, electricity, heat and magnetism. The ultimate purpose of the above-mentioned experiments is to verify the Zhineng Qigong Theory of Three Levels of Universal Matter recently put forward by the author.

In this theory, all matter in the universe is considered to possess three essential elements - mass, energy and information (the definition of information here is different than the conventional one). All matter can be classified into three levels - substance, field and Primordial energy. A substance at the first level has physical manifestation and mass, following the Law of Constant Mass, but its energy and information remain concealed within its mass. Modern science has already cognized the second level of matter - matter existing in the state of a field. This form of matter follows the Law of Constant Energy, with its mass concealed within its manifestations of energy and information. In the physical world studied by modern science, all types of matter follow the Law of Constant Mass and Energy.

In Zhineng Qigong science, the third level of matter - Hunyuan chi, is considered as possessing existence in the universe. This form of matter exists in the state of information, with its mass and energy concealed within its manifestation of information (or existing in a blended state of mass, energy and information). Although Hunyuan chi exhibits no manifestation of energy, it can be transformed into powerful energy. Through special training, the consciousness of man can alter the natural evolving process of the original Hunyuan chi and create matter, known or as yet unknown, directly from the original Hunyuan chi.

Although the above-mentioned experiments are not precise enough, they have virtually demonstrated that the basic theories of Zhineng Qigong are correct. It can be concluded that Zhineng Qigong theory is not merely a body of theory common to chigong science, but a theoretical framework stimulating modern science to explore new fields, to develop a new human culture and to promote the evolution of civilization.

39. The Hunyuan Concept of Change

In the Hunyuan Theory, everything is considered to be unceasingly moving and metamorphosing between two states: (1) The mutual transmutation between visible/physical substances and invisible/superphysical substances, and (2) the mutual transmutation between Hunyuan chi and Hunyuan entireties. This is termed by the ancient Chinese, "the mutual transmutation between being and non-being".

This process is the result of the gathering or dispersing of Hunyuan chi up to the point of reaching a critical threshold. This transmutational process takes place following its own natural laws with respect to all things in nature.

However, once mankind came into possession of the faculties of self-awareness, certain activities of human consciousness could then also result in transmutations wrought by the gathering (condensation) and dispersing (diffusion) of Hunyuan chi. One of the priorities of chigong practice is the strengthening of one's ability to both gather and disperse Hunyuan chi.

Although substances change from simple states into complex states, as well as in reverse, all changes take place against the background (or field) of the original Hunyuan chi. Everything is ceaselessly fluctuating and moving in seven ways: opening and closing, entering and exiting, gathering and dispersing, and finally, mutually changing and transmuting. Changes in all things are the result of the interaction, blending and unifying of these individualities with their surrounding Hunyuan entireties.

40. The Hunyuan Concept of Time

In the state of ordinary intelligence, time is understood to refer to the continuity of manifestation of the changes in things. The past, present and future of a thing are thought of as comprising a set of innumerable instantaneous manifestations, a view which is similar to the definition found in geometry of a line as being but a series of continuous points. This may well be the basis of the well-known "linear feature of time".

In the view of Hunyuan Theory, the temporal manifestation of anything is neither isolated nor absolute:

First, any momentarily existing thing embodies a record of its past transmutational history and data. Infrared post-photography is such an example - the activities of a person at a specific time in a specific place can be retrospectively photographed within a certain period of time after the person has left that place. This phenomenon is due to the past traces of change and the residual data of that person's presence still remaining in the atmosphere. In accord with the same principle, these past traces of change and residual data can also be accumulated and stored in the fabric of physical substance itself.

Second, any momentarily existing thing embodies its seeds of future change. Bio-photography is such an example - the morphogenetic field template (the embryonic energy pattern) of a leaf can be pre-photographed even before it blossoms from the branch of a tree, which indicates that the manifestation-patterns of its future growth are already embodied as a template within the form of the tree.

Because of the above two points, in view of the Hunyuan Theory, it may be said that the instantaneous existence of every thing is a Hunyuan state (a primordial energy state) embodying its own past, present and future. This is why people with superintelligence can, on the basis of the present, temporal existence of a thing, both foreknow its future and retrace its genesis and past.

41. The Hunyuan Concept of Space

According to the Hunyuan Theory, space is not a vacuum (indeed, there is no such thing as a vacuum). Space is a dimension in which original Hunyuan chi exists. This original Hunyuan chi possesses the capacity and property of containing all things; it also possesses the capacity and property of filling and permeating all things.

As stated in the Hunyuan Concept of Change, the individual Hunyuan chi fields of different things can mutually influence one another by means of the super-conductive/transitive nature of original Hunyuan chi (space).

The result of these properties is that the Hunyuan chi of differing substances may embody that of each other; at the same time, they are also "stored" (contained or "repositoried") in the original Hunyuan chi - the primordial being-ground of all things.

Because original Hunyuan chi is homogeneous and indistinguishable, it appears to exist in a state transcending sidereal time and physical space. All the other diverse levels of Hunyuan chi contained by it appear to be distributed throughout it.

Because of this characteristic, superintelligence can acquire the attributes of other substances from a single specific substance that embodies those former substances. Moreover, by means of superintelligence, the attributes of various manifest substances can also be acquired from the primordial void-nature, emptiness (*xu wu*), or multi-dimensional space in which original Hunyuan chi exists.

42. The Entirety Theory

The Entirety Theory expounded represents only one aspect of the Hunyuan Entirety Theory; it possesses many views identical to the Entirety Theory of modern science.

According to the Hunyuan Entirety Theory, an entirety is formed by the interactions of its inherent parts, and is completely, independently and individually manifested in its interrelationships with external things. It is based upon but not equal to the sum of all of its inherent parts. It is the composite unity of both its inherent structure and its diverse functions, in which is also included its dynamic balance. The characteristics of this entirety are embodied in all of its inherent parts in such a way that each of its parts also manifests the characteristics of the whole.

The inter-blending, transmuting and unifying characteristics of all things are set forth respectively in the Hunyuan Concept of Matter, the Hunyuan Concept of Change and the Hunyuan Concept of Time and Space. However, the "Oneness" formed by this triune process of blending, transmuting and unifying is itself none other than an entirety, so that the Hunyuan Theory and the Entirety Theory can not be separated from each other.

As an example, what is described in the Hunyuan Concept of Matter and the Hunyuan Concept of Change are the processes and states in which the physical existence of things, as well as the super-physical existence of things, are blended with their surrounding environments and transmuted and unified. This view is itself a complete entirety concept, because it is directly related to the entirety characteristics of a thing, as well as to the interrelationships among its component parts.

Thus, the Entirety Theory described here is only an extension of the Hunyuan Theory in relation to the aspect of the characteristics of its entirety. It consists of the Entirety Theory of the universe, The Entirety Theory of Man and Nature, and The Entirety Theory of the Human Body.

43. The Entirety Theory of the Universe

In Hunyuan Theory, the universe is regarded as an unceasingly evolving Hunyuan entirety; all the celestial bodies and all things upon them have evolved from original Hunyuan chi (Primordial Oneness), and will continue to evolve over a long period of time, to eventually be reabsorbed into the original Hunyuan chi. The following is a brief explanation:

The author is in accord with the views of modern astronomy that all celestial bodies (including the earth and the solar system) undergo the processes of growth and decline (death); even now, our flourishing earth and the ever-changing solar system are actively in the process of dying away.

When all of the hydrogen in the sun burns itself out, and as its central gravitation increases, the surface of the sun will implode, and this will result in yet a further explosion and the formation of a red giant star of immense volume. This red giant star will eventually reduce in volume and become a white dwarf star with extremely high density, huge mass and relatively small volume, in which atoms are ionized and electrons form loosely bonded electron clouds which are blended with atomic nuclei. Finally it will evolve into a neutron star, in which electrons and protons disappear and loosely bonded neutrons prevail.

At that time, there will be no differentiation among all existing celestial bodies; they will be virtually unified into one celestial body. The individual forms, chi fields and inner essences of all previously existing things will undergo extreme contraction within this unified form while, concurrently, the density, length and breadth of the Hunyuan chi expanding around such a celestial body will increase in inverse proportion to the contraction of its component forms.

As this universal body becomes infinitely small (for example, as small as an atom or a subatomic particle), the Hunyuan chi around it will undergo tremendous expansion. As soon as the body, the chi and the innate nature are inwardly concentrated to the point of reaching a critical state in which they can no longer be distinguished and divided, instantaneously will an internally and externally identical homogeneous Hunyuan state be formed. This is similar to the "critical non-resistance" phenomena found in the field of synchronicity.

At that point, a new primal order begins, and evolutionary transmutations and changes-of-state occur, all of which constitutes the equivalent of the great explosion (the "big bang") described in astronomy. Following this, the universe begins anew its cycles of condensation of substance, physical manifestation, and evolution (or self-perfecting), from the invisible to the visible (or from the superphysical to the physical) and from the simple to the complex - as described in the science of universe. All of the processes described in astronomical physics will also take place anew - the formation of new solar systems, the gradual creation of new planets, and the evolution of creation upon those planets, up through the emergence of mankind.

44. The Entirety Theory of Man and Nature (*Tian*)

Tian refers to both the natural environments and social environments found upon earth. The Entirety Theory of Man and Nature is another part of the Hunyuan Entirety Theory. It consists of the following insights:

    a. Man and nature comprise an organic Whole.
    b. Man and society comprise an organic Whole.
    c. The human body constitutes an organic Whole.

45. The unified entirety of man and nature

The basic understanding of the universe cannot be separated from the understanding of man himself, because man is the subject of this cognition. However, in the practical sense, the understanding of the "Self" is much more important than the exploration into the origins of the universe.

This is because, at its root, human life is a process of conscious or un-conscious self-preservation, self-understanding and self-perfection. How-ever, man is not separate from anything else. Man, nature and all things form a unified entirety. This can be explained in the views of both ordinary intelligence and superintelligence, as follows:

    a. The unified entirety of man and nature in the state of ordinary intelligence (in the context of physical time-space)

Man is the result of the evolution of nature at its highest level upon earth. While, in some respects, he has evolved directly from the higher animals, all the laws of evolution and the diverse aspects of the evolution-ary process of matter have been accumulated and incorporated into the human body. This process includes the progressive evolution of inorganic substances into organic substances, living beings, lower animals, higher animals and finally, man.

Every advancing link in this long, evolving chain is the result of the in-teraction between nature and the evolving form; thus, the human body has always been incorporated into an entirety with all other things, and with the universe itself. In this unified entirety, man, all things, the heavens and the earth, unceasingly interrelate with and act upon each other.

In order to deepen the understanding of the total unity of man and na-ture, in the following paragraphs further explanations are given from the view of diverse levels of matter.

Material exchanges in the natural cycle: a cycle of natural progression proceeds from inorganic substances to plants, which synthesize all types of nutrient substances, to animals, which consume these plant substances and excrete the wastes thereof, and then to microorganisms, which decompose these wastes, with the end products finally returning to the natural kingdom. Man is a link in the chain of this natural cycle.

Natural energy exchange: the essential energy of the earth comes from the sun, while man directly or indirectly absorbs this solar energy (for example, through the exploitation of chemical biochemical energy), and then releases this energy back to nature through all kinds of human activities.

Information exchange: The definition of information used here is not quite the same as that of modern scientific scholarship. The implications of the present definition of information are embodied in a principle referred to as the time-space structural principle (consisting of three key elements: basic substance and its essential quality, quantity and formation).

Everything possesses its own unique information. As man lives in the natural world, he continuously exchanges information with nature. This information exchange is subtler than the above-mentioned changes related to substance and energy; thus it is hardly perceptible, but nevertheless does have an effect on the human body.

For example, some people may naturally feel comfortable, relaxed and at ease in certain places while they feel uncomfortable, agitated, or awkward in other places. This may not always be due to the presence or absence of anions (or negative ions), because in many places the conditions are not present for the formation of anions. Of course, the ability to receive such information is also closely related to the inner state of the individual.

It must be pointed out that this entirety characteristic - the unity of man and nature - not only manifests in the exchange of both substance and energy, as well as information, but also manifests in the more important dimension - the activity of human consciousness. This is also the basic difference between man and other things in the natural world, and the most essential characteristic of man himself.

Human consciousness is not only able to passively receive external information and to cause related changes within the human body in order to maintain a harmonious relationship and total connection with the external environment; it can also consciously act upon nature in order to cause natural things and processes to conform to the needs of man. This manifests chiefly in the process by which, through industry, the human spirit (in combination with the totality of civilized knowledge) is creatively transformed into all manner of materials devised to meet the needs of mankind. Furthermore, innumerable substances from the natural world are processed and "humanized" in order to replace and immeasurably enhance the functions of man. All these have caused man and nature to become more closely connected.

In the comparison between modern man and ancient man, it must be pointed out that the entirety characteristics of the Hunyuan unity of man and nature present a remarkable difference in quality and breadth, as well as depth. This is an extremely important point which every Zhineng Qigong researcher must confront with the proper attitude.

> b. The unified entirety of man and nature in the state of super-intelligence (in the context of chigong science)
>> 1) Man and all other things arise from the same source - original Hunyuan chi, the original primordial energy- intelligence of the universe.

In both Zhineng Qigong science and traditional chigongology, chi is regarded as the source of both man and all other things. As has been stated in the above description of Hunyuan Theory, everything in the universe evolves out of original Hunyuan chi, thus an inherent mutual identity is retained between them.

Because man and all other things evolve out of the background of original Hunyuan chi, it constitutes the medium linking man and all other things. It is the medium through which all things are capable of interacting with and acting upon each other.

>> 2) Man absorbs external Hunyuan chi to nurture his own well-being.

The whole of human life is a process in which man unceasingly absorbs external Hunyuan chi, and blends and transmutes it into human Hunyuan chi. This manifests in the following processes:

> a) Absorbing and assimilating physical substances.

In view of Hunyuan Theory, every physical substance is gathered and condensed from Hunyuan chi. When physical substances (foods) which are consumed become decomposed into micro-elements into a condition in which they can be absorbed and utilized by the human body, they are assimilated by physical Hunyuan chi and become part of the body.

These new micro-components within the physical body neither retain nor lose all of their former natural attributes. In other words, every substance within the human body still retains a portion of its former natural characteristics (or characteristic nature). This is one of the mutually maintained aspects of man and nature in a unified entirety.

b) Fusion with external Hunyuan chi.

As in the case of other physical substances, there is also a thin layer of human Hunyuan chi of a specific density existing within a certain range around the human body. This externally distributed human Hunyuan chi is capable of co-existing with the external Hunyuan chi of other substances; they may also permeate each other and blend and merge with each other.

On one hand, external natural Hunyuan chi is taken in and transformed into human Hunyuan chi, which further influences the changes within the human body; this relates to the so-called "variation effect" described in modern science. On the other hand, human Hunyuan chi in turn acts upon the external environment, which influences external substances and causes change within them, leaving upon them the imprint of man. The human body and external environments mutually influence each other and unceasingly exchange Hunyuan chi; in the long perspective, a unified entirety, in which the Hunyuan chi of a man is mingled with the Hunyuan chi of things around him, presents itself.

46. The indivisibility of man and society

As all know, man is not only an entity of the natural world, but also a social being. According to the Entirety Concept of Man and Nature, and with regard to every individual, the life of an individual manifests both in her relationships with other individuals and within the social bonds by which she is constrained. Any individual who is absolutely independent of human society is not truly a human being.

All of man's life activities are carried out against the background of the whole society, which include not only the relationships between individual and individual, but also the basic activities of mankind - work activities and production activities, as well as activities whose purpose is the creation of outer circumstances. All these constitute external environments which interact with man; thus they represent important conditions acting upon and causing changes within the human Hunyuan body.

It is within this greater integral body, in which conditions of production and environment have been continuously improved, that mankind has progressed from the stage of ignorance to that of civilization.

As human civilization develops, many natural resources and materials have been utilized in the construction of human social environments; this has not only made such environments more complex, but has also profoundly influenced anew the development of mankind itself. All the moral codes, beliefs and philosophies, as well as customs and habits of humankind have come about within the framework of such social environments, and have become dynamics impacting the consciousness of every individual.

Moreover, the social behaviors of every individual create the circumstances which are responsible for influencing other individuals. All these have melded human society into an ever-advancing, blending and transforming totality, and every individual living within it is an expression of the synthesis of this continuously blending and transforming totality.

According to chigong science, one's state of consciousness and moral attitudes are intimately interconnected with all of one's life activities (both physical and spiritual, one's psychological conditioning being largely dictated by one's society). Thus it has been said, "The nature of man is not an innate attribute nor does it possess an objective reality, but is, in fact, the sum total of all his social conditionings." (Marx)

47. The indivisibility of the human body

Modern science and medicine are identical in their views that human life consists of complex and multi-leveled processes, including physical, chemical and biological processes, as well as the activities of human consciousness. While not all strata of life processes are on a parallel level with one another, they are all unified within the life processes of the whole.

There are certain differences between the characteristics of all the component substances present within the human body and the characteristics of the same substances present in the natural world outside of man. Taking the simplest and most basic shifting parameter of electrons as an example: the shifting parameter of the electrons in the human linear particle body of the respiratory system is from 10,000,000 to 100,000,000 meters per second, which is much higher than that of a non-organic system - the latter ranging from 0.01 to 100 meters per second. This is to say, the functioning of every part of the human body is subordinated to the totality of functioning of the whole life - the dynamics of the entirety.

What nature of entirety is the human body? According to the Hunyuan Concept of Entirety, the human body is an entirety formed by three key elements: the physical body, the chi and the spirit (consciousness), in which the body is the physical condensation of substance gathered from human Hunyuan chi, and the framework through which human life is manifested. Chi is a non-physical form of human Hunyuan chi, and is the manifestation of the life activities of the whole; it nourishes both body and spirit. The spirit (consciousness) is a special manifestation of human Hunyuan chi; it is the functioning of the unified field of awareness (the unity of consciousness), and is the controlling principal underlying all human life activities.

Although there are great differences in the respective forms of manifestation of these three aspects, they are nothing else but different dynamic states in which human Hunyuan chi exists, conditioned by the diverse characteristics it manifests within those respective states. These three rely upon each other, mutually transmute amongst and into each other, and comprise an organic entirety.

However, they do not exist parallel to or at the same level with each other. The physical bodily essence is the basis of human life. It is simultaneously nourished by chi and controlled by spirit (consciousness); it is the vehicle in which chi and consciousness dwell. In the early stages of the human life process, for example, at the stage of the human embryo, spirit (consciousness) and chi are consolidated into the physical body and submit (or are subservient) to the developmental requirements of the embryo.

Chi is incorporated into the physical body and into the spirit (consciousness); it is the medium linking the body and the mind, and it is the invisible substance that integrates and manifests the entirety characteristics of the human life functions. Chi can either be gathered and condensed to become part of the body, or it can be transmuted into spirit (consciousness).

The fundamental functions of ordinary intelligence are the transmuting of the physical body essence and the chi, as well as the carrying out of directions initiated by consciousness. In the state of superintelligence obtained through chigong practice, the first step is the unification of the body and spirit with chi. For example, one such manifestation of the state of superintelligence is the external generation of energy (the Chi-Transmission Method) and the effecting of changes within an object without benefit of physical contact. At an advanced level of chigong practice, the physical body essence and the chi can be unified with or transmuted into spirit (consciousness); then the form of the practitioner can either be visible or invisible as he or she pleases.

In short, there are different forms and levels in the human entirety. Every part of the human body is filled and permeated with Hunyuan chi, and these embody the entirety characteristics of the totality, so that every part may manifest the entirety characteristics of the human body.

48. The features of the Hunyuan Entirety Theory

a. It is a theory centralized upon man.

102

b. It is a unified spirit-matter world view, based upon the oneness of all substance.

c. It regards the chi of unified human consciousness as the highest level of Hunyuan chi, as a result of its higher position on the evolutionary spiral than original Hunyuan chi.

d. It possesses a distinguishing feature of levels.

e. It possesses a distinguishing feature of indeterminable time and space.

f. It possesses a distinguishing feature of subject-object-entirety.

49. The centralization of the Hunyuan Entirety Theory upon man

Hunyuan Entirety Theory is said to be centralized upon man because its key focus of study is man. Although many parts of the Hunyuan Entirety Theory concern the natural laws of the evolution of the entire natural world, it ultimately serves mankind, by helping it to attain liberty and freedom in the domain of living, and more directly, in optimizing the human life functions. Though it is of great significance in many other fields, the fundamental and ultimate goal of the Hunyuan Entirety Theory is the benefit of humankind.

50. The unified spirit-matter monist principle of the Hunyuan Entirety Theory

In the Hunyuan Entirety Theory, spirit (mind) is regarded as a special type of Hunyuan chi - the activity of the totality of consciousness. That is to say, consciousness constitutes the formative impulse of a special kind of substance.

This substance has identity not only with physical human Hunyuan chi, but also with the Hunyuan chi of the natural world. It can not only act upon internal human Hunyuan chi to bring about changes therein; it can also act upon external Hunyuan chi to transmute it.

The above mentioned concept has not only established the theoretical underpinnings for all of the subject matter embraced by Zhineng Qigong science; it has also provided a theoretical basis by which to understand the ancient method of chigong practice, the teaching of which is embodied in the phrase, "Transmute the physical bodily essence into chi and transmute the chi into spirit". If chi and spirit were truly two different elements, how could chi ever be transmuted into spirit?

51. The higher level of the chi of unified human consciousness (*Yi-yuan Ti*) above that of original Hunyuan chi in the evolutionary spiral

Original Hunyuan chi is invisible and formless, and its mass and energy exist in a concealed condition. It is an undiscernible, indescribable and homogeneous substance, but it can evolve into all forms of substance having mass and energy, and ultimately, into man.

Human consciousness is the activity of unified Hunyuan chi of the human brain, which is formed when, upon reaching a certain level, the cellular Hunyuan chi of the human brain is gathered and condensed. This substance possesses a close reliance upon the human cerebral organs - being a physical substance, yet with a certain independent quality of its own.

The chi of unified human consciousness is itself also invisible and formless, its mass and energy also existing in concealed form. When the consciousness is peaceful and tranquil, there is no differentiation throughout it, but when there is activity within it, it can gather and concentrate energy and even cause qualitative changes therein; this is quite similar to the working of original Hunyuan chi.

In addition, the chi of unified human consciousness can not only reflect external things, but can also reflect its own internal processes, resulting in transformations in all things. Through its own volition and initiative, it can cause nature to be transformed in accordance with man's wishes. Thus the chi of unified human consciousness occupies a higher level in the evolutionary spiral than original Hunyuan chi, which, by contrast, transforms itself in a completely natural and spontaneous manner.

Original Hunyuan chi is the source and basis of all forms of matter in the universe. It can permeate all things, proceeding from the simplest to the most complex, while conversely, the chi of unified human consciousness occupies the highest level amongst all kinds of Hunyuan entireties; it can penetrate all things, proceeding from the most complex to the simplest.

Moreover, the laws of motion and change of celestial bodies in the universe become altered because of the emergence of mankind. As, step-by-step, mankind frees itself, the destiny of a celestial body with mankind upon it will change correspondingly.

52. The distinguishing feature of levels in the Hunyuan Entirety Theory

According to the Hunyuan Entirety Theory, any Hunyuan entirety is blended and formed by two or more substances possessing different characteristics; thus Hunyuan entireties possess diverse levels.

In Hunyuan entireties, this characteristic feature of transmutational states manifests both in the substance proper and also in its way or process of evolving; that is to say, there are diverse phases within both the transmutational process and the substance itself. For example, the universe is formed by the interplay of two states of matter - the state of original Hunyuan chi and the state of physical manifestation; the latter can be further classified into non-organic physical states and organic physical states (including botanical organisms and animals). If we take the human body as an example, we see that it possesses many levels of diverse activities, such as physiological activities, chemical activities, general life-activities, and the activities of consciousness.

In summary, a Hunyuan entirety is blended and transmuted from the individual components embodied within it, or from those entities at diverse transmutational stages. Thus, we must pay attention to the following:

When studying the laws of change of a thing, the object of cognition is taken not only as a whole within itself but also as part of a higher-level whole. The object must be studied against the total background of all the higher levels of its entirety.

The so-called entirety is actually only the entirety within that component part, which is itself embodied within another entirety of yet a higher level; in addition, there are the influences of its surrounding environments. It is formed from all of the characteristics of the components, as well as from the new characteristics emerging from the interactions of these components.

Different levels of things require correspondingly different methods of study. In the field of science, there are physical methods, chemical methods and chigong methods. With regard to chigong, it is the understanding of human life according to the entirety views of diverse levels which provides the genesis of the different theories and practice methods of diverse chigong disciplines.

Because all component levels are embodied in a whole, there must be an identity linking each level and each part. If this identity - the essence - can be grasped, then the whole can be similarly mastered. The practice methods and theories of Zhineng Qigong are based upon this principle.

There are transmutations between substances of different levels. Lower-level substances can leap to higher levels, a principle which manifests in the evolutionary processes of all levels of matter, as stated above.

Matter of a higher level can also lose its unique characteristic features of that level and can fall to a lower level. For example, if a newborn baby cannot grow into natural human consciousness it may revert to the level of the animal (historically, children raised by wolves or tigers have not been able to successfully acquire natural human consciousness). In like fashion, the bodies of dead animals may dissolve, devolving to the level of non-organisms, and visible matter may be transmuted into the form of invisible energy. There are special qualitative rules which are operative for each level of a thing, and they do not equal the simple sum of its lower levels.

53. The indeterminability of time and space in the Hunyuan Entirety Theory

In the view of the Hunyuan Entirety Theory, in the universe, time and space are infinite. The contents of every level within it, though, have limitations in time and space, the boundaries of which are indeterminable.

In all things, original Hunyuan chi and the chi of unified human consciousness exist in a formless state beyond the parameters of time and space. However, the Hunyuan entireties of things are indeterminable in both time and space. The boundaries of Hunyuan chi around things are difficult to determine, and the time-frame of its evolutionary process is also indeterminable.

For example, the Hunyuan chi template of a leaf has already appeared before the bud emerges from a branch, a fact which has been proved by bio-photography. This is also the theoretical basis within which energy-sensitive people can foreknow the future and detect the past.

54. The unity of the subject and object of cognition

Here, the subject of cognition is referred to as the activities of consciousness (precisely speaking, the functioning of superintelligence) of the researcher. The object is that which is to be studied, which includes the researcher's own life processes and the objective existences in the natural world.

According to the Hunyuan Entirety Theory, there is a high-level identity between the subject of cognition and the object of cognition. In this regard, the entirety characteristics also manifest between them in the following ways:

When the researcher studies his own internal life processes, both the subject - one's superintelligence; and the object - one's own life processes - are parts of one's entire life function; they form an entirety on a higher level of identity. The subject and the object are unified within the life process of the researcher's own chigong practice.

When superintelligence (the subject) is used to study external things (various objects), superintelligence transforms the entirety of the object by means of its own state of wholeness; the subject and the object are unified within an entirety-related state. This is the essential condition in which and by which the researcher unifies the observing and thinking processes, and through which one can attain a "sudden enlightenment".

55. The External Observation Method

Mankind is the highest-level outcome of the evolution of the universe at its present stage. The individualized existence of human beings (including the brain and its diverse functions) is part of the evolution of the original primordial energy totality (Hunyuan entirety) of the universe. Mankind's ongoing process of understanding and creative re-forming of the natural world is actually the process of the universe's understanding and re-forming of itself. There are two approaches which are both antithetical and yet complementary to one another.

One is the way of chigong science, that is, relying upon superintelligence in order to understand and creatively re-form the world of nature (including man himself). Since in this process consciousness is introverted, it is called the Inner Perception Method (as described above). The system of science established for this process may be called Inner Perception Science (or the Science of Superintelligence).

The other approach is the way of modern science - relying upon ordinary intelligence (the human sensory organs, such as the eyes, ears, nose, tongue and body, as well as the organs of locomotion) to understand and creatively re-form the world of nature. Since, in this process, all the activities of consciousness are extroverted, it is called the External Observation Method (although this term may in fact encompass many specific individual methods). This system of science (including modern systematic science) is termed the External Observation Science or the Science of Ordinary Intelligence, and works in concert with the Science of Inner Perception.

The External Observation Method is not only the fundamental method upon which modern sciences rely for their formation and development; it is also the method by which man at every moment acts upon and interacts with the world of nature - a method that people are accustomed to commonly applying and skillfully using.

Although the technique of inner exploration - or the Inner Perception Method - emerged in ancient times as a scientific methodology, it was formalized in the 1980's when the science of External Observation arrived at a stage of high systematic development. It still remains largely unfamiliar to the majority of people. Because of this, and in order to apply the Inner Perception Method completely and correctly, it is of vital importance that one possess the necessary understanding of the External Observation Method and its relationship to the Inner Perception Method.

Although there are many methods embodied in the External Observation Method, in analyzing it from the vantage point of dialectical materialism, one finds that, in the overall process of the External Observation Method, man uses his ordinary intelligence in order to interact with the natural world; this process can be further classified into two aspects: the activities of outward practice and the activities of consciousness.

Practice is the process by which the subject – man - interacts with the object - the realm of nature; it includes active observation and experimentation. The observation discussed here in general refers to the use of various human sensory organs and instruments for the purpose of observing and examining natural phenomena and the conditions under which changes in these natural phenomena take place. Likewise, the experimentation discussed above refers to the planning and design of experimental means and equipment devised in accord with the realization of desired experimental goals, followed by implementation of these plans in the study and examination of the chosen experimental objects.

The data obtained from practice constitute only the raw materials for accurate cognition. In order to derive a correct conclusion thereby, correct principles of reasoning must be applied. Such reasoning methods chiefly include induction, deduction, and the process of tracing back into the initial causes of activities or phenomena.

The inductive method is a process of logical reasoning by which things are studied from the specific to the general, and from individual facts to the totality of understanding. It involves chiefly the extraction of common characteristics from a number of individual cases for usage as the basis for the process of classifying various species.

The deductive method is a process of logical reasoning by which things are studied from the general to the specific and from the general principle to the individual conclusion. For example, in the process of three-stage logical reasoning, the conclusion is derived from the interrelationship between the major premise and the minor premise.

The method of tracing back into initial causes is also called the method of logical recall. It is a less stringent method of reasoning applied to propositions which may be uncertain, and in which analogy and error-eliminating methods are applied in order to reduce the level of uncertainty.

In fact, these three methods are usually used in a mutually supplementary way, none of them being absolute. This is because, although the method of tracing causes is, in a sense, creative, it can provide only the possibility of verification, whereas the inductive method provides what may be considered a certainty, and the method of deduction provides a logical inevitability. Only when these three are organically integrated can theoretical thinking be implemented.

The above mentioned constitute the general reasoning, principles and practice activities employed. In practical scientific research, methods and modes of reasoning permeate each other and mingle with one another. Looking back into the history of science and studying its present state, two types of methods can be summarized: analysis and synthesis. With regard to these, there is a difference between the approach of logical thought and the methods of scientific research; in the following, only the latter is introduced.

Analysis is a research method by which the entirety of a thing or phenomenon is sub-divided into simple components (or essential elements) to be studied respectively. The guiding principle involved is contained in the premise that the structure and attributes of an entirety are constituted by its components. The emphasis of research is placed upon the individual element of the entirety, and its interrelationship with other discrete elements.

When one element is being studied, it is isolated from the entirety in order to retain its unique characteristics, and the interactions between this element and other elements are fixed into corresponding boundary conditions. By controlling the boundary conditions, their respective characteristics and laws are studied and understood in light of their varying processes. This is the implication of analysis.

In the context of its methodology, analysis falls into the category of constructionism; it constitutes the main stream of modern scientific research method. It is termed Reductive Theory when it is applied to research upon life phenomena.

The activities of human life are studied by retracing them from their psychological levels through to their physiological levels; the physiological activities are then further progressively simplified, level by level, through the activities present within individual systems, organs, tissues, cells and organic macromolecules, down to the level of biochemical and physical processes.

Through such processes of analysis and modern technology, great contributions have not only been made with regard to such achievements as the construction of the skyscraper, but also with regard to the most basic structure of life - DNA; the double helix spiral was also discovered by analysis. However, analysis has not revealed the mysteries of the life process itself because the structural attributes of life are not capable of embracing the dynamic process of life in its totality.

For example, while the DNA double-spiral structure is still present in a dead cell, the life-process of the cell is no longer capable of being activated. The life functions of even a single cell are not capable of being understood, to say nothing of those of a more complex organic body.

Although the method of logical synthesis was established in ancient times, it found favor in the eyes of modern science in its study of the complex entirety of things. The focus of synthesis is not upon the partial characteristics of things but upon the characteristics of their entirety, comprised of the totality of interconnections and interactions amongst the individual elements of that entirety.

The guiding principle of synthesis is one in which the entirety is greater than the sum of its components; an element within an entirety is different from an isolated element separated from the entirety. From this principle, it can be inferred that, first, an entire, true and complete understanding of a thing can not be obtained through analysis; and second, that the structural details of an entirety are irrelevant to the characteristics and laws of that entirety.

Thus, models can be established in accord with specific research objectives and goals without considering the detailed structures of the entirety object. Obviously, such models are arbitrary and created only in accordance with the specific aims of the research being undertaken.

Such a research method is called synthesis; system theory and control theory are synthetic methods. Thus, synthesis, in its methodology, falls within the category of entirety theory, or entirety concept.

Although tremendous and gratifying achievements have been obtained by synthetic method in the research into complex entities, it remains powerless in implementing research upon the activities of life itself. While they have widened the scope of research in the study of various fields of the natural and social sciences, even newly emergent theories such as structural dissipation theory, coordination theory and mutation theory can barely begin to play an effective role in the research upon life, especially human life. This is due to the fact that the unique capability of self-initiative and the spontaneous nature of human consciousness are too subtle and powerful to be encompassed.

It needs to be pointed out that, although analysis and synthesis are diametrically opposed to one another with regard to their means and objects of research, as well as with regard to the methodological categories to which they belong, the starting point of their methodology is identical - the dualism of spirit against matter. This world view stems from ancient Greek philosophy.

In this view of the world, the universe is divided into two parts - a spiritual world that is relegated into the keeping of the many gods in the heavenly realm, and a material world which is solely reserved for mankind. From then forward, with regard to the mainstream of research, the spirit and the body have been separated from one another and studied in different ways.

The separation and opposition between spirit and substance are the epistemological and methodological foundations of modern science and its basic standard of approach. Both structural theory (analysis) and entirety theory (synthesis) take as their prerequisite assumption the separation and opposition between spirit and substance. Precisely because of this, the view of modern science holds that, in any experimentation and research upon chigong science, it is neither scientific nor permissible to allow the recognition that the factor of human consciousness (spirit) may actively participate in such physical processes.

56. The relationship between the Inner Perception Method and the External Observation Method

As stated above, the Inner Perception Method and the External Observation Method seem as different as heaven and earth - even incompatible, as fire and water (the ancients also believed that only when External Observation was expunged could inner perception be acquired). In fact, the relationship between the Inner Perception Method and the External Observation Method is at one and the same time antithetical and mutually complementary. The Inner Perception Method and the External Observation Method both reinforce and supplement one another.

57. The antithetical nature of the Inner Perception Method and the External Observation Method

a. The Inner Perception Method and the External Observation Method are opposites because of the difference in their respective ways of understanding things.

In the Inner Perception Method, superintelligence is employed as a means of grasping the entirety characteristics of things, such as the entirety of space, the entirety of time, or the entirety of time-space. For example, while an individual is employing the External Observation Method, ordinary intelligence - the functioning of the sensory organs (including the extended sensing or sensory instruments created by science) is used in order to understand the isolated characteristics of things. As we know, no modern instrumentality can simultaneously obtain information about all the multifaceted characteristics of a thing.

b. They are opposites in their respective processes of cognition.

Because ordinary intelligence understands merely the partial characteristics of things, as mentioned above, one can only obtain a complete and essential knowledge of something through logical thinking in conjunction with the synthesizing of information. In the complete External Observation process, observing and thinking constitute two separate component processes.

Through the Inner Perception Method, superintelligence can absorb the entirety data of things. A complete and essential knowledge of something can be obtained without logical thought or the synthesizing of information. The observation process (which is, in fact, a process of both experiencing and observing) is unified with the thinking process.

c. They are opposites in their respective methodological basis.

The methodological basis of the External Observation Method is a world view characterized by a divided spirit-matter dualism, the science of which is spirit-exclusive. However, the methodological basis of the Inner Perception Method is characterized by a spirit-matter unity embraced within a world view of inherent entirety.

The Inner Perception Method relies completely upon the special spiritual faculties of superintelligence in understanding and acting upon external things. The power of the spirit is indispensable to the Inner Perception Method. This is the fundamental reason why modern science cannot accept chigong science.

58. The mutually enhancing and complementary nature of the Inner Perception Method and the External Observation Method

    a. The Inner Perception Method and the External Observation Method are mutually complementary in their respective ways of understanding things.

Although, in the process of understanding, the superintelligence of the Inner Perception Method has many advantages over the ordinary intelligence of the External Observation Method, its range of application is also limited (though the levels of superintelligence will continue to increase as chigong science continues to develop). The synthesis of both methods will deepen the knowledge of the partial characteristics in a whole, the entirety characteristics in a part, and the entirety characteristics inherent within the relationship of the parts of a whole.

    b. The Inner Perception Method and the External Observation Method are mutually complementary in understanding the mysteries of life.

In attempting to understand these mysteries, modern science has come across an insurmountable barrier. These problems concern the fundamentally unknown, indeterminable and superphysical dimensions of life, such as human initiative, the flexibility and creativity of non-logical thinking, and other uncontrollable, random and contingency-related phenomena.

By contrast, the Inner Perception Method possesses incomparable advantages in studying the processes of life, especially the processes of human life. Superintelligence can directly experience and observe the phenomena of the life processes. To be certain, the Inner Perception Method possesses the inherent shortcomings of all generalized perception - indistinctness and indeterminateness. However, these can be overcome by combining the knowledge obtained from the two complimentary sources - both the Inner Perception Method and the External Observation Method.

    c. The Inner Perception Method and the External Observation Method are complementary in their dynamic approach.

It is commonly known that the essential component aspects of the existence of a thing are mass, energy and information. When acting upon external things proceeding by way of the External Observation Method, man relies upon the perception of mass and energy, while information remains secondary. When employing superintelligence in acting upon external things, man relies mainly upon information, with energy and mass being secondary. The combination of both approaches will promote the development of an integrated dynamic approach.

        d. The Inner Perception Method and the External Observation Method enhance each other in relation to the process of cognition.

A correct judgment about a thing unknown cannot be obtained by ordinary logical thinking. A conclusion related to the understanding of something unknown, but derived through the principle of entirety, can only be obtained by using the faculty of super-thinking while one is functioning in the state of superintelligence - an entirety cognitive process in which no logical thinking occurs.

Many inventions and creations were achieved through inspiration (and at times, even through dreams). Inspiration should by no means be understood to emerge from a pre-condition lacking in foundations; rather is it the case that it is rooted in ordinary intelligence.

Ordinary intelligence gathers quantitative data about the partial attributes of a thing, whereas the super-thinking of superintelligence obtains the essential knowledge of a thing in its entirety. The former is a gradual change in the process of cognition, while the latter is a sudden one. When an understanding is gained, that conclusion returns to the field of ordinary intelligence.

This is the dual process of the human cognition of the objective world, possessing a synergistic relationship alternating between both ordinary intelligence and superintelligence.

If modern scientists and philosophers can understand the functions of super-thinking in the context of superintelligence, they will be capable of easily and skillfully solving complicated problems relating to the theories concerning the origins of science. In both its theories and its methods, chigong science has provided the groundwork and a convenient method of approach for this endeavor.

59. The emergence of chigong science as a requirement for the development of human civilization

As all know, since the 1960's, modern science and technology have developed rapidly and have made great progress. When adequate material conditions were achieved, and a certain degree of freedom was obtained in the spheres of both the natural world and the social realm, man began his exploration into the dimension of the science of life.

On one hand, comprehensive and multi-faceted research has been carried out in the study of mankind's physical existence. Though great progress has been made in biophysics, biochemistry, genetic engineering and other branches of science, the essential nature of the life processes is still unknown. All these conditions have formed an indispensable background and pre-condition for the birth of chigong science.

On the other hand, the masses began to seek methods of enhancing and optimizing their own life processes. In the West, beginning in the 1970's, there has arisen a vigorous movement focused upon the study of Eastern civilizations, and an unprecedented number of people have participated in the practice of many forms of meditation.

In China, many folk therapies were widely practiced by the masses, although today most of them seem absurd and unworthy of exploration. The thirst for both spiritual and physical health and the attainment of personal freedom had become the common incentives of the times.

After many failures on the journey of exploration, at long last chigong was discovered. Traditional chigongs have many shortcomings, such as abstruseness, over-elaborate theories and practice methods, the need for long-term practice before seeing results, the dangers of abnormal symptoms, private and esoteric instruction protocols, and other similar requirements. All these not only prevented the rapid spreading of traditional chigongs, but also fell short of meeting the needs of the masses.

This situation helped bring about the reformation of traditional chigongs, and in turn, the new reformed chigongs promoted the development of the contemporary situation. In meeting the needs of the times, chigong science emerged from and was synthesized out of these backgrounds.

60. The process by which traditional chigongs develop into chigong science

It took 20 years (from the early 1970's to the late 1980's) for traditional chigongs to develop into chigong science. A number of chigong masters with lofty ideals, one stepping into the breach as another fell, laid the foundation for chigong science.

There were two distinct periods during this span of time. The first was a ten-year period of reformation of traditional chigongs (1971-1980).

In China, for over the course of more than 5,000 years, traditional chigongs were secretly taught amongst small segments of the population. Though many chigong books were published after 1949, they were neither recognized nor accepted by the majority of the people.

In 1972, Ms. Guo Lin, a famous Chinese chigongist and one of the pioneers of chigong science, thoroughly reformed the traditional chigongs she had learned from her ancestors and teachers and created a new chigong - Guo Lin New Chigong (Walking Practice Form).

This new chigong was both easy to teach and to learn, as well as easy to practice. She put forward her new ideas with the purpose of helping practitioners to individually pass through the three barriers of practice – relaxation and tranquillity, maintaining an unwavering concentration of mind, and exercising effective breath control. All these factors caused traditional chigongs to take on a new appearance.

She not only solved the dangerous problem of avoiding abnormal symptoms, but also established a foundation for group practice. Moreover, she created pyramidal frameworks of instructor groups. This established diverse hierarchical levels of instructors, a policy which broke away from the esoteric teaching methods of traditional chigongs and which also provided an institutional guarantee - rather than a personal sanction - for the implementation of mass practice.

Her efforts were rewarded with success, for no sooner had her new chigong been born than were several difficult and complicated cases of diverse diseases - including cancer - successfully treated. The great attraction of her new chigong fascinated those who had been seeking ways to keep healthy and fit. From that point forward, chigong entered upon a new vista which spelled the beginning of the evolution of traditional chigong into chigong science.

In Beijing, large chigong groups were to be found all over the big public parks. By 1978 more than 10,000 people had joined the legions of chigong practitioners in Beijing. Concurrently, traditional hard-style chigongs were joining the world of sports. The demonstrations of hard chigong in the National 1978 Nanning Games shocked the country and the whole world, adding further momentum to the course of chigong's development.

The First National Chigong Conference Meeting was held in 1979, during which several high-ranking officials heard the reports presented and witnessed demonstrations of hard chigong. This meeting provided subsequent encouragement within chigong circles, and the term 'chigong' spread quickly amongst the people. Amid this new state of affairs, the practice of Guo Lin New Chigong became widespread throughout China.

At the end of 1979, the Beijing Qigong Association was formally founded. This was the first mass chigong organization, and under the leadership of both the government and the Science Association of China. This constituted an unprecedented event in the history of chigong. The knowledge of chigong, which previously was taught only privately, and which had remained the possession of a minority of itinerant showmen, was now brought out into the open and incorporated into the framework of science, with the purpose of serving the population as a whole.

As the advancement of chigong developed to a greater extent, the need for chigong theory became increasingly urgent. This was a key problem pivotal to the further evolution of chigong. Between 1979 and 1980, Professor Ming Pang and Mr. Jiao Guorui, as well as several others, began to reform the theories of traditional chigongs and gave lectures presenting their newly evolved theories in Beijing. Mr. Jiao explained the healing and health-enhancement mechanism of chigong practice from the medical point of view, especially that of Western medicine, and this constituted the first step toward the reform of chigong theories.

Professor Pang studied traditional chigongs from all available sources emerging from the background of ancient Chinese cultures and introduced the common principles of all chigongs - spiritual (mental) cultivation, moral cultivation, breath control, physical movement, and postural requirements. He summarized the essence of traditional chigongs, expressing this knowledge in a contemporary idiom. In 1980, Professor Pang also taught courses in Chigong and Traditional Chinese Medicine, and Chigong and Special Abilities for chigong students. In this way chigong science inherited the past while yet ushering in the future.

In the last half of 1980, the All-China Federation of The Trade Union held a national training class for staff-and-worker chigong coaches. The Beijing Qigong Association took over all of the teaching responsibilities.

Guo Lin New Chigong and Mind-Boxing Standing Practice Form (*Yi Quan Zhan Zhuang*) were taught in these classes. Professor Pang and Mr.

Jiao gave instruction in chigong theory. These classes were of great significance, confirming that a new stage had begun in the history of the chigong's development.

From 1978 on, numerous masters of chigong appeared, teaching their respective practice forms, but most of these were the original ancient-style forms. While the new practice forms may have been disdained by the traditional teachers, or viewed as departures from the classical forms and possibly even as rebellion against orthodoxy, they nevertheless spread rapidly all over China and came to assume a prominent position.

Although important reforms were carried out in Guo Lin New Chigong on both the practice methods and the theories, these still belonged to the category of the Inner Nourishing Practice Form (*Nei Yang Gong*) - in which one practices by oneself and derives benefits for oneself. For these reasons, this stage has come to be called the stage of reform of traditional chigongs.

The second period was the formative stage of popular chigongs as well as the Blueprint of Zhineng Qigong science.

The first stage was the formation of popular chigong. Popular chigong is not a synonym for low level chigong. It is referred to as that chigong in which both internal chi and external chi are mutually cultivated.

External chi is fully exploited for the purposes of improving one's practice, enhancing one's healing results, and shortening the time frame in which these benefits manifest themselves. Popular chigong does not possess as many strict rules as one encounters in traditional chigongs and thus is a suitable practice for the masses to undertake; it constitutes, as well, the basis of chigong science.

The period of the emergence of popular chigongs was from 1981 to 1985. The Soaring Crane Form - the first-level practice form of Zhineng Qigong, was created by Professor Pang and made public in 1980.

Earlier, One-Finger Zen (*Yi Zhi Chan*) was created by Mr. Que Ashui, followed by The Zen-Secret Practice Form (*Chan Mi Gong*) by Mr. Liu Hanwen, The Spontaneous Five-Bird Game (*Zifa Wuqin Xi*) by Mr. Liang Shifeng, The Empty-Power Practice Form (*Kong Jin Gong*) by Mr. Huang Renzhong, and there have been many others.

In the spring of 1981, a National External Chi Technique Training Class was given, in which the second level practice form of Zhineng Qigong was offered by the Beijing Qigong Association, and in which Professor Pang taught the External Chi Techniques. From that point on, external chi therapy has continued to become widespread.

From the latter part of 1984 to the early part of 1985, the Chi Field Technique (*Zuchang* - a monumental discovery by Professor Pang - X.J.) was implemented at a Zhineng Qigong Clinic in Shijiazhuang, where it achieved great success.

During this time, many chigong masters came out of seclusion and competitively contributed their own chigong treasures. A number of scientific experiments performed upon the phenomenon of external chi also succeeded in proving the existence of external chi and of its effects.

In 1985, Professor Pang systematized the Entirety Outlook Theories of traditional chigongs and openly taught the unique Hunyuan Chi Theory of Zhineng Qigong. The Crane Practice Form was reformulated into the Lift Chi Up and Pour Chi Down Method (*Peng Qi Guan Ding Fa*), and the second level practice form - The Body and Mind Form (*Xing Shen Zhuang*) was also widely taught.

The second stage was the prosperous period of popular chigongs.

In 1986, the China Qigong Association (an officially registered first-class institute) was founded. The Hunyuan Chi Theory provided the methods and theories of using external chi (rather than true chi from the Vital Center), for the practice of healing. In these ways the external chi technique began to be popularized.

The methods and theories of the Chi Field Technique were also unveiled to the public for the purposes of group healing and teaching. The Chi Field Technique is the best method for the dissemination and application for the mass practice of chigong. It is one of the Nine Characteristic Features of Zhineng Qigong. This method can be used by groups numbering in the hundreds or even thousands, for both healing and teaching. It has catapulted the technique of external chi to a new level.

The last stage was the formation of the Blueprint of Zhineng Qigong science.

In 1990, Professor Pang published *Brief Zhineng Qigongology*. In this book, he expounds in a preliminary fashion upon the principle of the Unity of Consciousness (the chi of unified human consciousness), as well as the Hunyuan Entirety Theory; this organized and completed the basic theories of Zhineng Qigong. More concrete work (especially theories of application in all fields) is still needed in order to perfect the whole chigong science.

61. The Blueprint of Zhineng Qigong Science

The Hunyuan Entirety Theory
↓
Oneness of Spirit-Matter World View
↓
The Inner Perception Method (Superintelligence)
↓   ↓   ↓

Receiving Information   Super-thinking Transmitting Information

↓   ↓   ↓

→   Applications   ←
↓

```
|                                  |
| -------Fishery                   | -----Geology
| -------Stock  Raising            | -----Astronomy
| -------Forestry                  | -----Physics
| -------Agriculture               | -----Medicine
| -------Industry                  | -----Biology
| -------All branches of           | -----Chemistry
|         natural  science---------- | -----Philosophy
|                                  |
|                                  | -----Law
|                                  | -----Education
| -------All branches of           | -----Psychology
|         social  science------------- | -----Literature
|                                  | -----Arts
|                                  | -----Sports
|
| -------Chigong Engineering (Integrated with ordinary
           intelligence and technology)
```

↓

Theories of Application in all Fields

Direction ↓   ↑ Perfection

Practice

62. The significance of the development of chigong science

    a. To promote the advanced development of modern sciences.
    1) To promote the modern sciences to develop in depth.

The superintelligence spoken of in chigong science can provide goals and resources for modern scientific research. Persons possessing the capacity for superintelligence can, to some extent, control and influence their own life processes as well as those of others; such human beings constitute a phenomenon which can provide resources that are not available in ordinary people.

The bio-phenomena of people of superintelligence, such as bio-electricity, bio-magnetism bio-luminescence, and other such phenomena, are totally different from those found in people of ordinary intelligence. The activities of consciousness of super-intelligent people can cause exogenous substances to change, both through displacement and reformation. Studies and investigations into these phenomena may deepen the understanding of the fact that there are diverse states of life processes, and that higher levels of life processes do exist.

Both the information obtained through the exercise of superintelligence - such as the entirety characteristics of a thing, or the characteristics of the individual components within an entirety - as well as cognitive abilities capable of providing virtually instantaneous rough-estimates - can provide focal points for modern scientific research. More detailed boundary conditions and experimental plans can be instituted for the implementation of analytic method, which can provide a multi-sided analysis; complete comprehensive plans and contents can also be provided to reduce the arbitrary quality of information derived through synthesis.

    2) To promote reformation in modern scientific methods of understanding.

Along with the development of science, philosophy likewise evolved also, progressing from a position of mechanical materialism to one of positivism, and then to positive doctrine or theory.

The methodology and methodological basis of chigong science have thoroughly reformed traditional modes of thinking, and this will result in the adoption of the philosophy of dialectical materialism by the field of life science.

    b. The synthesis of chigong science with the modern sciences is of vital significance in improving ways of living and methods of production.

1) In the future, chigong will help improve various methods of production.

Many chigong experiments geared toward increasing production have proved that, by combining chigong science with modern science, sophisticated, highly advanced technology may be developed, resulting in high technological achievements. In the future, chigong science may play an unimagined role in revolutionizing means and methods of production.

2) In the future, chigong will help improve humanity's traditional ways of life.

Through the practice of chigong it is possible to catalyze the internal process of chi-transmutation, greatly heighten the levels of human wisdom and ability, and mitigate humanity's needs in many areas of life.

There is an ancient saying "*Not sleepy when spiritual chi is abundant and plentiful; not hungry when physical chi is abundant and plentiful; no urge when essential chi is abundant and plentiful.*"

There are also many positive examples of people of superintelligence who are indifferent to heat or cold, who "dance in the boiling oil or fire" (who are resistant to extreme temperatures), who eat nothing for many days, or even years (*pigu*), and who possess other similar extraordinary endowments. All of these instances have demonstrated that the super-states of superintelligent people genuinely differ from those of ordinary people.

In view of the great influence of chigong science upon mankind's ways of living and production, a promising future can be predicted. As chigong science develops, and as superintelligence is widely applied, damage and pollution to natural environments will be greatly reduced, and man and nature will eventually be unified into one harmonious entirety.

c. The development of chigong science will help one to become "master of oneself - a free human being."

Chigong science is a science created with the purpose of studying, understanding, mastering and applying the laws governing one's own physical and spiritual being. The development of chigong science will, with certainty, quicken the realization of mankind's ultimate goal - "to become the master of oneself – a free human being."

63. Zhineng Qigong

In Chinese, *zhi* means wisdom and intelligence, the synthesis of functions performed by the cerebral cortex in dealing with external things; *neng* means ability and capability, in both their physical and spiritual aspects. Briefly stated, Zhineng Qigong refers to a chigong through the practice of which intelligence can be developed, and various abilities enhanced.

In other words, Zhineng Qigong is a chigong designed with the purpose of enhancing ordinary intelligence as well as developing superintelligence. It has become the specific term and a unique name for the chigong founded by author.

This name meets the essential requirements embodied in the description, "very effective in developing both ordinary intelligence and superintelligence". This name not only highlights the fundamental effects of chigong practice; it also raises chigong to a higher status. It will help alter the narrow concept that "chigong is no more than a healing skill."

The theories and practice methods of traditional chigongs are no longer found to be those of Zhineng Qigong. The author has extensively and thoroughly studied numerous classical monographs, books and records about various religions and ancient chigongs, as well as traditional Chinese medical texts. The present Zhineng Qigong is a fusion of the essence of many different chigongs emerging out of Confucianism, Buddhism, Taoism, Traditional Chinese Medicine, traditional martial arts, and folk religions.

The achievements of modern science, medicine and philosophy have also been integrated into Zhineng Qigong. It has been designed and created in accord with the rigorous standards that an independent science must possess.

The name, Zhineng Qigong, not only links this new chigong with modern science, but also embodies within it the specific science of Zhineng Qigong. In this regard, "Zhineng Qigong" constitutes a synonym for "Zhineng Qigong Science".

64. The guiding principles of the development of Zhineng Qigong

To guarantee the healthy development of Zhineng Qigong, the practice of the following four principles has been stipulated: One Aim, Two High Ideals, Three Teaching Principles and Four Cardinal Criteria.

One Aim: Under the guidance of dialectical materialism and historical materialism, deeply practice and probe into traditional chigongs, blazing new trails with sharpened minds. Render the ancient chigongs scientific and publicly accessible, encouraging participation by great numbers of people in their daily lives. Transform natural human instincts into conscious intelligence, advance the progress of mankind from the life realm of

123

necessity to the dimension of freedom, and promote human culture to leap to a higher level.

Two High Ideals: Hold high the ideal that "Zhineng Qigong is a science"; hold high the ideal of "Unity".

Three Teaching Principles: Create conviction within students by power of reason, set a good example by demonstrating the virtues in your own life, and win the confidence and trust of the students through the attainment of skills and practice results.

Four Cardinal Criteria: These are used in evaluating the levels of development of both teachers and students, and include the Zhineng Qigong theories, practice methods, skills, and morals and virtues.

65. Zhineng Qigong science - a totally new science

Zhineng Qigong science has opened totally new fields of research. Zhineng Qigong science studies the entirety of life (in both its physical and spiritual aspects) and the related natural objects thereof; these are subjects which have not been touched by modern sciences.

Zhineng Qigong science involves a totally new focus of study, studying the space-entirety, time-entirety and time-space entirety of various life processes and natural things. These are brand-new research objects for the entirety concept of modern sciences.

Zhineng Qigong science uses superintelligence as its research means; this constitutes a radically different approach from the research methods, methodology and methodological basis of modern science.

66. Zhineng Qigong science - a complex science

The human body is an open, complex and super-giant system. It is the most complicated aggregate of all material processes, including physical processes, chemical processes, life processes and the activities of consciousness.

Zhineng Qigong science studies the laws of the activities of human life based upon objective existence, including the many types of activities of the human body, the interrelationship between man and nature, and the activities of consciousness. While Zhineng Qigong science takes the findings of modern science as a closely related body of basic knowledge, it also possesses unseverable connections with philosophy, religion and ancient Chinese culture.

All of these have laid the cultural groundwork for Zhineng Qigong science, and without them it could not have been created.

67. Zhineng Qigong science - a highly advanced science

Because it has been established upon foundations that are both broad and comprehensive, Zhineng Qigong science is a highly advanced science. In Zhineng Qigong science, the emphases of study are the activities of human life and human consciousness; these constitute activities of a higher-level than those of a physical and chemical nature which are studied by modern science.

The research means of Zhineng Qigong science is superintelligence - which also functions at a higher level than does ordinary intelligence. Its aim is the advancement of the evolution of mankind into the dimension of freedom. The fulfillment of the aforementioned goals will make it possible for mankind to realize the highest values of human life.

Zhineng Qigong science sets its sights upon the life activities of man himself. In the Hunyuan Entirety Theory, the emphasis is upon benefiting oneself while engaged in benefiting others, an approach which unifies the researcher's social values with the totality of his or her life values. All of these endeavors raise the values of human life to their summit.

68. The distinctive features of Zhineng Qigong

Zhineng Qigong possesses nine major features:
  a. A unique system of theory - The Hunyuan Entirety Theory.
  b. A system of practice methods - Three practice forms and three stages of practice.
  c. A number of practice secrets collected from wide-ranging sources.
  d. Three simultaneously adopted teaching methods: 1) teaching through intuitive transmission, from mind to mind or spirit to spirit (as opposed to employing activities of direct observation, or information-gathering); this is best embodied in the Chi Field Technique, and represents the highest level of instruction; 2) teaching through oral communication (explaining the theories and methods); this represents a lower and less subtle instructional method; and 3) teaching through active physical demonstration, which represents the lowest level of instruction.

e. A technique of non-specific mental concentration.
f. The use of the Chi-Attraction Method (*Yin Qi*) for mobilizing chi.
g. An open-type chigong style.
h. The transmission of chi to others without damage to one's internal essential chi.
i. Distinct reactions as a result of practice.

69. The system of Zhineng Qigong practice methods

This system consists of three practice methods or forms - dynamic practice forms, static practice forms and dynamic-static practice forms. Each of them consists of three stages - the External Hunyuan stage, the Internal Hunyuan stage, and the Central Hunyuan stage. This process is a progressive one, moving from a lower level to a higher level.

70. Dynamic Practice Forms of Zhineng Qigong (Zhineng Dong-gong)

The dynamic practice forms of Zhineng Qigong consist of three stages - the External Hunyuan stage, the Internal Hunyuan stage, and the Central Hunyuan stage, as well as six levels of practice curriculums.

Level one - The Lift Chi Up and Pour Chi Down Method (*Peng Qi Guan Ding Fa*), which stresses the process of gathering, blending and transmuting of external Hunyuan chi; this constitutes the External Hunyuan stage of practice.

Level Two - The Body and Mind Form (*Xing Shen Zhuang*), in which emphasis is placed upon the mutual blending and transmuting of the body with the mind; this constitutes the Internal Hunyuan stage of practice.

Level Three - The Five One Form - the making of the five internal organs into one unity - (*Wu Yuan Zhuang*), in which emphasis is placed upon the blending and transmuting of the true chi (essence) of the internal organs. This also constitutes the Internal Hunyuan stage of practice.

Level Four - Central Channel Hunyuan, Step Five - Central Line Hunyuan, Step Six - Return to the Original Self-nature and become one with the universal nature (*Fanben Guiyuan*). Level four, five and six all occupy the stage of Central Hunyuan practice. These six levels of form practice are arranged according to diverse levels of activities of human life.

The Three Centers Merge Standing Form (*San Xin Bing Zhan Zhuang*) - a standing practice - also occupies a place amongst the six levels in the practice process. This is both a basic practice and a transitional practice, moving from External Hunyuan practice to Internal Hunyuan practice, and also from Internal Hunyuan practice to Central Hunyuan practice.

Proceeding from the Lift Chi Up and Pour Chi Down Method, the Three Centers Merge Standing Form is a transitional practice by which to absorb external chi within the body. It is also a necessary practice by which to proceed from the Five One Form to Central Hunyuan practice, in which the merging position and meditation technique differ from their former counterparts.

71. The Lift Chi Up and Pour Chi Down Method - an External Hunyuan practice

The human life processes are carried out upon different levels. All the various layers of skin, muscles, blood vessels, the vital internal organs (heart, liver, spleen, lungs, and kidneys) bones and cells have membranes around them. In those who never practice chigong, the major flow of internal Hunyuan chi is solely through these membranes. The process of exchanging internal chi with the external chi of the natural world is also carried out within these membranes, layers of skin and other shallow surface layers of tissue.

The goal of the first level - the Lift Chi Up and Pour Chi Down Method - is to enhance these innate functions in order to clear and open the channels along which the chi of the internal membranes is exchanged with the external chi of nature, and to blend the chi of the skin, fascia and tissues with natural Hunyuan chi in order to render them into a seamless unity.

This is a process of employing the mind, imbuing it with the idea of blending and transforming the chi existing mainly outside the physical body; thus, this stage is called the stage of External Hunyuan practice. The main idea of this step is releasing one's internal chi and taking in and absorbing more external Hunyuan chi. By doing so, not only is the quantity of internal chi increased, but there is also an improvement in quality of the chi as well. Moreover, the practitioner can develop the ability to treat others by the Chi -Transmission Method.

Because the functions of the membranes and the sensory organs are enhanced, other levels of superintelligence may also be tapped. For example, chi-vision (the ability to see chi), super-vision (the ability to see through the body and distinguish muscles, bones, internal organs and even nerves and cells), mind-sensing (the ability to know what is going on within the minds of others) and other such abilities may also be accessed.

However, superintelligence obtained through External Hunyuan practice is limited. This is because chi flows mainly through the shallow surface layers and the collateral channels of the body, where the texture of the organs is looser; neither the discharge of, nor the strength of, the chi is great enough to obtain higher-level abilities.

It should be clear that when one does reach the level of External Hunyuan practice, the normal functioning of one's life processes can be insured, and one is completely capable of remaining healthy and preventing oneself from experiencing illness.

72. Body and Mind Hunyuan Practice

The practice of Level Two - the Body and Mind Form - places its emphasis upon the mutual blending and transmutation of the body and mind. It is essential to interconnect or merge the body with the mind, a process which can cause Hunyuan chi to pass completely through the body, from its shallow surface layers to its depths.

In this process, chiefly physical Hunyuan chi is cultivated. The human body has five structural levels - skin, muscles, tendons, arteries and veins, and bones. If the chi can pass through all of these, then the chi in the main and collateral channels can be blended with both the chi in the physical body and the chi in the blood, which ultimately come to form a unity. Thus, chi can nourish the whole body in increased amplitude and depth. When all parts of the body are full of Hunyuan chi, its respective functions can be enhanced and a graceful figure can be acquired.

Because, during the practice of the Body and Mind Form, the tendons and bones must be pulled and stretched, it constitutes the most difficult form among the six levels. Through the practice of this form, chi is driven to penetrate muscles, bones and other physical structures.

As the sensitivity of these parts is heightened, the practitioner will be able to feel and to become aware of the condition of the muscles and bones. Although internal organic true chi is, in part, also involved in the practice of this form, the practice of the Five One Form is still required in order to fully cultivate it.

It should be understood that when one successfully reaches the level of practice of Body and Mind Hunyuan, one's level of health is already higher than that of ordinary people.

128

73. Internal Organic True Chi Hunyuan (*Zangzhen Hunyuan*)

In Internal Organic True Chi Hunyuan practice, not only is there the cultivation of the true chi in the five vital organs - the heart, liver, spleen, lungs and kidneys - but at the same time, there is the cultivation of the related spiritual and emotional activities.

In Chinese medical theory, these five vital organs are closely linked to five emotions: the heart is linked to joy, the liver to anger, the spleen to thinking, the lungs to worry and the kidneys to fear. The five vital organs are also related to five spiritual activities. The spirit (*shen*) is concealed within the heart, the conscious soul (*hun*) in the liver, the consciousness (*yi*) in the spleen, the non-conditioned reflex nerve activities (*po*) in the lungs, and the will (*zhi*) in the kidneys.

Through the practice of the Five One Form, the vital organs are filled with true chi, their functions are enhanced, and the spiritual and emotional activities related to them may be properly balanced. The ability to mobilize both internal and external chi may also be heightened.

At the Internal Hunyuan stage of practice, the internal chi is cultivated and blended with the internal organs, main and collateral chi channels, bones, external musculature and, in fact, all other parts of the body, which come to compose a unity.

When a practitioner reaches the level of Internal Hunyuan practice, the internal chi is abundant and plentiful, the mind is peaceful and tranquil, the body is strong and healthy, the figure is beautiful, the body and mind are in harmony, and the overall level of health is greater.

To some extent, the practitioner is able to control the internal life processes, such as the speed of the heartbeat, the blood pressure, the peristaltic motion of the intestines, and other functions. The ability to control the mind can also be strengthened.

In order to speed up the transition from this stage to Central Hunyuan, the Eight Methods of Cultivating Chi were made public in the fall of 1998. This eight-posture extra form is mainly designed to enhance the entirety of physical chi within the human body and help deepen the cultivation of superintelligence.

74. Central Hunyuan Practice

As external chi continues to permeate the body, the degree of penetration by both internal and external Hunyuan chi is greatly increased. Based upon the foundations of External and Internal Hunyuan practice, if chi permeates deeper yet, it arrives at the stage of Central Hunyuan practice.

The Central Hunyuan stage of practice consists of three levels - Central Channel Hunyuan practice, Central Line Hunyuan practice and Returning to and Becoming One with Nature (*Fanben Guiyuan*). The Central Channel is a special channel in the human body, and will gradually appear only when a practitioner reaches a certain level.

The special abilities obtained will be greatly heightened after the practice of Central Channel Hunyuan. As chi is further concentrated upon the central line of the Central Channel, it arrives at the stage of Central Line Hunyuan practice. The final level is the complete unification of man and nature.

75. Why only three of the six levels have been made public

Zhineng Qigong serves the many rather than the few; in order for Zhineng Qigong to become popularized, a strong, expansive and powerful chi field is required for every stage of practice. Before and unless a specific chi field is established for a specific stage of practice, it is quite difficult and painstaking to make progress.

76. Reactions due to chigong practice

As soon as one starts to practice Zhineng Qigong, one will begin to see the result of its effects. Through practice, as the level of one's health improves, various discernible changes will take place within the body.

In the process of moving toward a higher level of health, both spiritual and material impurities which have been accumulating inside the body over a long period of time will be gradually discharged. During this period, various uncomfortable or possibly even painful sensations or experiences, which are termed reactions due to chigong practice, may occur in related areas of the body. There are several kinds of such reactions:

     a. Disease-discharging reactions.

After a period of chigong practice, there may be some disease-manifestations which are not capable of being directly normalized or dispelled. These harmful internal substances need to be discharged immediately through alternate physical pathways in order that many different kinds of necessary cleansing reactions may occur.

The common reactions include: diarrhea, blood or pus in the urine or excrement; in women, increased menstruation and discharge; coughs, increased sputum, vomiting, vomiting blood or pus, a running nose, an issue of blood or pus from the nose, increased mucus in the eyes, fevers, sweating, rashes, sores, symptoms similar to beriberi, and related symptoms.

All these are disease-discharging symptoms. They are usually related to their original diseases. For example, diarrhea may take place in the patients with intestinal diseases; coughs are related to lung disease; fevers may occur in those whose diseases were caused by fevers.

When reactions do take place, one should neither be worried nor anxious, nor cease practicing. If one cannot tell whether the symptoms one is experiencing are those of a disease or a reaction, these too can be dispelled, so long as one has a firm faith in chigong and continues practicing.

If one doubts the healing effects of chigong, and continues to suspect the possibility of an illness, it is permissible to take appropriate medication, but the use of antagonistic or inappropriate medicine is forbidden.

    b. Reactions due to the intensive concentration of chi upon the illness.

It is sometimes possible for the patient to feel even more uncomfortable after chigong treatment than before, due to the effects of chi which has been intensively focused upon diseased areas.

This is a unique phenomenon which occurs when the internal true chi has been cultivated and becomes plentiful enough for the healing of the illness to be implemented, but not yet full enough for a complete healing to take place.

This occurs because the cultivated true chi breaks through the former abnormal balance between the body and the illness. The affected area then becomes more - rather than less - sensitive. This reaction is actually a signal that the function of the injured site has begun to recover. If one keeps on practicing, pains and soreness will eventually disappear.

There is also another kind of reaction, in which various hidden weaknesses or old traumas are revealed by chi, and cause reactions. This indicates that, although the illnesses seem to have been cured, their roots have not been completely eradicated. These are signs that the body is gradually being purified.

    c. Reactions denoting improvement.

It is possible for a healthy practitioner to experience various kinds of reactions as he or she experiences higher levels of health through the practice of chigong. Their related impurities need to be discharged in order to reach these higher levels; thus reactions similar to disease-discharging reactions will also take place. Some reactions purely related to one's progress may be even more severe than disease-discharging reactions. These kinds of reactions are not unique to Zhineng Qigong. They also occur at high-level stages in other chigongs, with only their respective manifestations being different.

It is important to face these reactions calmly and to know that they are only temporary phenomena in the healing process. A glad heart and positive affirmations to oneself for swift and strong recovery may improve the situation and help in developing a favorable result; otherwise things may become worse.

If one is clear about the fact that one may experience distinct reactions during Zhineng Qigong practice because these are one of its characteristic features, one should then face these reactions in the spirit embodied by the axiom "No painstaking efforts, no rewards".

77. The main differences between Zhineng Qigong and other chigongs

a. Zhineng Qigong starts from the blending of man and nature.

Most of the traditional chigongs are chigongs of the closed type, in which the physical essence, chi, and consciousness, or spirit, are confined within the body until all of the internal parts become a unity.

In the final step of such practices, the internal chi is released and exchanged with the external chi of nature. This practice procedure is first internal, then external. The internal chi permeates the body from the inside toward the outside.

Zhineng Qigong is a chigong of the open type. The practice procedure here is just the opposite of that of traditional chigongs. From the start, the internal physical chi is fused with the external chi of the natural world. The individual practitioner is unified with the greater environment and forms an entirety with it. The forces of the man/nature entirety and the self/others unity are fully exploited for the purpose of attaining their specific related benefits.

Chi passes through the body from the outside to the inside. The aim is to cause chi to flow transversely, penetrating across the channels instead of moving along specific channels. In this way, both the main and collateral channels are linked together and unified, chi fills the whole body, and man ultimately becomes one with nature.

b. The emphasis is placed upon the practice of dynamic forms.

In traditional chigongs, static forms are stressed, and regarded as advanced practices, while dynamic forms are looked down upon as practices of a lower level. Zhineng Qigong holds that there exist low levels and high levels in the practice of both dynamic and static forms. The practice of dynamic forms is especially emphasized.

This is due to the fact that a state of true emptiness and tranquillity is too difficult for ordinary people to achieve. According to the requirements of Taoist practices, a genuine high level of tranquillity consists in the cessation of the arising of ideas within the mind, the discontinuance of breathing, and the stilling of the heartbeat. Buddhist practices also require the practitioner to dispel the five vital activities in order to reach advanced state of tranquillity. However, such a state can be reached only when the chi and the blood are plentiful, unimpeded and unobstructed in every part of the body. A single point of blockage may disturb the brain and cause irritation.

In fact, as long as chi can be evenly distributed completely throughout the body without obstruction, a state of clarity and intelligence can be attained. Zhineng Qigong emphasizes a completely unobstructed and unimpeded flow (*tong*), and the practice of dynamic forms through which the chi and the blood can become plentiful and unimpeded throughout the body.

The practice of dynamic forms can, on the one hand, increase the flow of chi within the existing open channels, and, on the other hand, open new channels; this aids in cultivating more true chi and in causing it to function effectively.

At the beginning of Zhineng Qigong practice, the body, the chi and the mind are opened up to both the human realm and the realm of nature. The practitioner is required to cultivate chi in quiet places, and in noisy places required to cultivate the mind, which helps to more rapidly raise one's level of development.

      c. Emphasis is placed upon using one's mind through one's own initiative.

The difference here is that "Voidness, Quiescence and Tranquillity" are not the focal points of practice, but emphasis is placed rather upon the using of one's mind through one's own initiative. This requirement involves being concentrated, focused and singleminded.

This strategy is much easier to understand and to practice. Sometimes the unified mind is focused upon one point, sometimes upon the combination of the activities of consciousness and the life processes, and sometimes upon the union of the body and the mind.

The fusing of body and mind is a flexible application of a systematic approach of "singlemindedness". The aim of chigong science is to actively and

133

in a positive manner exploit superintelligence, and to understand the laws of human life and their correlation with the laws of nature. Thus, in the entire process of Zhineng Qigong practice, from its rudimentary levels to its higher levels, the emphasis is placed upon creatively using one's mind through one's own initiative.

     d. The concept of the effects of group dynamics is stressed.

The old method of teaching traditional chigongs involved the passing on of specific knowledge and skills, in privacy, from a teacher to an individual student. Even among fellow students of the same teacher, it was forbidden to accidentally hear what one should not have heard. By contrast, in Zhineng Qigong, the effects of group dynamics are emphasized - in both the processes of teaching and treating illness by the Chi Field Technique. This method is based upon the Hunyuan Entirety Theory and meets the needs of our contemporary world.

A Zhineng Qigong teacher can build up a chi field for a group comprising dozens or even thousands of students. In this orderly, unified and powerful Hunyuan chi field, under the direction of the teacher, all participants simultaneously perform the same physical movements while holding identical ideas in mind. The effects of this practice upon teaching and healing are inestimable.

     e. The chi of the Vital Center is not harmed when one treats others by the Chi - Transmission Method.

C. THE OPTIMAL PRACTICE OF ZHINENG QIGONG

1. Reaping the best rewards from Zhineng Qigong practice

It is easy for everyone to learn how to practice chigong, but in order to reap the richest rewards, efforts need to be made to embody the following requirements of practice:
     a. Build up a firm faith and confidence.
     b. Be clear about the aims of Zhineng Qigong practice.
     c. Do away with unenlightened beliefs.
     d. Follow the laws of Zhineng Qigong.
     e. Build up a profound Zhineng Qigong (energy-intelligence) consciousness.
     f. Adopt an appropriate attitude towards the reactions that may occur during Zhineng Qigong practice.
     g. Give attention to re-aligning one's way of life.

2. Building a firm faith and confidence

A firm faith and confidence can be transformed into an indefatigable determination, and thus bring about great power. This power may become a motivating force and a reservoir of stamina by which to reach the goal, heightening the wisdom and the courage to overcome difficulties, and enhancing one's ability to withstand both spiritual and physical hardship. It is impossible to succeed in any arduous endeavor without confidence and a firm faith.

This faith contains two implications: the first is believing that physical, mental and spiritual health can be attained through Zhineng Qigong practice; the second is believing that one is capable of becoming an effective practitioner and that one can attain great achievements.

This faith must be rooted deep in one's mind; one cannot undertake a successful practice while maintaining an attitude of mind which is half believing and half doubting. How does one build up such a firm faith and confidence?

a. Deepen one's understanding of Zhineng Qigong.

As explained in the former sections, Zhineng Qigong is not a simple single method or skill; it is a complete body of learning, a profound and advanced science. It has its unique theoretical system, specific methods, objects and aims, as well as its own ranges of research.

Although Zhineng Qigong is completely new to most people, its validity has been and is being proved by millions of practitioners. Every practitioner should avoid worship of and blind faith in chigong, but should seek rather to obtain a complete rational understanding of chigong.

Only when one has a real understanding that Zhineng Qigong is an authentic science can one establish a genuine trust in it. One is then able to see the great power of this faith in one's own practice.

Only when one studies and masters the theories of Zhineng Qigong in depth is it possible to rid oneself of the limitations of general knowledge (including the general knowledge of modern science), and only then is it possible to accept the seemingly miraculous phenomena of chigong as normal, natural and proper.

It is not enough to study theories only; one needs to prove them through one's own practice. Amongst the multitudes of Zhineng Qigong practitioners, what each sees and hears can not only deepen their understanding of these theories, but also helps to build up a power of faith in one's consciousness, which will become an internal motive power during one's practice and application of chigong. One's power of faith is closely related to the levels of one's achievement.

As soon as a firm faith is established, neither doubts nor suspicions will arise, even in the event that one does not completely understand the various extraordinary phenomena that may be experienced. One will conscientiously seek to conform to the principles of practice, and to do what is required; this accords with the spirit of those engaged in various fields of scientific study, who refrain from exhausting themselves in a mad pursuit to comprehend everything, and who instead patiently continue on with their studies in a spirit of acceptance.

For example, when a patient sees a doctor, she will take the medication seriously and conscientiously, according to the doctor's instructions, even if she doesn't know the exact ingredients of the doctor's prescription, its anticipated effects on her, or how these ingredients work. Relatively few people would go out of their way to search for the answers to questions such as which illnesses this medication treats, or how long it will take to cure these illnesses. The reason that patients seldom ask such questions is that medical science is a generally recognized and accepted, and that they believe in their doctors. Nowadays, many people frequently question the effectiveness of chigong practice; in such situations, the key problem is that they believe that chigong is unscientific and untrustworthy. It takes time to change such people's view of chigong.

b. The tempering of one's self through sustained endeavor.

It is easy to have a generic faith in chigong, but a process of consistent effort is needed in order to build up a firm faith. The time and effort needed to see results differ from person to person.

When no effects appear after a period of practice, it constitutes a critical moment in the testing of one's faith. At this time, if one loses confidence and stops one's practice, one will not be able to complete the journey of the remolding of one's body and mind; conversely, if one continues to believe in chigong, remains without doubts, and continues practicing without ceasing, one will achieve what one wishes.

Upon seeing signs of recovery, most patients have been filled with confidence. But, when symptoms returned (most of these being reactions to practice), they have commonly lost confidence and stopped practicing, which spoiled all they had achieved, whereupon the symptoms experienced sometimes worsened.

This is due to the fact that, at the time they undertook their chigong practice, most patients seized upon chigong as their last hope as a means of curing the incurable. A truly scientific faith had not been established in their minds. When they experienced the first effective results they ignored the need of further understanding chigong. Moreover, they were not well prepared for the reactions attendant upon the practice of Zhineng Qigong.

When the symptoms returned, they would succumb to a state of utter bewilderment. They lost their ability of directing the body with the mind, and completely overlooked the evidence of all their former achievements.

At this critical moment, it is of vital importance to hold firm to one's faith and to keep on practicing; in this way, the illness can be eventually eradicated and health finally restored.

3. On "It works if one believes" and "It doesn't work if one doubts"

The saying, "It works if one believes", is regarded as the standard of practice in chigong circles. It is also greatly stressed in the practice of Zhineng Qigong.

This is because in chigong practice the power of faith in one's mind can play an important role in generating positive initiative. It is also a truism that firm believers obtain better and more rapid results than doubters (even so, there does not exist a one hundred percent corresponding rate of cure).

The author agrees with this thesis, but disagrees with the statement - "It doesn't work if one doubts". Chigong is a science having its own unique laws, and faith is only one of the components of its effectiveness; although it is a very important one, it is not the only one.

Even if one does not believe in chigong, as long as one follows the laws, and practices in strict accordance with the correct requirements, it will still be effective. However, the results may be slower to come or tend to be discounted due to the conscious antagonism of those who may not believe.

4. Being clear about the aims of Zhineng Qigong practice

The ultimate aim of Zhineng Qigong is to advance the development of human culture to the point of making a leap to a higher level of living. There are different requirements at different stages in the overall process of reaching this goal.

Whether for the prevention and healing of illness, the maintenance of health, or the development of intelligence, the ultimate aim of Zhineng Qigong should be to promote the heightened development of human civilization, to create a better world, and to benefit the whole of mankind.

Only when one unifies one's own aims with those of the whole of mankind is one capable of practicing more conscientiously and not giving up in the face of difficulties. It is impossible to attain a high level if one practices only for one's own benefit, even if one succeeds in improving one's health and develops various rudimentary abilities. There is an ancient saying - "Virtue (morality) is the mother of merit (or achievement)." Also, "One's chi is pure when one possesses high moral character." When a systematic and complete life science and chigong science is established, it is also possible for a practitioner to then become a chigong scientist. It is a reasonable goal to pursue such lofty aspirations and great ideals.

Different kinds of chigongs stemming from different sources have different standards by which to evaluate the practitioner's achievements and levels of ability. Every Zhineng Qigong practitioner should establish a correct conception of what constitutes merit.

From a subjective point of view, one can attain such diverse qualities as strength and health, high energy, good-temperedness and noble-mindedness, brightness and intelligence, high efficiency and resourcefulness, and so on. From an objective point of view, the criterion is one's ability to achieve better, greater, more immediate and more economical results both in relieving patients from their sufferings and in raising the productivity of life in different areas, such as the industrial and agricultural realms.

Overall, in Zhineng Qigong science, the levels and accomplishments of a practitioner can be evaluated by objective standards. This conception of merits is founded upon objective reality and upon the interests of the majority of the people involved.

5. Doing away with unenlightened beliefs

Throughout the history of China, for over the course of more than two thousand years, chigong was connected with various kinds of religions. The extraordinary abilities developed through the practice of chigong were explained as the superpowers of Buddha or of the gods. In order to develop the science of chigong, these unenlightened beliefs must be dispelled.

If one wishes to be a practitioner of attainment, one must likewise expunge these unenlightened beliefs from one's consciousness. Otherwise, one can never attain a high level; even worse, one may be led down wrong and dangerous paths.

We can restore the essence and scientific aspects to chigong only by tearing away the feudal and religious veils covering it. On one hand, we must take a clear-cut stand in dispelling unenlightened beliefs; yet on the other hand, we should not negate everything pertaining to them, but seek, with a rigorous and scientific attitude, to prove their truth or falsity.

For example, many of the remarkable abilities of practitioners of the past were thought to be the gifts of Buddha or of the gods. In fact, such abilities were the fruits of the practioner's own practice of chigong. When one reaches a certain level of ability, various related vital points, paths, and channels in one's head can be cleared and opened, followed by the manifestation of various supersensory abilities transcending those of the ordinary five sense organs (eyes, ears, nose, tongue and body).

In such cases, one may be able to see through objects, to see remote locations, to hear at distances, to sense the thoughts or ideas of others, to foreknow, and to perform similar feats. Even many ancient practitioners of great accomplishment privately knew - as the adage goes - that "Buddha and the gods are actually human beings." (By this it is meant that phenomena long attributed to supernatural powers were seen by the initiated to be extensions of the deeper functions of human consciousness.)

6. Abiding by the laws of Zhineng Qigong

    a. Respect both the teacher and the Tao.
    b. Practice conscientiously and seriously.
    c. Be relaxed, natural, and tranquil.
    d. Integrate practice (*lian*) with rest and nourishment (*yang*).
    e. Apply the faculties of both concentration (*ding*) and observation in a complementary fashion (*hui*).

7. Respecting the Tao

One of the principles of chigong practice is the necessity of respecting both the teacher and the Tao; this is not contradictory to the new teaching-learning relationship advocated by Zhineng Qigong. In the process of teaching and practicing, students and teachers co-exist as equals. Teachers should not think themselves as superior to their students, nor even as rendering charitable service. From the point of view of optimal learning, however, it is strongly recommended that both the teacher and Tao be respected.

In the past, chigong practice was called cultivation of the Tao (*xiu dao*). What is the Tao? The Tao is the most fundamental principle/substance in the universe, as well as the dynamic laws pertaining thereto. There are essential differences between the Tao and various skills found in chigong. Such simple specific chigong techniques or methods are only peripheral issues in the practice of chigong; the Tao only is of utmost importance.

Zhineng Qigong is a science. Its practitioners should not become fixated upon its simple methods and erroneously take Zhineng Qigong to be nothing more than a single simple skill. To respect the Tao is to respect Zhineng Qigong science, and both its theories and practice methods.

The practice of chigong is a matter of great importance for the practitioner's own state of physical and psychospiritual well-being. It is a process of remolding both the body and the mind, and also a process by which to alter the practitioner's destiny, whose course is determined by the functional levels of her life activities.

In what way is the Tao to be respected? The key point is to practice Zhineng Qigong with whole-hearted devotion and never to change one's mind. Zhineng Qigong can meet the needs of different levels of practitioners. As soon as one has learned Zhineng Qigong, one more surely maintains a firm and unshakable practice, and does not alter one's original intentions.

8. The inadvisability of combined chigong practice

Every type of chigong has its own characteristics. In order to achieve a certain goal, a practitioner must observe its special requirements. Different chigongs may cause different changes in the body.

Being committed to only one chigong causes the body to be harmonized with this particular practice, and helps in producing a natural functional rhythm and a good balance. If one practices several chigongs at the same time, different functional rhythms may be generated, resulting in disorder in one's life processes and preventing one from making progress.

If one deems Zhineng Qigong to be good, one should not at the same time practice other chigongs. If one thinks another chigong is good, one should not at the same time practice Zhineng Qigong.

It is usually dangerous to be simultaneously involved in several chigongs. Practitioners of a single chigong can make faster and better progress than practitioners of multiple chigongs.

9. Respecting the teacher

Those who are in the position of helping to guide one in making progress should be accepted as one's teachers, and deeply respected. To respect others is to respect oneself. To respect others as one respects one's teacher can help to maintain a respectful and sensitive state of mind. To be concentrated, focused, tranquil and neither impetuous nor aggressive will help one to better receive instructions from the teacher, as well as from the surrounding external environment. It will help in allowing one to become conscious of a greater number of things, in activating one's vitality and in making more rapid and greater progress.

This respect should also be extended to nature, including both natural environments and all living things within the field of nature. One should fully exploit the vigor of nature in activating one's own vitality. All these abilities and qualities flow from the attitude of being calm and tranquil within, and respectful and humble without.

10. Practicing conscientiously and seriously

In order to benefit oneself more effectively and more rapidly through one's personal practice, one must rely upon one's own self. The teacher can only teach theories and methods, and offer advice and help at various critical moments, which then may have the effect of encouraging students to attain higher levels of achievement.

However, if one does not practice at all oneself, it is not very likely that receiving the teacher's instructions would result in relevant changes in one's own body. How, then, is one to practice?

a. Practice assiduously and perseveringly.

First of all, one must be clear about the postures and the essential requirements thereof, and also about the functions of each movement. Zhineng Qigong places emphasis on both its theories and practice methods, and only by studying both of these can further progress be made.

There are two foundations of practice that yield the best rewards: one is to practice conscientiously (using one's mind through one's own initiative) for a considerable period of time; the other is to cultivate one's moral nature and to transform one's own being.

As all know, rewards come after arduous practice. One may wonder, "How hard should I practice?" That is all up to you, according to your own mental and physical conditions. The standards are different from person to

141

person because each person has his or her own personal nature and physical conditions.

To do a little bit more than one thinks one is able to do is appropriate, and can be called "working hard". A practice schedule should be carefully worked out with consideration for all aspects of one's life, such as one's work, studies and daily life.

It takes time and effort to attain results. The more one practices, the sooner one is rewarded. In terms of results, one should not constantly compare oneself with others; one should only compare oneself with one's former self.

Perseverance is also very important. It is impossible to make progress if one practices a dozen hours one day and does no practice forms on other days. It is also harmful to one's health to practice in fits and starts. It is impossible to mend the omission if one misses one's practices even for just one day (for example, if one happens to experience discomfort of one kind or another), especially when one is making progress. As soon as one stops, all one's former efforts may be in danger of being lost, and may be discovered to have been done in vain. It will take further time and effort to restore this shortfall.

It is recommended that the practice of chigong become as important as the axiomatic "three-meals-a-day"; it is essential to form a practice-habit, so that it becomes a part of one's daily life.

The fruit of perseverance is the tempering of one's willpower. An indomitable willpower is the decisive factor in bringing chi fully into play.

  b. To reap results, practice in proper order, step by step.

Perseverance, patience, and determination are all needed in one's chigong practice, but one should not be too earnest, too eager or overanxious for quick success. One must follow a proper sequence: from the simple to the complex from the easy to the difficult, and from the few to the many. One should work out a suitable daily practice schedule for oneself. Progress can be made only step by step and little by little.

For part-time practitioners, it is recommended that one learn Level One - the Lift Chi Up and Pour Chi Down Method, and the Three Centers Merge Standing Form first.

After a period of three months of external Hunyuan practice, they may then be able to learn Level Two - the Body and Mind Form. If one practices all of them at the outset, the body cannot immediately accustom itself to all of the different practices. One may become exhausted and overtired, and one's practice will not be very effective. Two or more years may be needed to meet and complete all of the requirements of the blending and transmuting of body with mind.

In the beginning, the practice time can be shorter, twice a day, for 15 minutes or half an hour each time. Then the time may be gradually extended.

At first, it is important to be familiar with the movements and clear about the practice requirements. One should try to do the physical movements as accurately as possible. When one can practice correctly with skill and ease, it is then requisite to focus one's mind upon the physical movements and to merge body and mind. This is described by the saying, *"Mind is focused on body, and chi moves as body does."*

One's accomplishments in chigong practice are also attained in a natural sequence, from the few to the many. One should not always expect prematurely quick success.

The correct attitude towards accomplishment is to practice assiduously and perseveringly, in accord with the theories and methods of Zhineng Qigong, and to be concerned only about efforts rather than rewards. Unceasing efforts will yield certain success.

An over-eager desire for results may divert one's attention and distract one's mind from the necessity of maintaining a calm practice. Excessive enthusiasm with regard to achieving results may spoil one's efforts, resulting in setbacks. The principle to heed is *"neither forget to practice nor push oneself too hard"*. When conditions are ripe, success will come.

c. Fully actualize the group dynamics effects of Zhineng Qigong.

This qualifies as the most fundamental of the Nine Features of Zhineng Qigong. Establishing and building a chi field is applied in the areas and activities of teaching, practicing and healing.

Everyone should contribute chi to the chi field; then one is able to absorb a greater amount of chi. The basic principle involved is serving the group as a whole as well as serving others individually. Benefiting others will in turn lead to the benefiting of oneself. It is difficult to receive and absorb chi from the field if one only wants to absorb chi and makes no contributions to the chi field (that is, if private interests preoccupy one's mind). Moral caliber is also of prime importance in practicing in a group chi field.

11. Relaxation

What is referred to here is the relaxation of the body. During chigong practice, neither tighten the body nor resort to using brute force, but instead relax the body in a conscious and natural manner. The ideal is, *"to be*

143

relaxed but not slack, to be poised but not stiff." The essential point is to allow the idea "Relax" to penetrate that part of the body that is to be relaxed.

The mind governs the chi, and where the mind arrives, the chi follows; conversely, where the mind does not arrive, chi cannot penetrate. Wherever in the body chi can freely penetrate, there is necessarily a state of relaxation. To be truly relaxed, one must relax one's mind as well. A relaxed mind is the presupposition of a relaxed body.

There are several ways of relaxing the body:

a. Pronounce *Song* moving from a level tone into a falling tone, with the falling tone being longer. The two tones of *Song* can cause chi first to rise and then fall, thus relaxing the whole body.

b. The practice of the Lift Chi Up and Pour Chi Down Method also helps relax the body.

c. Follow the teacher's instructions to relax from the crown of the head to the soles of the feet during the process of establishing a chi field.

d. In one's daily life, for the purpose of opening various specific parts of the body, repeatedly dwell upon the idea "Relax", and gradually the respective tensions can be dispelled.

12. Tranquillity

This refers to the mental and spiritual state. A state of peace and tranquillity can be attained by focusing one's attention upon only one point or upon only one idea.

It is not easy to harbor only one idea and to maintain this idea for a given period of time, uninterrupted by other ideas. In Zhineng Qigong, the precondition for tranquillity lies rather in focusing upon the movements of the body instead of drifting off into wild flights of fancy.

13. Naturalness

During Zhineng Qigong practice, the movements of the physical body should be natural, unrestrained and unforced. Some people may feel unnatural in the beginning; this is because old bad habits have yet to be corrected through chigong practice.

It is important to address the requirements in a manner appropriate to one's own physical condition. One should not compare oneself with others.

As more chi is enabled to pass through it, the body becomes more relaxed and the movements can be perfected.

14. Integrating practice with nourishment and rest

Zhineng Qigong stresses both *lian* and *yang*. *Lian* means hard practice, while *yang* means taking nourishment or tonic, and proper rest. To integrate both *lian* and *yang* is to organically synthesize chigong practice with one's daily life.

There are times when one feels tired, or short of energy and vigor. This occurs when various new channels are being opened and a greater amount of plentiful and higher quality chi is needed to fill them in order to achieve a higher level of health. In meeting this need, the taking of nourishing foods, and sometimes, tonics, is also necessary. This temporary phenomenon is a sign of progress. Proper practice and good nutrition are both needed at this time, and proper rest is also necessary.

To "practice hard" does not mean practicing 24 hours a day, in spite of fatigue. The proper standard of practice is that one feels energetic and relaxed, rather than tired, after practice. It is, however, normal to feel tired at the beginning when one is learning how to practice.

15. The complementary application of concentration and observation (*ding* and *hui*)

Concentration (*Ding*) is the ability to dispel irrelevant thoughts and ideas, through which one can become singleminded. This skill is usually employed at the elementary stage. Observation (*Hui*) is the ability to focus one's attention on experiencing and observing various internal changes after one attains a state of peace and tranquillity.

These changes include the sensation of pins and needles in various places in the body, soreness, the flowing of chi, the circulation of chi in the channels, the opening and closing of energy pathways and vital points, variations in consciousness and other similar phenomena.

At this time, all of one's attention should be concentrated within the body with the intention of experiencing and observing only, rather than reasoning and thinking. The deeper one's attention is focused, the more detailed will be whatever one experiences and observes, and gradually various supersensory abilities may be developed.

145

These two skills are not contradictory - but rather mutually complementary - principles, and they are often alternately and repeatedly employed in practice.

16. Cultivating a deep Zhineng Qigong consciousness

a. Enhance one's study of the theories of Zhineng Qigong.

The purpose of chigong practice is not merely physical movement, but also the transformation of the mind through self-cultivation, and the enhancing of the mind's ability to direct the body. A profound energy-sensitive consciousness must be established in order to achieve beneficial effects.

Most people possess no chigong consciousness within their minds. When chigong is mentioned, they may superficially evaluate it according to their own scientific knowledge. Such an approach will rob chi of its vital, flexible and self-sufficient qualities, causing it to play only a limited role within the body.

Only when one studies the theories, impresses one's mind with the deep imprint of chigong, and establishes a chigong field within one's consciousness, will one be able to conscientiously practice in accordance with those theories, and to study things according to the laws and principles of chigong. As soon as an energy-sensitive consciousness is created and formed into a habit, one may become capable of directing one's own unconscious and subconscious life processes.

The theories of Zhineng Qigong can, in a unique way, help both the sick and the healthy, as well as those who want to develop various special abilities, to obtain their desired goals. Only by understanding both the theories and the methods of Zhineng Qigong can one better experience their essence in one's practice.

We may not understand what we are experiencing and sensing, but we can perform the practice better when we understand why we are performing it. This principle is of special importance in Zhineng Qigong practice.

b. Create a Zhineng Qigong consciousness through practice.

This point is as important as the study of theory. In order to deeply root the theories in one's mind, and to build up a true chigong consciousness, one should plunge oneself deeply and consistently into practice.

c. Practice at a fixed time and place.

Work out a schedule (time, place, and practice curricula) and do not change it no matter what may happen (bad weather, fatigue, sickness, or

146

anything else). If one can continue practicing even under unfavorable circumstances, a great power of will can gradually be cultivated, and this will enhance one's spiritual power in directing the body and the life processes overall.

The practice of Zhineng Qigong must not be confined only to the cultivation of chi, for the essential principle involved is the tempering both of one's mind and of one's willpower. Practicing at a fixed time and place will help achieve this effect.

In addition, this is also helpful in forming a chi field - something which is of additional importance for those who may practice alone. A further benefit of so doing is that one's chi can be blended with that of one's surroundings to form a unified field of chi.

d. Putting chigong practice into one's daily life.

It is not required that one cultivate chi all day long, but it is required that one implement the essence of chigong in one's daily life, work and studies.

First, extend the qualities of chigong practice into one's daily life: always maintain an attitude that is peaceful, relaxed and comfortable. Second, incorporate the various chigong movements into one's daily life wherever one is and whenever one can. Third, maintain an energy-sensitive spirit and frame of mind in one's daily life - keep calm and tranquil even in the face of irritation and disturbance; this forms the focus of yet a higher level practice.

e. Live a chigong life.

This implies embodying the essential spirit of chigong in one's daily life, work and studies, and governing the activities of daily living while maintaining an energy-cultivation consciousness.

First, permeate one's daily life with a chigong consciousness. The essential point of chigong practice is to merge the mental (spiritual) activities with the movements of the body, so that one's entire life is actively informed by and permeated with the presence of chi.

In addition, one should always maintain an awareness of being a Zhineng Qigong practitioner. One should seek to make various contributions to Zhineng Qigong; in this way one can be easily connected with the powerful chi field of Zhineng Qigong and can make rapid progress.

Second, pay attention to the rhythms and dynamics of the world of nature, discern their principles of function, and follow these laws in order to enhance one's own vitality.

Third, try to understand the implications of chigong in various Chinese idioms and words, such as *"Hunyuan Ling Tong!"*, *"tong,"* and *"song."*

17. The meaning of *"Hunyuan Ling Tong!"*

"Hunyuan Ling Tong!" is the most frequently repeated saying for all Chinese Zhineng Qigong practitioners. *Hun* means to blend and transform, *yuan* means one; thus, Hunyuan means to blend and transform, becoming one or a whole. This saying refers to the original Hunyuan chi. That is to say: to be blended, transformed and to become one with the original Hunyuan chi.

Ling means effective - Hunyuan chi works. *Tong* means open, unobstructed and throughgoing. It indicates that Hunyuan chi can fill the whole body without being obstructed; it functions as one wishes so long as one can blend one's body and mind with it and become one with it. This is one of the tasks and goals of Zhineng Qigong practice. It is also a very good high-level practice method - a practice of mind cultivation.

The pronunciations of the last two words *ling* and *tong* can also vibrate the middle and upper vital centers. So it is better to pronounce this saying correctly in standard Mandarin Chinese. While its effect is essentially vibrational in nature, and on that level independent of linguistic or cognitive meaning, it does possess a psychological and spiritual resonance as well, due to its ability to empower one's faith and to focus and enhance one's awareness, thereby simultaneously heightening one's inner perception of the chi-flow in direct proportion to the purity of one's concentration.

18. Adopting a correct attitude towards reactions in practice

In the process of chigong practice, a practitioner may encounter many kinds of reactions; these can be classified into two types: reactions related to illness and chi-reactions.

    a. Reactions related to illness.

These reactions have symptoms similar to their original illnesses, as explained above. They may bring various pains and sufferings upon the practitioner. Some may suspect these to be the recurrence of an old illness, the manifestation of a new one, or abnormal symptoms of various kinds, while at the same time not knowing just what to do. The following are some countermeasures:

        1) First of all, eliminate the possibility of misguided or incorrect practice.

Carefully and thoroughly check the theories and practice methods according to the correct requirements with reference to the postures, movements, and operative ideas (activities of consciousness, such as techniques of visualization and concentration). The addition of other types of chigong practices to the practice of Zhineng Qigong is not permitted. If nothing is amiss, one can be assured that no corrupted practice will take place.

If the discomforts are caused by incorrect postures and physical movements, one should make an effort to try to perform correct movements and maintain correct postures during practice. If one does not know what to do, one can treat all kinds of reactions by the Wall Squatting Method (*Dun Qiang Fa* – referring to the practice methods part for instructions).

2) How can illnesses (whether old or new) be distinguished from reactions?

Generally speaking, although normal reactions may bring about various kinds of suffering, in such instances both the mind and chi are clear; this differs from the heavy and sluggish sensations experienced as a result of illness. Some pains do not have much influence on normal functioning, but at times it is difficult to distinguish practice reactions from illness.

When symptoms appear, an unbalanced mental or spiritual state may worsen the symptoms, transforming the condition into a serious illness. Many cases have demonstrated that even serious diseases can be cured if one is able to maintain a calm and stable spirit and to focus one's mind on one's practice; on the contrary, a worried, doubt-ridden mind may transform a slight illness into a serious one, or even worse.

The best approach is not to attempt to analyze whatever it is, but rather just to wholeheartedly devote oneself to practice; in this way both reactions and illness can thus be treated. Those who find themselves unable to focus effectively on their practice may consult a physician and follow his or her advice. From the point of view of Zhineng Qigong, an effective solution would be to ask a Zhineng Qigong teacher to give treatment using the chi-transmitting method.

For those who have serious or "incurable" illnesses, or for cancer patients, the process of recovery is not an immediate one, but rather the result of sustained practice. Through unremitting practice and effort, the prevalence of illness can be completely dispelled.

This is a unique principle of chigong therapy in which, in a recurrent cyclic manner, symptoms appear when sick (pathogenic) chi converges upon a specific location and disappear when sick chi disperses. When one experiences a relapse, one should be clear about the fact that this is a sign that the sick chi is being dispelled from the whole body and that one is becoming well. One should gladly and enthusiastically continue practicing with even stronger determination, thereby ridding oneself of the new convergence of sick chi.

   b. Reactions from transformations of internal chi.

Healthy practitioners may also experience various reactions which are manifestations of internal chi transformations. The highest and most essential axiom in such a situation is to "ignore it and leave it alone." Maintaining a calm and peaceful mind and adhering to your practice will gradually and smoothly raise you to a higher level. The most common chi reactions are as follows:

   1) Physical sensations.

When one reaches a certain level, one may experience many extraordinary sensations, falling into one of approximately eight categories:

Expansion and contraction: During practice, one may feel as if the whole body or part of it is growing larger or smaller. The flow of true chi in the *yangqiao* channel causes one to feel bigger, while such a flow in the *yinqiao* channel will cause one to feel smaller.

Heaviness and lightness: One may feel lighter - seeming to float up, while another may feel heavier - seeming to descend. These sensations can be modified by adjusting the breath, lightly inhaling and deeply exhaling, or simply by allowing the condition to remain as it is until the end of the practice. When the true chi is accumulated in the Governor Vessel channel, one may feel a lightness of body, while, when it is accumulated in the Conception Vessel channel, one may feel a sense of heaviness.

Coolness and warmth: One may feel coolness or warmth flowing in an unceasing periodic circulation through various parts of the body, such as the Vital Center, the back, or even over the entire body. A sensation of warmth usually appears in the initial stage of practice, while that of coolness appears when one reaches a certain further level.

Tingling and itching: When true chi reaches the skin layer and tries to pass through it, one feels an itching, while a tingling sensation is caused by the obstruction of true chi in the collateral channels. When such sensations appear, never scratch, otherwise true chi will retreat inside the body and the process of passage will be arrested.

One should have an accurate and thorough knowledge of the above eight sensations, so as to avoid being unnecessarily frightened in the event that such phenomena should occur; one should instead keep a natural and indifferent attitude, whether or not they appear or disappear during one's practice. Even if one experiences itching and tingling too intense to ignore, the best course is to avoid fidgeting, and to remain centered, while lightly touching the itching or tingling area with the fingers. These reactions appear only at certain stages and will soon disappear if one continues practicing.

In the event that a violent rocking of the body takes place during the Three Centers Merge Standing Exercise, one should take special care to control one's mental poise in order to prevent oneself from performing a practice of spontaneously generated movements.

  c. Reactions in the main and collateral chi channels or pathways.

After sufficient true chi has been cultivated and accumulated within the body, the interior sensory abilities will become enhanced. When one enters a state of tranquillity, one may become aware of the existence of the main and collateral chi channels, seeing many large or small passages within the body. Do not make any particular fuss over it, but continue to ignore it, and leave it alone.

Some may also feel the chi pathways and vital points within the body, with a sensation of chi flowing out from various openings. This is a good sign, showing that these pathways or vital points have been opened, but chi is not actually flowing out of them; dispel the notion that chi is flowing out. The most easily opened pathways are as follows: the crown-point (*Baihui*), the navel, the door of life (*Mingmen*), the center of the palm (*Laogong*), and the center of the sole (*Yongquan*.). Do not be frightened by these phenomena, because they are good signs and they indicate that one is making progress.

  d. Reactions in the five vital organs.

As chi penetrates further into the body, changes may take place in the five vital organs. Because the physical structures of the five vital organs are all different, various chi lights may appear, some being red, some yellow, and some white. All these phenomena are due to reactions in the five vital organs.

According to Zhineng Qigong theory, white light is related to the lungs, yellow light to the spleen, red light to the heart, indigo light to the liver, and dark blue light to the kidneys. Black light is an abnormal manifestation.

We do not perform a special practice of observing such lights, so simply leave them alone and continue practicing. If a light of mixed colors irritates you, just give it a puff (pronounce *chui* and *xu* together) and it will disappear.

  e. Reactions due to the purification of the mind.

At an ordinary level, distracting thoughts may emerge during one's practice, even if one has already established oneself in a state of quietude and tranquillity. These are reactions in one's field of awareness.

151

As soon as distracting thoughts are dispelled from the surface layer of the mind, new thoughts from deeper layers may appear, which may cause further disturbances. One should make up one's mind to persist in practicing until the completion of one's normal allotted practice time.

As the mind is further purified and one becomes more sensitive to things in one's surrounding, various illusions or hallucinations may emerge, caused by the interaction and reactions of the internal energies in the process of interfacing with innate concepts held in the mind. These illusions are anomalous reflections of past experiences.

At such moments, whatever one hears and sees during chigong practice is of a completely false nature, and one should neither believe in its reality nor pursue it further with one's thoughts.

Amongst all the various kinds of hallucinations, special care should be given to understanding and dealing with illusory imagery and the contradictory interactions of real and false sensations and perceptions, as described above. These are discussed in detail in *The Essences of Zhineng Qigong Science*.

19. Adjusting one's way of life

In order to be best rewarded in one's practice one needs to adjust one's lifestyle in order to maintain what has been achieved. Give special attention to addressing the following four areas of life:

a. Increase the nutritive quality of one's food and drink.

It is necessary to increase the nutritive value of one's food and drink concurrently while practicing chigong. However, the concept of nutrition in Zhineng Qigong is a bit different from that of modern science.

In modern nutrition, great attention is given to vitamins, proteins, microelements and similar substances. What is of greatest concern is whether or not the particular food in question contains plentiful chi. Generally speaking, fresh foods from wild, vigorous, and flourishing sources contain greater chi. Plants growing in adverse circumstances and in poor soil take in more nutrition (chi) from nature. The actively moving parts of animals contain more chi than other parts.

One should attempt to include all the various flavors of foods rather than limiting oneself to just a few. Choose foods for those who are sick according to their specific situational needs. For common practitioners, besides taking care to partake of a careful selection and combination, allow yourself neither to be famished nor too full, avoiding foods that are too fatty, too cold or too hot.

An appropriate amount of wine is all right so long as the mind, the chi and the blood are not disturbed. The guiding principle is that, after drinking, one appears as if one had drunk nothing at all.

Dress properly in order to keep the internal physical environment balanced with the external environment of nature. The essential principle of remaining in good health is using one's energy, essence and spirit sparingly rather than expending them carelessly. With regard to clothing, there is no need to go to foolish extremes, such as wearing less in the cold weather or more in warm weather.

During practice, the wearing of loose, comfortable and casual clothes is recommended. There is no need to be elaborately dressed and richly ornamented.

Flat-bottomed shoes are recommended, especially for female practitioners, as high-heeled shoes are harmful to health. The internal organs are closely connected with the channels and energy paths in the feet, and the uneven stimulation on the feet in high-heeled shoes may cause imbalances, or even chronic diseases in the internal organs.

b. Create favorable living environments.

One's house should be full of fresh air and well-ventilated, with an appropriate temperature and humidity. Although Hunyuan chi can be gathered in regardless of the directions, places or times of practice, it is better to practice in a favorable setting. Places near green hills, clear waters, dense pine woods, cypress groves, or other scenic spots are good for chigong practice. If there are no such places available, select a relatively good place within your access.

The reason for doing so is to inspire a positive frame of mind and a pleasant mood for the purpose of a more effective practice. If no such favorable places are available, there is no need to be too particular about it.

In the practice of Zhineng Qigong, the importance of building of a chi field is emphasized. No matter where you practice, first build up a chi field before you start your practice.

As you practice day after day, this place will continue to become stronger in chi. It is better to periodically establish a chi field at home; thus all family members, pets and even flowers can be benefited.

c. Conduct oneself openly and honestly.

One should follow the three principles of Zhineng Qigong - not only in teaching and practicing, but also in one's daily life, and one should observe the social moral principles:

1) Be open and above board; think and act in one and the same (integrated) way.

153

2) Treat friends and fellow practitioners frankly and honestly.
3) Have a loving heart and find pleasure in helping others.
4) Raise the quality of one's teaching ability, and, day by day, through the treating of others, gradually make progress in the cultivation of one's chi and one's moral nature.

One should try to fulfill the above requirements from the depths of one's heart, even if one finds oneself alone and unsupervised by others. In this way, one's chi may become purer, one's mind may become sharper and clearer, and one's spiritual and physical health can be more rapidly brought to a higher level.

One should take the following admonitions carefully:

First, in order to avoid a disorder in one's chi and blood, one should never nurse evil thoughts or hatred in one's heart.

Second, hold noble values so as to make one's mind clear, and never be greedy for money or other material wealth.

Third, to consolidate one's essence and preserve one's spiritual chi, properly control one's sexual desires. The reason for doing so is that the out-flowing of one's essence may cause a loss of one's vital chi.

In the beginning stages of practice, when the essential chi is plentiful within the body, a strong sexual desire may appear. This is a critical moment in which to exercise control; otherwise, it is difficult to make further progress. All one's former efforts will have been expended in vain and wasted, and greater harm may then be done than had one remained an ordinary non-practitioner of Zhineng Qigong.

When a very sick person starts to practice chigong, it is appropriate for that person to have no sex during the initial 100 days, or for the first year. Even if one has become a skilled practitioner, one should not indulge oneself in sexual pleasures. This is a biological law of the Tao. When one reaches a certain level, one can enjoy higher-level pleasures beyond those of sex, food and sleep.

D. CHIGONG, TRADITIONAL CHINESE MEDICINE AND SPECIAL ABILITIES

1. The relationship between Traditional Chinese Medicine and chigong

Zhineng Qigong medical science is a branch of Zhineng Qigong science. However, in Chinese history, traditional chigongs and Traditional Chinese Medicine are two bright pearls in the treasure chest of Chinese culture. In the long river of history, they illuminate each other with dazzling brightness.

What is the relationship between them? To a considerable extent and within certain parameters chigong constitutes an important part of, and provides the essence and foundation for, Traditional Chinese Medicine.

The extraordinary applications of chigong - such as practices involving the breaking of metal and stone, rendering the body impenetrable to blades or firearms, and various health-enhancement effects - have won universal praise. There may be no philosophical opposition if chigong is merely regarded as an integral part as well as the underlying essence of sports. But there are relatively few people who agree that chigong plays such an important role in Traditional Chinese Medicine as has been stated above. There are two reasons for this lack of agreement.

First, there are various types of chigongs in China, each having its own applications (for example, martial arts chigongs, acrobatic chigongs, chigongs for maintaining well-being, calligraphic chigongs, and others). The recent propaganda of chigong has placed particular emphasis upon demonstrations of hard-style chigongs (hard chigong is only one member in the chigong family, though it has splintered into many sects). A fragmentary opinion - such as one which regards chigong as nothing more than a single special technique, rather than a comprehensively based opinion - such as one realizing that hard chigong has little relationship with Traditional Chinese Medicine - tended to pervade the public mindset.

Second, in China, chigong was originally closely allied with Traditional Chinese Medicine, their paths diverging only after the Tang and Song dynasties. Among the present echelon of leading authorities in Traditional Chinese Medicine, few have expertise in chigong; at the same time, masters of many schools of chigong know nothing about the theories of Chinese medicine.

Because of the two above-mentioned points, it is decidedly difficult to clearly delineate and reconcile the relationship between these two fields of practice. More than theoretical analysis alone is needed; historical exploration is also necessary. In this book, we can only present a number of superficial views.

What is the relationship between chigong and Traditional Chinese Medicine? In the view of history, the doctrine of chigong and the theory of Traditional Chinese Medicine are two fresh blossoms from the same stem; in view of their respective contents, they are companion volumes in the science of human life. Both of them are rooted in the philosophy found in classical Chinese cultures of nurturing the spirit for the conservation of life.

Starting with the physiological and pathological manifestations of the human body, Traditional Chinese Medicine reveals the relatively superficial and ordinary laws governing the processes of interaction between body, chi and consciousness, the foundation upon which the traditional teachings of diagnosis, treatment and health-enhancement have been based.

However, chigong places its emphasis upon the interrelationships between these three - body, chi and consciousness; upon this a complete system of methods has been developed with the aim of promoting the comprehensive and healthful development of both body and mind, with the purpose of inspiring and enhancing human potentialities, and deepening the mind's ability to control the body.

Although there are obvious differences between the chigong and Traditional Chinese Medicine, their respective subjects of study are one and the same - human life. Only when these two bodies of knowledge are closely integrated can the theories concerning the human life processes be unified into a totality (including such areas as physiology, pathology, diagnosis, treatment, healthcare and longevity). Only then will man be able to understand the laws underlying his own life processes.

2. The Entirety Concept of Life as the common theoretical foundation of both chigong and Traditional Chinese Medicine

In ancient Chinese cultures, through the process of directly observing and experiencing both his own life and the world of nature, and through comparison, synthesis and deduction, man gradually established a unique understanding of human existence - The Entirety Concept of Life. This

156

concept is the cornerstone of both chigong and the theories of Traditional Chinese Medicine, and manifests in the following ways:

a. The Entirety Concept of Man and Nature

Man was regarded as a part of nature, and the life activities of man were studied against the entire evolving background of all things in the universe. This concept was presented in detail in the classical works of Traditional Chinese Medicine, such as *The Yellow Emperor's Classic on Internal Medicine* (*Huangdi Nei Jing* - second century B.C.).

For example, the influences of the variations of the seasons upon the activities of life were stated in the following words: "*The yin and yang - spring, summer, autumn, winter are the beginning and ending of all things, the nature of life and death. If one acts contrary to this law, one suffers illness and misfortune; if one accords with this law, one enjoys health and fitness.*"

The application of this principle for the preservation of health evolved into the sage's secret of maintaining well-being: "*Nourish yang in spring and summer; nourish yin in autumn and winter, rise and fall together with all things at the gate of growth, adapt oneself to the changes of the seasons, and to the cold and the hot.*"

In the practice of Chinese medicine, this principle, in its application in the areas of physiology and pathology, evolved into concepts such as "*Man's responses to Nature*". In therapeutics, besides taking medicines in accordance with the seasons and the time of day, there existed also the meridian method of acupuncture.

For a long time these theories were deemed worthless, and discarded. However, recent studies have shown that these initially unbelievable ancient doctrines and methods actually embraced profound scientific implications.

For example, between 1967 and 1972, at two principal hospitals in India, among the emergency heart attack cases, the statistics showed an obvious direct relationship between heart attacks and fluctuations in the earth's magnetic field, due to the magnetic activities of the sun. Complete physiological examinations were carried out upon 43 volunteers, with the results showing that the rise and fall of blood pressure and the increase and decrease of the number of white blood cells coincided with the cycles of variation in the earth's magnetic field within a given time-frame.

All of these studies have proved that the view that man is responsive to nature is not a groundless heresy, but rather an accurate reflection of the relationship between the human body - this "small world" within - and the universe - that "giant world" without.

With respect to the meridian method, it may be said that it is the summarized, distilled experience of the ancient Chinese obtained through long-term observation of the phenomena of the human biological clock. It is rooted in the various biochemical processes within the human body, and possesses undeniably scientific implications. It has drawn serious attention from scientists outside China.

b. Entirety Concept of Mind (Spirit) and Body

In the view of this concept, the human spirit (consciousness) and the physical body were regarded as an indivisible whole, and upon this basis the life processes of man were studied. The ancients thought that man was the unity of spirit, chi and body.

In an ancient work - *Huainanzi's Fundamental Teachings on Taoism* (*Huainanzi's Yuan Dao Xun*) - this concept was explained as one in which the physical body is the basis of human life, the spirit is the director of the human life activities, and chi is the manifestation of encoded life information, filling the whole body and unifying the body and the spirit into a totality. With regard to this totality, the ancients especially stressed the importance of the controlling role of the spirit, which maintains stability and change within the human body, as well as the safety of human life.

This entirety concept - which regards the spirit as the controlling element in the unity of body, chi and spirit - differs in essential ways from the modern Western concept of life.

In modern medicine, a considerable amount of extensive research has been conducted upon the study of the human body in the areas of anatomy and histology (tissue science), but the study of the psychospiritual dimension has been ignored.

Neurology places its emphasis upon the processes by which signals stimulated in accord with internal and external environmental changes travel within the nervous system, as well as the reactions of the central nervous system to these signals; but in so doing it has ignored the volitional, initiatory nature and dominant role of the spirit or consciousness in the total human life process.

Psychology has studied human moods and behaviors, as well as their relationship to the observable nervous system, but it has known nothing of chi.

Although the above-mentioned research has been quite extensive and accurate, the understanding of human life obtained from it is still quite partial and fragmentary. The explorations of the ancient Chinese into the human body, though not as accurate and detailed as those of modern medicine, reflect the laws of human life processes in their totality. This is why the understanding of human life found in ancient Chinese cultures has attracted great attention from modern scientific research throughout the world.

c. The Entirety Concept of the Human Body

First, the human body is regarded as an organic whole. In Traditional Chinese Medicine, all of the component parts of the human body - the layers of skin, the muscles and bones, and the internal organs - interrelate with each other and interact with each other, forming an organic totality centered within the internal organs.

Within this unity, there are organic relationships between every internal organ and all of other parts of the body. There are many statements with regard to this subject in *The Yellow Emperor's Classic on Internal Medicine*, which became the source and basis of the doctrine of the vital organs and the classical theory of organic/visceral interrelationships in healing.

Second, in the views of the ancient Chinese, the human body - this organic whole - is formed and maintained by the coordination of the main and collateral chi channels, comprising 12 main channels and 15 collateral channels, which are connected internally to the viscera and externally to the bones and muscles. The processes of human life are carried out by means of chi, which circulates and flows along these channels and their points of intersection, or vital points.

Moreover, every part contains the capacity to reflect the life-condition of the whole; this constitutes another manifestation of the entirety of the human body. Due to the fact that chi binds together the entirety of human life processes, and that it fills and flows through the whole body, one single partial component can to some extent relay information reflecting the state of the whole body.

For example, the state of the viscera can be reflected both in the color and the coating of the tongue, and in the contours of the eyes.

Any abnormal changes in the internal organs can be detected from the hand's ulnar artery. The state of every part of the body can be reflected in the manifestations of the corresponding reflexology points of the face.

Are these statements correct? From 1976 to 1977, at Longhua Hospital in Shanghai, 1,251 surgeries were made with acupuncture anesthesia applied through reflexologically related points, raising the success rate to 96%, which provided overwhelming evidence for the accuracy of these ancient doctrines.

All said, human life is a totality of body, chi and spirit. This human life is controlled by the spirit and is a body/mind unity existing within the context of a man/nature dynamic. The life of the physical body is centered within the internal organs and maintained by the flow of the chi through the main and collateral chi channels. The spirit (mind or consciousness) "resides" in the heart. The chi circulates and flows along the main and collateral chi channels, filling all parts of the body and unifying the spirit or consciousness with the physical body.

This concept is the theoretical basis of both chigong and Traditional Chinese Medicine. The Theory of The Main and Collateral Chi Channels as well as The Theory of Chi and Its Transmutation are the respective manifestations of this concept of the entirety of life.

3. The theory of chi and its transmutation as the essence of traditional Chinese medical theory

The Theory of Chi and its Transmutation and the Theory of the Main and Collateral Chi Channels are the two pillars of Chinese medical theory. Medical doctors of every dynasty attached importance to the theory of the main and collateral chi channels. In one chapter of *The Yellow Emperor's Classic on Internal Medicine*, the following statement is found:

> *These twelve channels decide life or death, heal all illnesses, control strength and weakness, and must be clear and unimpeded.* (See Appendix A – Kaneko Shoseki: The Nature and Origin of Man)

In another chapter the vital role of the main and collateral chi channels in the life processes of man is further emphasized in the light of both the theories and practice of Chinese medicine.

> *These twelve channels are the basis upon which man is able to sustain life, by which illness either appears and disappears, from which one commences to learn . . . , it is an easy matter to grasp crudely but a difficult one to perfectly master.*

However, in comparing the Theory of The Main and Collateral Chi Channels with the Theory of Chi and Its Transmutation, we see that chi is the essence and content, while the main and collateral channels are merely the paths (and, of course, more than just paths) along which chi travels. These channels conduct the activities of the chi.

In a sense, the main and collateral chi channels are the servants of the chi. Because of this, the Theory of Chi and Its Transmutation should be placed in the cardinal position in Chinese medical research. As Professor Yuan Hongshou put it, "What is the core-essence of Chinese medical theory? Only one word - chi."

In Traditional Chinese Medicine, chi is classified into many distinct types, as stated above. What we describe here refers to true chi, which actually includes both chi and its active transmutation.

The role that chi plays in the life activities of man has been described above in a general manner. Here let us further discuss the role it plays in the physiological and pathological processes, as well as its controlling influence in traditional Chinese medical diagnosis and treatment.

The basis of all life activity is the metabolic process at diverse functional levels. The organic entities at these respective levels unceasingly absorb the nutrients they need and incorporate these nutrients into their own cellular structure. At the same time, they also individuate themselves and release energy to meet the needs of their various functional processes.

These processes of assimilation and individuation function in proper balance and good order within organic microstructures of the same level or among biological tissues at different levels.

In fact, this is the "chi-into-matter" - "matter-into-chi" process of transmutation functioning at diverse levels within the human body. As stated in another chapter of *The Yellow Emperor's Classic on Internal Medicine*, all metabolic processes rely upon chi for their initiation, sustenance and completion (as energy is transmuted into matter). At the same time, the entirety of chi expended in the human life processes is generated through the metabolic process (as matter is transmuted into energy). Thus, the processes transmuting energy into matter and matter into energy are the primal activities of the life processes within the human body.

Moreover, chi is the essence of the activities at work within the internal organs as well as within the main and collateral chi channels; chi also constitutes the body's defense against unhealthy interference from external sources. In *The Scripture of Calamity*, it is stated that the birth, growth, flourishing and decline of chi within the human body decide the birth, growth, strength and aging of man. In *The Yellow Emperor's Classic on Internal Medicine*, the life process of man was summarized as the increase and decrease of both consciousness and energy. As soon as "*the spirit and chi are both gone*", though the body may be intact, the life of man is at its end.

The above-stated functions characterize the role that chi plays in the physiological process of the human body. In the area of pathology, Chinese medicine holds that illness is caused by various pathogens (attacked from without by one or more of the 'six evils' - unhealthy environmental changes - and injured from within by one or more of the seven moods - emotions - which result in a disorder in both the chi and the blood within the human body.

In *The Yellow Emperor's Classic on Internal Medicine*, illness is described as the result of the interaction between the healthy and the unhealthy. It was further stated that every internal change caused by pathogens or disturbances of the spirit would result in an abnormality in the chi:

> *Anger leads the chi up, joy slows the chi down, grief dissipates the chi, fear brings the chi down, coldness contracts the chi within. . . . fright disturbs the chi, fatigue expends the chi, over-thinking knots the chi.*

However, man may not necessarily fall ill even if he is infected by unhealthy factors; if the healthy chi is plentiful and abundant as well as able to circulate and flow in an unimpeded way, he will not fall ill even when unhealthy invasive influences attack him. Not only are the causes of illness related to chi, but so also are the functional, organic or psychospiritual aspects of illness related to the transformations in both the chi and the blood.

Overall, although there are various diseases having many complex names and manifestations, the common pivot of all causes of disease is the abnormal circulation and consequent disorder of both the blood and the chi; this results from the imbalance in yin and yang, and affects the internal organs as well as the psychospiritual states of man.

Because of this, the principle of therapy in Traditional Chinese Medicine is to activate, generate and balance the patient's chi, as well as to facilitate the transmutation of that chi in order to restore the body to normalcy. Although there are many methods of treatment in Traditional Chinese Medicine, their common purpose is to dispel the unhealthy, to augment the healthy, to balance yin and yang, and finally, to bring the disordered chi and blood into balance.

With regard to the important role of chi in Chinese medical therapeutics, the author has had many personal professional experiences demonstrating their clinical application. The following is one case in which bacterial inflammation was treated with acupuncture.

In 1978, a worker named Liu Zhenrong felt pains in her swollen left breast fifty days or more after she gave a birth to her baby. The infected area was a hard knot about three centimeters by three centimeters; the body temperature was 38.2 C.

She was diagnosed as suffering from acute mastitis (inflammation of the mammary gland due to liver stagnation and sluggish chi) and was treated with acupuncture. The needle remained in the body for one hour during which the hard, swollen knot disappeared and her body temperature returned to normal. The patient recovered with only this one treatment.

During the course of over twenty years (prior to 1980), the author treated dozens of patients with acute mastitis with acupuncture; 90% of them experienced immediate relief. This can not be explained in terms of Western medicine, but represents the type of condition for which Traditional Chinese Medicine has its own system of principles and treatment. This is only a small glimpse of the miraculous effects of such chi and chi channel balancing therapy, providing some evidence for the verification of the vital role of chi and its transmutation in the life activities of man.

4. The scientific confirmation of chi and the main and collateral chi channels

Both The Theory of Chi and Its Transmutation as well as The Theory of the Main and Collateral Chi Channels have existed for more than 2,000 years. But what is chi? What are these channels? These are still insoluble mysteries for most people, even in our era of highly developed scientific research.

The most advanced electron microscope can distinguish micro-matter as fine as 0.3 angstrom (A). Not only can macromolecules be seen, but so also can micro-molecules and even non-organic hydrate ions; yet no trace of either chi or chi-carrying channels can be found. Because of this, there are a number of people who doubt the existence of chi and the network of chi channels.

The following are our views:

First, the samples which have been observed are only those of dead tissues or tissues excised from the body proper by anatomic method. To seek both chi, which is a living manifestation of life functions and information, and the pathways along which it flows - the main and collateral chi channels - in dead things may well be likened to "climbing a tree to catch fish". It is unreasonable to negate the existence of chi and the network of chi channels due to the fact that they can not be found in dead bodies. (See Appendix A – Kaneko Shoseki: The Nature and Origin of Man.)

Second, in the view of modern physics, matter exists in two forms: one is called physical existence, formed by basic particles such as molecules and

163

atoms; the other form is that of a field, such as an electrical, magnetic or gravitational field. The sounds from a radio or the images on a television prove the existence of an electromagnetic field, but ordinary people can neither see nor feel such fields. Of course, we have not been certain that chi and the chi channels exist in the form of fields, but we are nearly certain that it may not be relevant to explore the existence of chi and the chi channels by traditional methods of anatomy, tissue science or physiology.

As a result of the achievements of acupuncture anesthesia, the chi channels have been subject to considerable study both in China and throughout the rest of the world. New methods of research have been developed, and unprecedented progress has been made.

Not only have meridian-sensing and chi-transmitting phenomena been observed, but in addition several objective parameters which may be instrumental in proving the existence of chi channels have been detected and measured; an example of these would be the unique phenomena observed when electricity, microwaves and radioisotopes were conducted along the chi channels. Although these studies are only in their inception, they have proved that chi channels are special systems existing within the human body, contrary to the view espoused by some, that "…. The theory of chi channels is no more than an expedient reasoning tool to explain the life phenomena of the human body."

On the other hand, recent experiments on the physical effects of the external chi of chigong have provided direct scientific evidence for the existence of chi. When chigongists Lin Housheng and Zhao Guang gathered and accumulated chi in their hands, Professor Gu Hansen and Professor He Qingnian detected and measured infrared radiation in front of their *Laogong* points (acupoints in the palms). This infrared radiation differed from that of ordinary people in its obvious and regular low-frequency amplitude modulation.

We hold that this is a partial external effect of the information embodied in the internal chi of these chigongists. The information recorded from externally generated chi has proved the existence of chi that moves by means of a specific mode of operation.

Beyond this, the experiments have also verified that the physical characteristics of external chi differ from each other in accord with the chigongists who practiced different chigongs. Some of these manifested electrostatically, some in unusual magnetic fields and some in physiological plasma. As we know, the internal chi of a chigongist is the source of chi generated outwardly, so that these experiments studying the physical effects of external chi have provided positive evidence for the theory that chi is a form of matter.

Special attention should be paid to the fact that scientists in Beijing and Qingdao have developed an infrared information-therapy instrument in accord with the external-chi information provided by some chigongists. When this instrument was applied in clinical treatment over a period of five months upon 121 patients with conditions ranging over more than 20 different illnesses including high blood pressure and rheumatagia, the overall healing effectiveness rate was as high as 85%.

It must be pointed out that this instrument is different from infrared physiotherapy instruments in the following aspects:

First, the power of the infrared information-therapy instrument operates at a level of microwatts, while the power of the infrared physiotherapy instrument operates at the level of hundreds of watts. It is obvious that, in the case of the former, information, rather than energy, played a dominant role. From this, we infer that information is one of the essential elements of chi.

Second, the infrared physiotherapy instrument is used upon various areas or parts of the body, while the infrared info-therapy instrument should be applied according to the theories of Traditional Chinese Medicine (dialectical treatment specifying precise points along the chi channels). For example, if there is a pain in the small of the back near the spine, the effect will not be good if this instrument is applied directly to the painful part, but immediate relief will be obtained if it is placed upon the *dazhui* point below the spinous process of the seventh cervical vertebra. Obvious transmission phenomena along the chi channels can also be observed if this instrument is applied to the limbs.

Information-therapy is still in its exploratory stages. However, it has convincingly demonstrated that chi and chi channels do exist. As science develops further and as the research into chigong deepens, the mysteries of The Theory of Chi and Its Transmutation, The Theory of The Main and Collateral Chi Channels, and even the entire theory of Traditional Chinese Medicine will eventually be brought to light by modern science.

5. Chigong practice as the vital source of Chinese medical theories

The theory of Traditional Chinese Medicine is so profound and subtle that even modern science cannot plumb the full measure of its profundities. How, in the pre-technological era of the ancients, did China's forefathers come to know and to gradually evolve the Theory of the Main and Collateral Chi Channels, the Theory of Chi and Its Transmutation, or even the entire theoretical system of Traditional Chinese Medicine?

We hold that the theories of Traditional Chinese Medicine were formed gradually both through the process of long-term struggle against illness and through the chigong practice of the ancients. As in the evolution of other valid theories, it also progressed respectively through both experiential and rational stages.

In the process of man's ongoing struggle with nature, the ancients gradually accumulated experience in healing. For example, various illnesses might have been healed when someone was accidentally cut by stones or branches, thus developing into a primitive form of acupuncture ('stone-needle-acupuncture'); the knowledge of taking a substance in specific response to a certain illness could be developed into a primitive form of medical therapeutics.

There is no doubt that the medical knowledge obtained in this way was both incomplete and fragmentary, embodying merely a simple repetition of the initial response experienced. Such understanding was acquired purely through objective observation and could neither reveal the essential laws of illness nor unveil the mysteries of the human life processes, so it remained at the level of merely perceptual understanding.

However, the theory of Traditional Chinese Medicine - at least the theory stated in *The Yellow Emperor's Classic on Internal Medicine* - was established not simply by synthesizing, analyzing and abstracting the experiences of those who came before, but also by gradually distilling the formation of those theories through the practice of chigong. In order to explain this point, it is necessary to discuss the fundamental theories and practice methods of chigong briefly and succinctly.

The theories of traditional chigongs touch upon unwieldy and complex aspects such as yin and yang, the five elements (*Wu Xing*), the Heavenly and Earthly Stems (*Tian Gan Di Zhi*) as well as the Eight Diagrams (*Ba Gua*) and mathematics. Moreover, the theories vary as the practice methods differ.

However, if changes within the human body are what is referred to, these cannot be effected without the transmutational "matter-into-chi" - "chi-into-matter" process within the internal organs, nor without the main and collateral chi channels and their components. Since there are numerous sects of chigong in China, the practice methods as well as the sensations experienced by the respective practitioners during their practice differ from one another.

166

Life chigong (*Zhoutian* chigong) is the main traditional chigong; during its practice the practitioner can directly experience and perceive the chi channels, various changes in the internal organs as well as the transmutation of matter into chi and chi into matter. The practitoner can further explore the mysteries of her own life processes. Various ancient Taoism chigongs belong in this category.

There are two main schools among chigongs in Taoism - the School of Seclusion (*Qing Jing Fa Men*) and the School of Transportation (*Ban Yun Fa Men*). According to the theories of Taoism (which are also the theories of Chinese medicine), the true nature of human life is embodied in the three "treasures" - essence (*jing*), energy-intelligence (*qi*) and spirit (*shen*). The essence is gathered in the lower Vital Center, which is both the biophysical basis of human life and also the source-supply for the transmutation of chi. Chi is gathered in the middle Vital Center, which is the general of blood circulation, and used for nourishing the whole body. The spirit resides in the upper Vital Center, which is the commander or ruler of both the essence and the chi, and controls human intelligence. All the subtleties of chigong are embodied within the interactive transmutational processes occurring amongst these three principles - essence, chi and the spirit.

In general, there exist the following steps of practice: the accumulation of saliva to generate essence, the transmutation of essence into chi, the transmutation of chi into spirit, the transmutation of spirit to return into the void-nature, and the transmutation of the void-nature to return into non-being. All these transmutational processes are implemented through means of the chi channels, and through "matter-into-chi" transmutations. Now let us take the School of Transportation as an example.

The rudimentary skills of the Transporting Method (also called *Zhoutian* Transportation, or River Vehicle Transportation) consist of two steps: one is the transmutation of chi and another is the cultivation of the channels.

The skill of chi-transmutation is to stimulate the generation of true chi through a combination of specific breath controls and psychospiritual activities. As soon as the true chi is plentiful and abundant, the place upon which consciousness has been focused will become warm. When the accumulation of warmth reaches a certain level, it begins to flow within several specific pathways. Then awareness closely but passively follows the movement of the warm sensation. This is called the practice of channel-cultivation.

The Conception Vessel Channel and Governor Vessel Channel are usually the first to open, followed by another eight channels, until finally all twelve channels can be observed and experienced. If the practitioner practices further, the activities of the internal organs, variations of the seven moods (emotions) and the interaction of the human body with the natural world can be experienced and observed. These internally-sensed paths along which the true chi flows are the chi channels, while the various changes within the human body are the result of chi and its transmutation; all these are classified under the joint terminology 'internal geography'.

It is through the observation of such internal geography during chigong practice that those who have a relatively complete understanding of the chi channels, the internal organs and the phenomena of chi-transmutation, have acquired such skills.

In this way, and based upon the perceptual knowledge obtained through outer observation and the subtler process of inner vision, the understanding of the human body and the prevention and treatment of illness have risen further, to the status of rational knowledge. This is not the superficial understanding of "seeing inwardly" but is a special and unique sensation experienced during chigong practice - the process called Inner Perception. The theory of the main and collateral chi channels, the theory of chi and its transmutation and the entire theoretical system of Traditional Chinese Medicine were thus gradually established through repeated verification and exploration during the practice of chigong and medical therapeutics.

Can the above-mentioned internal geography really be observed and experienced? Most assuredly it can. For the present we would not discuss that which was recorded in various classic works on chigong (such as *Huangting Scripture of Internal Scenery* and *Huangting Scripture of External Scenery*.) A number of medical doctors living in past dynasties also confirmed them. A famous ancient doctor - Li Shizhen (author of *Compendium of Materia Medica*), said, *"Only by inward seeing can one perceive and experience the internal geography and chi channels."* Many modern works on chigong have also described the unique sensations experienced when the chi channels were opened. A number of chigongists of great attainment have experienced such mysterious sensations.

Were these sensations just illusions? No. As we know, under certain kinds of stimulation, various sensitive people may perceive the existence of the chi channels. Recently, in Shanghai, Wang Buxiong and several other researchers applied a method of inducing relaxation and tranquillity, through which ordinary people could become sensitive to chi channels; the method's rate of success was 88%. The level of tranquillity of the chigong practitioners was much deeper than that of ordinary people.

It is entirely possible to perceive and experience internal geography through the practice of chigong because the true chi is concentrated, its circulation is enhanced and the faculties of internal sensing are sharpened.

Some may wonder: Since there are also energy practices (such as Yoga in India), why didn't others create theories of chi and its transmutation, as well as of the chi channels? The answer is that not all forms of energy practice enable one to observe and experience internal geography, an ability which is closely related to the particular aims of respective approaches.

For example, the aim of Confucian chigongs was the abnegation of one's personal self and the purification of the mind for the purpose of performing one's proper social responsibilities, an attitude which was stressed in order to aid in the governing of society. In their exploration of the fine points of self-cultivation, the practitioners of Confucianism were enjoined to practice self-restraint and to manifest uprightness of heart. The aim of Buddhist chigongs was to completely awaken and to realize the truth, and to get rid of "the fleshly body"; its practitioners focused their attention upon "dispelling misunderstanding and verifying the truth".

Although great changes can also take place within the human body through the practice of these chigongs, the main and collateral chi channels can hardly be cleared and opened because the focus of the awareness is not concentrated upon the respective vital points and apertures along the chi channels. Even if the whole body is already clear and unimpeded, the presence of the chi channels may still not be observed and experienced because the awareness is in a state either "dormant" or "indifferent" to chi and its transmutations.

Although these chigongists may have acquired great virtue and attainment, even they knew very little about "internal geography". The fact that there is neither any theory of chi and its transmutation nor any theory of the main and collateral chi channels in other countries has conversely provided appropriately convincing evidence for our conclusion that the ancient chigong practice of past Chinese dynasties was the vital source of the theories of Traditional Chinese Medicine.

6. Chigong as the basis and essence of Chinese clinical medicine

In the preceding section, the interdependent relationship between Chinese medical theory and chigong practice is thoroughly explained. In order to further discuss the important role chigong has played in Traditional Chinese Medicine, let us present here a brief introduction to the relationship between chigong and Chinese clinical medicine.

It is stated in *The Yellow Emperor's Classic on Internal Medicine*:

> *There are five qualifications for one to be universally accepted as an expert doctor: The first is to know how to cure psychospiritual illnesses; the second is to know how to keep healthy and fit; the third is to know the value or ineffectiveness of drugs; the fourth is to know how to apply stone-acupuncture; the fifth is to know how to diagnose illnesses of the internal organs through observing the condition of the blood and the chi.*

The goal of chigong - the maintenance of spiritual and physical health - was placed first among these five conditions. Indeed, the great ancient masters of Traditional Chinese Medicine such as Bian Que, Hua Tuo, Sun Simiao and Li Shizhen all had a good command of chigong. Why did Traditional Chinese Medicine also develop chigong?

First, chigong is the basis of Chinese clinical medicine.

As mentioned above, the theory of Traditional Chinese Medicine was formed through repeated empirical confirmations both during the practice of chigong and the medical clinics. Until modern science reveals the actual nature of these theories, especially the Theory of Chi and Its Transmutation and the Theory of the Main and Collateral Chi Channels, if one does not practice chigong and does not undergo the experience of the various internal sensations personally, it remains difficult to understand their essence. Because one possesses no real personal experience with regard to the traditional Chinese medical theories concerning physiology, pathology and pharmacology, one can either arrive at only a superficial understanding of the concepts or else abide by the "experimental treatments" accorded patients.

It is possible for such Chinese medical doctors either to parrot others or to misunderstand the correct statements of others, but this cannot demonstrate the unique physiological models of Traditional Chinese Medicine. There exist further and similar fundamental misunderstandings with regard to the Theory of the Main and Collateral Chi Channels. For example, there is also Traditional Chinese Medicinal theory, which may be too arcane to elicit any great interest from the average reader; but recent research has revealed that it is not only the theoretical basis of Chinese pharmacology but also the objective reality underlying both the applications of Chinese drugs as well as the biochemical activity of those drugs within the human body.

It can be concluded that great ancient medical masters could not have understood the human body so precisely without the help of empirical knowledge of internal geography yielded by the practice of chigong. Because of this, in a sense, chigong can be looked upon as the foundation of Traditional Chinese Medicine. Only when this foundation had been established was it possible for the skyscraper of Chinese clinical medicine be erected.

Second, chigong occupies an important position in Chinese clinical medicine.

Great skill in chigong can to a remarkable degree refine the techniques of diagnosis and treatment used in Traditional Chinese Medicine. The early exposition of chigong diagnosis and treatment appeared in *The Yellow Emperor's Classic on Internal Medicine*.

In this book, physicians were classified into two categories - ordinary physicians and brilliant doctors. Ordinary physicians might know the pathological mechanisms present through questioning, pulse-testing and analysis, but yet remain unclear about those conditions with regard to the details of the illness within the patient's body. Brilliant doctors could be clear about the condition and pathological mechanism present without the need of questioning and testing the pulses; this is the skill of intuitive perception, in which consciousness could be as clear about the nature of the illness as if it were watching a blazing fire, yet still be incapable of explaining how such knowledge was obtained.

This is not mythology, nor are such miraculous doctors rare nowadays. In a documentary film "Miraculous Chigong", the incredible diagnostic skills of various chigongists (most of whom are known personally by the author), are so miraculous and subtle that one would claim them as absurd if one had not seen the facts with one's own eyes.

If chigong is seminal in the genesis of Chinese medical diagnostic technique, it becomes even more vital in therapeutics. The means of treatment in Chinese medical practice are not beyond the scope of pharmacology, acupuncture, massage, and the guiding or directing of chi.

Among these methods, with the exception of pharmacology, all are closely related to chigong. It is well known that the treatment results of massage therapy (including the setting of broken bones), as well as those of chi-directing therapy, hinge upon the abilities of the healer. Even highlevel acupuncture also relates to chigong.

The personal clinical practice of the author repeatedly verified the principles of chigong-acupuncture set forth in *The Yellow Emperor's Classic on Internal Medicine*.

As far as investigation reveals, there are a number of therapists who use "chigong-acupuncture" in their clinical practices. It has also become a favorite anecdote that some chigongists can relieve the pains of their patients in seconds and dissolve tumors in a instant by means of chi alone. In this sense, it is not an overstatement to praise chigong as constituting the essence of Chinese clinical medicine.

In summary, the theories of Traditional Chinese Medicine and chigong are two important components of human life science. They relate closely to each other and help each other forward.

In history, ancient medical grandmasters made great contributions to the development of chigong. Chigong practice is not only the vital source of the theory - but also the foundation and essence - of Traditional Chinese Medicine. Both at present and in the future, the modernization of Traditional Chinese Medicine will further promote the development of chigong science. At the same time, only through the mass practice of and future research upon chigong science can Traditional Chinese Medicine take the formulations of modern science and create a contemporary synthesis of the two for the benefit of mankind. This is the historic vocation of both chigong and Traditional Chinese Medicine.

7. Special abilities of human beings

In recent years, various abilities not possessed by ordinary people have been discovered in some children, such as the ability to read figures or words without the use of the eyes. In order to distinguish them from ordinary human abilities, they are called special abilities of the human organism.

The discovery of special abilities has opened a new chapter in the research into the mysteries of the physical life processes of mankind. On one hand, the special abilities of these children can be used as a means of exploring the mysteries of the human body; and on the other hand, such special abilities have revealed new aspects of these mysteries.

As in the nearly identical case of research into chigong and Chinese medicine, the exploration of mankind's special abilities will powerfully advance the science of the physical body.

The results of research in the past few years have revealed that the occurrences of such special abilities have gradually been increasing, and that the parameters which they embrace have widened. The range of these has developed from reading through non-visual means to seeing through the human body, from remote-vision and thought-transmission to telekinesis. It is difficult to predict the limits of such special abilities.

How should we understand such inconceivable phenomena? What is the relationship between these phenomena and those equally mysterious effects of chigong? In what directions and in what ways should they develop?

Professor Qian Xuesen, a well-known Chinese scientist, said that research should be conducted on the combination of chigong, human special abilities and Chinese medical theories. With regard to this issue, in view of the Hunyuan Entirety Theory, a comprehensive exposition has been presented in another book *The Technique of Zhineng Qigong Science - Superintelligence*. A brief analysis and statement is given here from the point of view of traditional chigongs.

In ancient Chinese cultures, chigong and special abilities, along with Traditional Chinese Medicine, are embraced in a unity in which each is related to the others. The close and inseparable relationship between chigong and Chinese medicine has been presented above. Some issues related to the special abilities and their relationship to chigong will be explored in following sections.

8. The universality of human special abilities

Since March 1979, when the first child who could "read through the ears" was discovered, a number of such children have been discovered all over China, whether in the south or north of the Changjiang River, or within or beyond the Great Wall. Many scientists have been involved in experimental research on such special phenomena. The experimentally confirmed special abilities generally include the following:

Super-vision includes reading without the help of the eyes, seeing through the human body, remote-vision, micro-vision (perception at the cellular level), and light sensitive vision (perceiving the colors of chi sent from a chigongist).

Extrasensory perception means having knowledge of the thought processes of others without the use of language, words or other informational clues.

Telekinesis means causing a specimen to move macroscopically, without physically touching it, for example, using the mind to move the hands of a watch, to open a lock, or to cut a cake. Even the mind alone is used to transport marked specimens from one place to another (such as aluminum strips, watches, magnetic bars, micro tracing elements, micro radio transmitters, sensitization films, insects, and other objects.) In this process, no physical traces of such transporting can be found.

Other supersensory abilities include directly sensing the earth's magnetic field, and perceiving the movement of others' activities of consciousness.

Are these merely strange things that only happened in China in the eighth decade of the twentieth century? Not at all! Such unusual things also occurred in ancient times and were documented in many historical records and books. The most detailed descriptions appeared in both Buddhist and Taoist books and records. The special abilities involved were classified into two levels.

At the advanced level, the Buddhists called them the "six openings", such as the opening of the heavenly eye of remote vision, the opening of the heavenly ear of remote hearing, the opening of the ability to know another's heart. They also include the interchangeable usage of the six abilities (in which the functions of the six sensory organs, the eyes, the ears, the nose, the tongue, the body and the mind, can permeate each other and substitute for each other). In Taoism, such special functions were regarded as natural results in the successive steps of practice, such as "the opening of the heavenly gate" and "emerging out into the void-nature", after the transmutation of chi into spirit (consciousness).

At the lower level, special abilities may emerge in the form of one's consciousness reflecting the scenery of the external world after a state of tranquillity has been established. Based upon preliminary investigation, most of the special abilities of the present chigongists are at this level. It is not proper to frequently exercise extraordinary abilities at this stage, because much spirit and chi will be consumed in their application, and this may affect further self-cultivation.

Since the advent of the 19th century, various Westerners have attempted to study such unusual phenomena by means of scientific methods. This science has been termed as psychic research, and studies the following phenomena:

Psychospiritual abilities: The abilities enabling one to psychically affect the characteristics and conditions of living and non-living things.
Clairvoyance: The ability to see that which is distant or hidden the use of the eyes.
Clairaudience: The ability to hear that which is distant or hidden without the aid of the ears.
Precognition: The ability of foreknowing future happenings by means

of an unknown source of information.

Telepathy: The ability to transmit thoughts between two or more individuals.

A number of highly respected scientists, including Einstein, have inferred the validity of such supersensory perception and suggested possible methods of its study. Although opposed by a number of people, the research on supersensory perception has since the 1960's attracted the attention of a growing number of scientists.

For example, as reported in the French magazine - "Viewpoints", Stanford University carried out a number of experiments on the baritone singer Ingo Swann, who has a miraculous ability to see remote locations. As long as he was told the latitudinal and longitudinal coordinates of a place, he was able to describe its conditions; he has also been able to observe Jupiter and Mercury. What he saw has been verified by space-exploration data.

As stated above, the incidence of special human abilities is not a rare occurrence at any time or in any county. It can be concluded then that special abilities are indeed universal.

9. Innate special abilities in mankind

All experiments related to special abilities have shown that it is only when the subject has concentrated upon and devoted her full attention toward an object that special abilities were capable of being demonstrated. Whether or not an experiment was successful depended greatly upon the psychospiritual state of the demonstrator, the respective experimental environment in question, and whether the individuals involved were comfortable and in agreement or not. As can be inferred from this, the particular point regarding special abilities is that their performance greatly depends upon the vital role played by the mind of the subject.

These special abilities are not unique discoveries that only specially endowed persons possess; they also exist in ordinary people. Experiments have shown that special abilities can be induced and actualized through training. As reported at Beijing University, forty ten-year-old children were randomly selected to undergo a short-term training together with special children, and were trained to distinguish figures without the aid of the eyes; 60% of them acquired the ability to read by non-visual means to varying degrees. Experiments at Beijing Teachers' College have also proved that the ability of telekinesis can be tapped through training.

It needs to be pointed out that this psychic ability also exists in ordinary untrained people. At the College of Engineering and Applied Science, Princeton University, the United States, a series of experiments were carried out observing the supersensory abilities of ordinary people.

Such experiments have proved that these randomly selected volunteers could psychically raise the temperature of a thermal resistor to from three to four one-thousandths of a degree, and move the mirror of an interferometer to a distance of one ten-thousandth of a millimeter.

From this it can be inferred that so called special abilities are actually parts of mankind's innate intelligence potential. The fundamental difference between these abilities and other "normal" human abilities underlies the fact that man's consciousness directly acts upon external things without the aid of the physical organs. However, this intelligence usually remains in a dormant or latent state.

10. The relationship between special abilities and chigong

In another book, *Exploration into the Profundities of Chigong*, it has been pointed out that, through chigong practice, "the innate potentialities of the human body can be activated and enhanced, and various faculties of superintelligence can be developed".

At first sight, after painstaking and arduous cultivation, the special abilities acquired through chigong practice seem different from the inborn or spontaneous special abilities of children. In fact, they are identical in nature; both are the application and manifestation of the potential intelligence of mankind. This relationship is stated in the theoretical and practical aspects of traditional chigongs as follows:

a. There is a close identity in practice.

They are identical in their manifestations. For example, until the present time, all of the outwardly observed and measured external chieffects of chigong practice have followed the same working model parameters. The chigongist uses her mind to generate external chi and causes this chi to act upon some specific instrument to cause it to move in a regular way.

In fact, this is also a form of telekinesis. A number of chigong masters can observe and be aware of the occurrences within others' bodies without the aid of any instruments. Some can directly see through the human body; others take samples of information from an object and reflect the condition of that object within their own body. It is not rare among chigongists who have obtained great skill to find that they are also in possession of other special abilities, such as thought-transmission, remote psychic control, clairvoyance and precognition.

They are generally identical in their internal reactions. This manifests in the following ways:

First, only when the mind is concentrated upon an object with whole-hearted devotion can special abilities emerge. As described by a child endowed with special abilities, whether "reading" by non-visual means, or performing telekinetic transportation of objects, the desired ability emerges only when he devotes his mind to thinking of the object and making it appear on the "screen" within his forehead.

Almost the identical situation presents itself with regard to chigong masters. Ancient chigongists also said, *"be concentrated and single-minded"*; then one is able to *"know things far away"*, and to *"know by reflection,"*

Second, with regard to various supersensory abilities, neither chigongists nor specially gifted children can tell just how they sense things. These children at present can only say "it appears" or "it does not appear" in their brain.

Third, in both cases, plentiful and abundant true chi is the prerequisite for bringing about special abilities. Experiments have shown that the rate of success is much higher when children with such special abilities are happy, content and energetic. After a series of tests, they would feel mentally and spiritually - rather than physically - exhausted.

According to the theories of chigong and Traditional Chinese Medicine, true chi plays a vital role in nourishing the spirit. In the performance of tests such as these, the children's happy, contented and energetic psychological and physical states are the conditions which guarantee clear and unimpeded chi channels, smooth and fluent circulation of both chi and blood, as well as plentiful and abundant true chi.

Only when the spirit is nourished by plentiful true chi can the sensory abilities be enhanced and lead the experiment to a successful conclusion. On the other hand, the true chi has another characteristic: in performing hard work it spreads out and disperses.

Since bringing special abilities into play is also a kind of work or activity, it certainly disperses and consumes true chi; then the spirit loses its source of nourishment and becomes slow in reacting and understanding (reflecting external things).

Thus, the ancient chigongists maintained that the conditions in which to acquire special abilities through chigong practice were contained in the axioms: *"Keep chi and blood within rather than letting them spread be-*

yond the five internal organs. . .This causes the five internal organs to be balanced, peaceful and filled with chi"; and *"Guard against any leakage of chi"*. In this way, one is able to ". . . *have sharp eyes and ears, to see and hear whatever one pleases"*; one can even know what has happened in the past as well as predict what will occur in the future.

When the present chigong masters apply their special abilities, they also feel tired in a way similar to the sensations described by those children with special abilities. It can be inferred from this that the generating mechanism involved and the changes caused in the human body are basically the same in both cases.

There is an obvious affinity between chigong masters and special-ability children. A number of experiments have shown that special-ability children can "see" external chi generated by chigong masters - chi which is invisible to ordinary people, and which in many cases is undetectable by instruments.

In this vein, when children with special abilities do non-visual reading or perform psychic transportation of objects, neither recording instruments nor ordinary sensory organs can detect any evidence of such processes, but chigongists can perceive every detail. Furthermore, it has also been verified that chigongists of great attainment can both stimulate and enhance - or restrain - the special abilities of children, as they please.

In noisy environments, chigongists can provide protection of both the spirit and the chi for special-ability children, helping to render their abilities sharp and stable. They can also use their minds to obstruct the special abilities of such children. The existence of this interaction further verifies that the two cases are identical in nature.

b. There is a close identity in theory.

The close identity of the inborn special abilities of special children and the acquired special abilities of chigongists has been stated above; while this is inconceivable to modern science it is nonetheless reasonable in light both of the theories of traditional chigongs and the classic Entirety Concept of Life. The following relates to the profound and subtle theories of chigong. Only a preliminary introduction can be presented here.

In view of the ancient Entirety Concept of Life, man is the unity of the physical body (including essence), chi and spirit. Each of these three vital elements has its own unique functions; they rely upon, nourish and transmute out of and into each other.

At the same time, man is also the condensed form of the omnipresent Tao (the original Hunyuan chi). The spirit is not only the director of these three, but is also the key link connecting man and the Tao.

By virtue of the existence of this critical faculty, the consciousness of man is capable of directly exchanging information with and also interacting upon all things in the universe. Various supersensory abilities are largely the manifestations of such informational exchanges, while all kinds of telekinesis caused by externally generated chi are manifestations of those interactions.

Thus, special abilities are the manifestation of the intelligence inherent within the human body. In ordinary people, they remain latent and have yet to be tapped.

The aim of chigong practice is to promote and enhance the transmutations between these three principal entities - essence, information-encoded energy (chi) and spirit. The theories of traditional chigong hold that the essence, energy-intelligence and spirit of a human embryo exist at a congenital stage. The vital essence and vital chi only weigh about 30 grams after birth.

As an individual matures, she continues to take in external nutrients and to transmute the acquired essence and chi into vital essence and chi until she is 16 years old. By that time her true vitality (a term embodying both vital essence and vital chi) reaches 500 grams. This true vitality nourishes the five internal organs and is concealed within the kidneys.

When she reaches puberty, the vital essence is transformed into reproductive essence and flows downward, and the vital chi is also lost as the vital essence flows out (serious illness and exhaustion can also damage the vital chi). After this, approximately 60 grams of the true vitality is consumed every eight years until it is all gone; then a human being dies. (While the number of years may not be entirely accurate, it is important to understand the underlying principle conveyed.)

The process described above controls the birth, growth, decline and dissolution of the vital essence and vital chi in the overall life of human beings.

Although the vital essence and the vital chi nourish the vital spirit, the latter does not change as the true vitality grows or declines because the sensory function of the vital spirit is innate. After birth, its "pure and simple" unconditioned nature is gradually veiled by increasing knowledge.

Man begins to use concepts and words in his thinking process. The consciousness conditioned by knowledge begins to act and to control the physical body. The dynamic and perceptive nature of the vital spirit is gradually repressed and veiled by the conditioned mind.

Because the instinctual sensory functioning of the vital spirit is repressed and submerged by acquired knowledge, the key link connecting the vital spirit and the ever-existing Tao is obstructed or impeded. This is why ordinary adults do not possess special abilities.

Through chigong practice, the vital chi becomes plentiful and abundant, the vital essence and vital spirit are strengthened and conserved within, and the previously obstructed vital link connecting man and the Tao is once again opened and re-established. Thus, the submerged potential intelligence can be tapped and re-emerge in the form of various special abilities.

This is one aspect of the so-called "*stage of returning to the innate*" in traditional chigongs. Because chigong practice methods differ in thousands of ways (some first cultivate the acquired essence and chi in order to nourish the innate vital chi, then nourish the vital spirit with this vital chi, while others directly cultivate the vital spirit), the potential intelligence tapped and the results of these practices also vary greatly. Thus there are differences between practices focusing upon intelligence, general activities of living, fitness, and other dynamics.

Why do special abilities emerge in children even if they do not practice chigong? This is because, in comparison to adults, the cognitive intelligence of children is not strong enough to obstruct access to such abilities; the pure, unconditioned nature has not been overlaid with the acquired consciousness and can therefore have a direct action upon things. Even if the natural character of the vital spirit has already been veiled, it is not solid enough to resist the inducing effect of the special abilities training, and these native abilities can still be easily restored.

Some may wonder why infants, who hardly possess the faculties of a comprehending consciousness, do not have special abilities, even while they can, through their vital spirit, also act directly upon external things. There are two reasons for this:

First, a clear and unimpeded vital link is only the necessary prerequisite for the manifestation of special abilities; sufficient vital chi and vital essence are needed to nourish the vital spirit. As stated above, the vital chi and essence of an infant weigh no more than "250 grams", and mainly serve the growth processes of the body.

Second, at the infant stage, there is not sufficient conceptual knowledge in a baby's brain to allow special abilities to manifest. Although its vital spirit possesses sensory ability, it cannot distinguish the things sensed; the external world is no more than a simple material world to the vital spirit of a newborn baby.

Thus, the demonstration of special abilities is out of the question in this case. In this sense, there is a range of application in which children may demonstrate special abilities and in which the faculty of understanding plays a part, but also in which the vital spirit has not been completely veiled.

The child possesses at the same time both the sensory capacities of the vital spirit and the distinguishing capacities of the cognitive mind; in addition, her vital essence and vital chi must reach a certain level of sufficiency. It is in fact the case that most special-ability children range five to sixteen years old.

In summary, it may safely be said that special abilities and abilities derived by the practice of chigong are both theoretically and practically identical. They may be called "twin lotus flowers on one stalk".

11. Combining the research on special abilities with the modernization of Traditional Chinese Medicine and scientific research on chigong

Both the seemingly miraculous special abilities and the effects of chigong are both unacceptable to modern medicine and science; but chigong and special abilities have their own native home to which they can return - the respective theoretical systems of chigong and Chinese medicine - embracing the classical Entirety Concept of Human Life. The undertaking of scientific experimentation upon both special abilities as well as upon the external effects of chigong have provided positive contemporary scientific evidence for the classical Entirety Concept of Human Life. This concept has now been proved valid; it will both provide clues and open a shortcut to the understanding of mankind's life processes.

It is not difficult to conclude from the above statements that special abilities, Traditional Chinese Medicine and chigong comprise an entirety; they are all unified under the aegis of human life science. This was, is and will be true - in the past, at present and in the future.

The relationship between chigong and Traditional Chinese Medicine has been set forth above. Here, let us seriously discuss the relationship between the research on special abilities and the development of chigong science. This is an issue vital to the future of research into special abilities.

Whether in China or elsewhere, research on special abilities (or supersensory perception) has received mixed responses. There are two reasons for this situation:

One reason is that the existence of special abilities (supersensory perception) has broken the frame of existing scientific knowledge. A deep breakthrough must be made on the level of underlying paradigms in order to understand these special phenomena. At present, it is still too early for this to be accepted by the great majority of ordinary people.

Another reason is that both special abilities and the experimentation upon them possess inherent variability, which manifests in the following ways:

First, the special abilities of children endowed with them from birth are not stable. As these children grow older, or as other physiological or psychological changes take place, their special abilities may regress or even be completely lost. There were and are a number of such cases both in the past and at present, both in China and in other countries.

If this were to occur, these psychic persons would certainly be labeled as "swindlers", and those who had conducted research upon their special abilities would also be seen as fools cheated by these "swindlers", and lose all standing and reputation. The future of research on special abilities would be uncertain if this problem were not to be solved.

Second, the experimental results obtained may still differ greatly even if the subject is the same person demonstrating them at the same place, and is observed under the same physical, chemical and biological conditions by the same methods as previously. This possibility exists because the result of an experiment not only depends upon the psychospiritual state of the demonstrator, but also relates to the attitudes and energy fields of the laboratory technicians and onlookers present.

There have been many experiments, the methodologies of which were universally regarded as reliable, which were subjected to severe questioning simply because the results were unpredictably divergent at different times and with different demonstrators. These reproaches made those "believers" involved hesitant to explore further, because in modern scientific experimentation, such intangible factors are deemed unacceptable.

For the future of research on special abilities, it is of life-and-death importance to solve the problem of the variability of the experimental results on special abilities. Indeed, the results of such research may greatly vary at different times and with different demonstrators. The approach to solving this problem may be undertaken from two directions.

One is to have a proper understanding of the reasons for this variability, which will not be stated here in detail. The other is to solve the problem of the regression of abilities in special children, and to create controllable experimental environments, so that the experiments are reproduceable. The solution to this problem depends upon chigong.

In fact, chigong, which has been distilled by the ancient Chinese from their thousands of years of practice, is the most effective way to stimulate and enhance the potential intelligence of mankind. Zhineng Qigong possesses even more remarkable effects in this regard.

In addition, it is the spirit, the consciousness and the chi of human beings that play an important role in bringing the external effects of chigong (special abilities or higher sense perception) into play. Thus, the most vital elements among these experimental environments, which at the same time form component parts of these environments, are the spirit, consciousness and chi of the practitioners and the onlookers. In order to guarantee stable experimental results, the demonstrator should be protected in some manner from the interference of the mind-field and chi- fields of others in those environments. Only chigongists of high attainment can provide such protection.

In summary, in order to unveil the mysteries of special abilities (supersensory perception) and to understand the subtleties of human life, not only is objective observation (the synthesis research of modern science) necessary - but also indispensable is the process of Inner Perception - thereby improving the levels of human intelligence, developing the intelligence potential and bringing about a qualitative leap in the intelligence of mankind. Only when these two approaches are integrated can the mysteries of life be revealed. In order to achieve such a qualitative leap in the intelligence of mankind, there is no other way than through the development of chigong – the cultivation of energy-intelligence.

BOOK III

THE
PRACTICE
OF
ZHINENG QIGONG

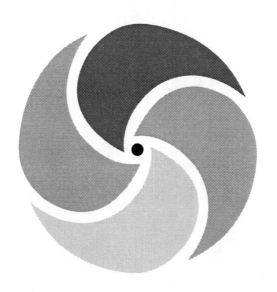

Caution: Before starting the practice of any of the following forms, it is advised that one consult with one's physician for advice. The authors are not responsible for any injuries caused by incorrect practice or departures from the forms. Study the relevant foregoing parts of the book first in order to be well-prepared for any reactions due to chigong practice.

Note: With reference to the practice of the Lift Chi Up and Pour Chi Down Method and the Three Centers Merge Standing Form, the following explanations are integrated from Professor Pang's book - *Practice Methodology of Zhineng Qigong* and later lectures given by him following the publication of this book. The explanations of the extra forms following these two regular forms, as well as of Professor Pang's teachings, are distilled from my training at the Center, as well as from the experiences of my fellow practitioners. (- X. J.)

A. LIFT CHI UP AND POUR CHI DOWN METHOD *(PENG QI GUAN DING FA)*

1. Introduction

   a. Literal Interpretation
   Peng - to hold and carry in both hands.
   Qi - herein chi is referred to as:
   1) The chi of the external universe, the Hunyuan chi of nature.
   2) One's own external chi distributed around one's body.
   3) One's own internal chi.
Emphasis here is placed upon the cultivation and mobilization of external chi.

   Guan - to pass through, to pour chi down through.
   Ding - the top of the head; herein the Lift Chi Up and Pour Chi Down Method, refers to the Crown-point (*Baihui*), though it has various special definitions and positions in the context of other forms.
The whole import of the Lift Chi Up and Pour Chi Down Method, which also constitutes the fundamental essence of this form, consists in holding and carrying the gathered natural Hunyuan chi up above the head with both hands, then pouring chi down through the top of the head into

the whole body (from crown to toe), filling the entire body with a ceaseless stream of chi.

b. Aim and structure

The first practice level of Zhineng Donggong - the former Soaring Crane Form - was made public in the autumn of 1980, and it was this which was later transformed into the Lift Chi Up and Pour Chi Down Method. It exists at the stage of External Hunyuan practice.

This is a basic practice for the prevention and healing of illness, as well as the enhancement of health. Through both physical movements (the opening and closing of the body) and the guidance of one's thoughts, internal chi is released and external chi is absorbed, thus clearing and opening the pathways and channels which connect the chi of human beings and the chi of nature. In this way, man is more closely unified with the natural world. This form is very effective for purposes of both gathering and absorbing chi; through the practice of it, one can quickly learn the Chi Transmission Method and understand how to treat others using external chi.

The Lift Chi Up and Pour Chi Down Method consists of five postures: 1) the Beginning Posture, 2) Posture One - Starting From the Front and Lifting Chi Up Laterally, 3) Posture Two - Starting From Sides and Lifting Chi Up Anteriorly, 4) Posture Three - Lifting Chi Up Diagonally, and 5) the Ending Posture, which repeats the Beginning Posture, but along reversed paths; Posture Two also repeats Posture One in a reverse manner. Though there are many movements, the form possesses virtually only two substantial aspects: Pulling Chi (*la qi*) and Transmitting Chi (*guan qi*).

c. Features of practice

The fundamental practice principle of the Lift Chi Up and Pour Chi Down Method is the connecting, combining and merging of the mind with the chi, using the mind to direct the mobilization of the chi by means of targeting its point of destination rather than by forcibly directing its path of travel; here, the emphasis is placed simultaneously upon both the mind and the chi. While the physical movements of opening and closing enhance the opening and closing of the mind, this effectively appears to be placing emphasis upon both the body and the mind. The main idea, in fact, is not the enhancement of the body per se, but the releasing of the internal chi and the absorbing of the external chi through means of physical movements.

To achieve the above goal, one should:

1) Be perfectly relaxed, peaceful and tranquil, content with oneself, calm, and at ease.

2) Perform the movements smoothly and skillfully, without restraint or excess, opening and closing to the appropriate degree.

3) Keep the movements soft and mellow, continuous and uninterrupted, moving in a fluent and effortless manner. In terms of the movements, there should be no breaks in a fast moving practice and no interruptions at a slower pace; instead the flow of practice should remain perfectly agile and smooth.

4) The key point of this form is the opening and closing of consciousness. When the mind opens, the farther afield (into the center of the universe) it expands, the better; when the mind closes, and the deeper within (the body) it penetrates, the better.

d. Benefits

1) By opening the blockages within the energy system linking man and nature, the collateral chi channels running across the membranes, energy paths, and key vital chi points of the body can be cleared and opened, and the smooth, unimpeded flow and circulation of chi can be achieved; thus human vitality can be enhanced.

2) Through the practice of this form, the practitioner can quickly become aware of the existence of chi. The sensation of chi will be strong, and this chi is very effective for the prevention and healing of illness, as well as the enhancement of health.

3) Various potentialities can be tapped and sensory abilities can be enhanced.

4) This is an effective method for gathering and absorbing chi. The student can quickly learn to apply the skill of treating others with external chi, as in healing; it is also helpful in leading group practice by means of the creation of a field of intelligent energy.

Note: For beginners, it is better to become proficient in the physical movements first. After a considerable period of regular practice, the ideas and visualizations may then be incorporated into the practice of the physical movements; otherwise, one will not be able to attend to the former aspect without losing sight of the latter.

2. Preparatory Posture

General postural requirements: *Put the feet together, keeping the whole body upright, centered and well balanced, naturally allowing both hands to hang down at the sides; gaze forward at eye level, withdrawing one's vision within oneself; gently close the eyes, and relax the entire body.* (As shown in Figure 1)

Put the feet together: As soon as one hears this instruction - "put the feet together", one should adjust oneself, both spiritually and physically, moving from a natural state of mind to a chigong - or energy sensitive - state of mind in order to fulfill the requirements of practice. With the inner side of one foot naturally touching that of the other, closely connect the kidney channel with the *Yinqiaomai* (an extra channel originating from the inner side of the heel and running upward beside the kidney channels to meet the canthus); in this posture, the juxtapositioning of the feet plays a special role in cultivating and nourishing the kidney chi. In addition, the lower part of the body forms itself into a totality, which also unifies the chi throughout the entire body.

Keep the entire body upright, centered, and well balanced: The key point lies in allowing the head to be borne upright, straight, and in a correct position, neither bending forward nor backward, nor tilting to the right or to the left. One should feel as if one's crown-point (*Baihui*) is being lifted from above, and at the same time, as if one is also gently heading upward from within, much at the same thrusting angle at which a soccer player head-butts a ball into the air. While implementing these instructions, one should also take care to:

    (1) First, withdraw the Adam's apple; then tuck the chin, as if the chin were searching for the Adam's apple; while the attention continues probing further backward and upward to the occiput (*Yuzhen*), and finally to the crown-point (*Baihui*), maintaining it in an upright position. In this manner the head assumes its correct position, as does the entire body.

(The above is sufficient for beginners. Skilled practitioners may wish to further adjust the head and body by following (2) and (3).)

    (2) Focus upon the mid-eyebrow point (*Yintang*), then bring the focus within, to the center of the head, and then up to the crown-point, maintaining it in an upright position.

190

(3) Focus upon the tip of the nose, moving the focus down to the perineum (*Huiyin*), then backward across the perineum and upward along the spine to the crown-point, holding it upright.

Allow both hands to hang down naturally at the sides: First relax the shoulders, then gently and effortlessly lift them slightly outward and upward, as if chi is supporting them from within. Let the armpits become naturally empty and relaxed. Relax the whole of the upper limbs, from the shoulders down to the fingers. Allow the fingers to naturally close together, positioning the middle fingers at the seams of the pants; in this way chi can flow smoothly and unimpededly throughout the upper limbs.

Gaze forward at eye level, withdrawing one's vision within oneself, and gently close the eyes: Passively gaze forward at eye level for a while, merging one's awareness into one's vision, following the mind into the distance and to the horizon. The focus of the mind and the vision may also be concentrated upon an imagined space immediately surrounding oneself, and occupying an area of one meter to the front. Gradually focus the attention and vision upon an imaginary point within this circumscribed area. Withdraw the vision, gently closing the eyes: the vision following one's awareness and withdrawing within the mid-eyebrow point (*Yin-tang*); commencing at the outer corners of the eyes, gently and gradually allow the upper and lower eyelids to close together. The eyes can be completely closed or narrowly opened. The former is helpful in maintaining one's concentration upon the practice and in maintaining a peaceful and tranquil mind, while the latter is helpful in mobilizing, enhancing one's connection with, and absorbing the chi of the natural world. As soon as the eyes are closed, allow the eyeballs to remain in the forward-looking position, and moving them neither up nor down, nor to the left or to the right.

Relax the whole body: The principle here is to relax the whole body from crown to toe, from the inside to the outside, and finally, to relax one's entire being, from the body to the mind.

Head: Smooth the eyebrows and focus on the mid-brow point, relaxing it from within. Focus the attention upon the inner corners of the eyes and relax them; then widen the attention to the ends of the eyebrows, relaxing them as well, moving down to the cheeks; mentally connect the two corners of the mouth and lift them up slightly, creating a pleased, softly smiling expression. A happy mood is helpful in facilitating the smooth flow of the chi and blood. Gently close the lips, the upper teeth aligned with the lower, softly touching the upper palate with the tip of the tongue (for beginners, the position is at the juncture connecting the root of the upper front teeth and the gum).

Neck: Relax the neck from within, taking care to not stiffen it as the *Baihui* is being supported.

Middle Part (chest and back, waist and hips): First, inhale deeply and, and the same time, lift the shoulders, rounding them. Second, as one breathes out, lower the shoulders backward and downward, dropping them, then slightly close them in a forward direction, hollowing the chest, and immediately lift the shoulders upward and outward, opening the chest. Finally, relax the shoulders and lower them naturally, emptying the armpits. Withdraw the abdomen slightly, expanding the Door of Life (*Mingmen*) outward, and allow the tip of the tailbone to be vertically suspended, as if anchored from below by a plumb line, maintaining the perineum lifted in an upright position.

Upper limbs: Relax the upper limbs - from the shoulders, to the upper arms, to the elbows, to the forearms, to the wrists, to the palms and fingers.

Lower part: Relax the lower part of the body from the innominate bones (the pelvic girdle), to the thighs, to the knees, to the calves, to the ankles, to the soles and the toes. Place both feet flat on the floor. Place the weight towards the forefoot; this not only reduces fatigue but also helps open the centers of the feet (*Yongquan*). Leading with the crown-point (*Baihui*), slightly rock the whole body forward and backward for a little while; this allows the body as a whole to relax and mobilizes the chi field around oneself; this also benefits the practitioner in other ways.

Internal organs: Relax the internal organs, then relax the whole body from the skin layer to the muscles, to the tendons and veins, to the bones and bone marrow.

Inner adjustment - The Eight Key Ideas:

(1) Extend upward into the sky and step down into the earth

(2) Relax the entire body and expand the awareness
(3) Be tranquil within and respectful without
(4) Clear the mind and maintain a reverent attitude
(5) Dispel all distracting thoughts (unify the mind)
(6) Permeate the mind with the void-essence.
(7) Introvert the awareness to observe the entire body -
(8) - Which is now warm, comfortable, and completely relaxed

Before the practice of the Lift Chi Up and Pour Chi Down Method, these Eight Key Ideas help adjust the mind in achieving an energy-sensitive state of mind. The overall requirement of practice is the unification of oneself with the void-essence and the blending of the human chi with universal chi in order to experience and observe the state of calmness or the sensation of tranquillity within a relaxed body; this will further adjust the states of body, mind and chi in achieving an energy-sensitive - or chigong – state.

Extend upward into the sky: As the crown heads upwards from within, imagine the head reaching the void-nature of the blue sky instantly; do not attempt to analyze how high or distant the blue sky may be; rather, conceive that it is immediately above the head. The color blue embodies the vital radiance of all flourishing things; this will in turn evoke the practitioner's own life-vitality.

Step down into the earth: As the feet step down into the earth, imagine that both the mind and the body expand downwards, deep into the void-realm upon the opposite side of the earth. Do not confine the mind to the awareness of standing firmly or steadily upon a solid floor; this may keep the practitioner's chi on the surface of the earth rather than allowing it to expand down, deeply into the earth.

We should allow ourselves to "zoom out" to view the earth against the vast background of the universe; it is a tiny sphere within the void-nature. If we view ourselves this way - on the one hand rooted within this tiny sphere in space, and on the other hand, surrounded by universal chi in all directions, through the mind's power of imagination, human chi can be unified with universal chi. Only through such visualization can we lay a foundation for the practice of "blending and transmuting man with nature". By way of metaphor, the earth may be seen as the yolk of an egg (the universe) with ourselves existing within this "yolk"; it is surrounded by the chi of the void-essence, which may be understood to represent the white of the egg. In this way, we are also engulfed by universal chi in all directions, and naturally unified with it. If one can conceive in this manner, the body and mind are not confined to the sky and the earth, but are blended with the void-nature, and become a oneness with the universe. As soon as one can successfully attain such a visualization, the sensation of chi (the natural and slight swaying of the body) becomes strong. The aim of this visualization is to blend one's own chi with the original Hunyuan chi, in order to gather and take in this most basic source-energy.

Relax the whole body: Relax the mind first, then relax the whole body, from the skin to the muscles, to the tendons and veins, to the bones and marrow, to the internal organs. One may also imagine that the pores and the capillaries are loosened and opened; this may further help chi to flow in and out.

Expand the awareness: There are two implications to expanding the consciousness. First, fill the relaxed body with the mind - "scan" or try to be consciously aware of the relaxed body. In this way, chi will follow the awareness, filling the whole body. Second, expand the mind out into the void-nature in the six directions (up and down, front and back, left and right). If a successful visualization is conducted, both the mind and body are felt to be expanding in all directions. The aim is to open one's heart and to embrace the universe with an open mind-field; thus one's spiritual chi can be easily blended with the original Hunyuan chi of the void-nature.

"Relax the whole body" and "expand the awareness" are directives which mutually supplement each other; one must do both at the same time in order to reach a state of 'relaxation-without-slackness', and 'poise-without-stiffness'. This is essential to the practice of the Lift Chi Up and Pour Chi Down Method. The benefits of this practice are the maintaining of a peaceful and tranquil mind, the causing of the chi to flow smoothly, and the enhancement of the practitioner's chi-transmissivity. The process is "to relax the body, to permeate and fill the relaxed body with spiritual chi and, with chi following thought, to reach every part of the body".

Be tranquil within and respectful without: All know that, in the practice of chigong, tranquillity - a state of concentration and singlemindedness – is important. But few know that a respectful inner state is also essential. In actuality, a respectful spiritual state is helpful in achieving a tranquil condition. For example, at the moment when one meets a person whom one has long adored, are there any distracting thoughts in one's mind? Those moving feelings which emerge from a reverent state are beyond description. According to chigong theory, a respectful mood will result in a concentrated mind (tranquillity); this can stimulate human vitality. Ancient chigongists required their students to respect their teachers. In fact, students enhanced their own cultivation in the process of revering the teacher. We guard against the cult of the individual, and we do not require the students to respect their teachers as the ancient students did. However, we do require that every practitioner respect Zhineng Qigong Science, and revere one's own practice. Only when one maintains a reverent and serious attitude can one practice conscientiously and meticulously; this may lead one to reach a chigong-state in a relatively brief period of time.

Clear the mind and maintain a reverent attitude: Maintaining a clear mind and reverent attitude is a further extension of the above-mentioned conditions of respect and tranquillity. Clarity is the continuity of tranquillity, which indicates that not only are there no distracting thoughts in the mind, but also that the mind is as clear as water and as bright as a mirror. Reverence is the extension of respect, which allows the condition of internal respect to be expressed with a corresponding reverent external demeanor. Thus one reaches a deeper state of energy-sensitivity.

Dispel all distracting thoughts (unify the mind), permeate the mind with the void-essence: Because it is often too difficult for ordinary people to keep the mind clear of thoughts, we enjoin the practitioner to concentrate one's attention upon (and into) the great void-essence, and to merge one's mind with the blue sky and the bright, clear panorama of the universe. In this way, the practitioner will become more deeply calm and maintain a mind which is unoccupied and tranquil, clear and bright. This is a spiritual cultivation of a high level.

Introvert the awareness to observe the whole body, which is now warm, comfortable, and completely relaxed: With one's spiritual chi already unified with the universal chi of the void-essence, upon bringing that unified chi back within oneself to observe the whole body, the universal Hunyuan chi will naturally flow throughout the body following the path of one's awareness. This will cause the body to be filled with Hunyuan chi, leading one to experience a sensation of warmth and relaxation throughout the entire body.

In order to better retrieve the mind, together with more Hunyuan chi from the void-essence, one may wish to recite a key phrase which embraces the major dynamics involved: *kong* (meaning 'empty', articulated from the rear of the throat and pronounced 'kong', with the final sound more nasal than glottal), *qing* (blue), *lai* (pronounced 'lie', meaning 'come'), *li* (meaning within', and pronounced 'lee', but with a brief final vowel sound). This phrase serves two purposes: one is to vibrate the vital chi centers and points through the pronunciations of these Chinese words. (Note: The pronunciations of the corresponding English words will not produce this effect, however, due not to the fact that English is lacking in words, sounds or of vibrational power, but rather that these particular words as translated - "empty", "blue", "come" and "within", do not happen to employ them.) The other purpose of this saying is to bring the energetic potential of this formula into active play - bringing chi from the blue, (in reality colorless and formless) void-essence, back into one's body.

Reflection upon these eight axioms is, in fact, itself a very good chigong practice method. Conscientious experience and observation of its content constitutes in itself a complete process of practice. Through the adjustment of both the mind and the body, the practitioner is led into a chigong state, which harmonizes the practitioner and unifies her with the universe. In traditional chigongs, the above-mentioned state is already considerably auspicious. However, in Zhineng Qigong, we must actively perfect our body and mind further, so that the mind is gathered back from the cosmos and merged with the body in order to practice Zhineng Donggong; this will further maintain the practitioner in a state of "me-within-chi-and-chi-within-me", as well as "self-unified-with-nature".

3. Beginning Posture

a. *Rotate and point up the hands, press down and pull the chi: push forward, pull back; push, pull; push, pull.*

Physical movement: Leading with the little fingers, rotate the hands and arms inward 90 degrees so that the palms are facing backward (the little fingers rotate first, the wrists second, the elbows third, then the shoulders), as shown in Figure 2. With the wrists fixed, leading with the middle fingers, raise the hands up with the palms facing the floor, fingers pointing forward, forming a right angle between the hands and the wrists and forearms; at the same time, keep the arms naturally stretched and relaxed, as shown in Figure 3. With the shoulders as axes, push the hands and arms forward and pull them back three times. When pushing forward, cause the arms to form a 15-degree angle with the body (the distance of one hand's length), as shown in Figure 4. When pulling back, the roots of the thumbs arrive at the seams of the pants, as shown in Figure 5. Keep the palms facing the floor during the whole push-pull process.

Imaginal Technique: When rotating the hands and arms, imagine that they are stirring deeply down into the Hunyuan chi in the void-essence beneath the earth. As the hands are raised, bring this chi back into the body, allowing the chi to be guided by passively targeting its destination-point rather than by forcibly directing its path of travel. As the hands are pressed down, release the internal chi (without totally relinquishing the root of chi within the depths of the body, as a far-extended kite is still anchored to its owner) and blend it with the Hunyuan chi deep down in the void-nature. As the hands are pushed forward and pulled back, the awareness opens and closes in synchronicity with the opening and closing of the body; this leads to the releasing of the internal chi and the absorbing of the external chi.

Skilled practitioners may wish to practice the push-pull movements along an elliptical pathway. The paths of pushing forward and pulling backward are the longer arcs of an ellipse (releasing internal chi into the void-nature with the palms pressing down while pushing out the palm-centers (*Laogong*). At the far end of the ellipse, slightly release the pressure upon the palms (absorbing the external chi from the void-essence with withdrawn or hollowed palm-centers). When pulling back (releasing internal chi), employ the same thought as in pushing forward. At the back end of the ellipse, slightly release the pressure upon the palms (absorbing the external chi with withdrawn palm centers), then begin another cycle of push-pull. As the palms are pressed down and withdrawn upwards, the body also opens and closes (while both the internal and external physical chi also expand and contract). This idea can also be applied to the vertical movements of lifting and lowering, as well as the horizontal openings and closings found in the following postures.

   b. *Relax the wrists, rotate the palms, hold and carry chi upwards anteriorly in both hands until they reach the level of the navel; transmit chi back into the navel. Rotate the palms downward and spread both arms sideways to the back, transmitting chi into the Door of Life (Mingmen), while visualizing the navel beyond.*

Explanation: Leading with the little fingers, relax the wrists and rotate the palms 90 degrees, with the palms facing the sides of the body; at the same time, both the elbows and shoulders also follow the rotation of the palms. Relax the arms, slightly hollow the palms with the little fingers slightly bent inwardly, keeping the wrists at shoulder-width, and lift chi up anteriorly, as shown in Figure 6. When the hands are at the level of the navel, hollow the palms and transmit chi into the navel, while visualizing the Door of Life beyond, as shown in Figure 7.

Then, leading with the little fingers, rotate the hands, with the palms facing down, and the arms naturally relaxed and stretched, at the level of the waist, and spread the hands and arms sideways, as shown in Figure 8-9. As both the hands and arms spread to the back, turn the elbows outward, withdraw the forearms toward the back of the body, hollow the palms, slightly bend the little fingers inward, and transmit chi into the Door of Life, as shown in Figure 10.

The lower Vital Center is an area between the navel and the Door of Life, slightly closer to The Door of Life. The function of the chi in the lower Vital Center (the gathering place of the internal physical chi) is essential for maintaining and stimulating vitality; it is the basis of life. All weakness and illness are caused by the shortage of this chi. Thus, the actual purpose of transmitting chi into the navel and The Door of Life is to fill the lower Vital Center with chi. The hands should not be lower than the waist.

Imaginal Technique: As the wrists are relaxed, hands rotating and lifting chi up, imagine that the hands and arms are reaching down deep into the depths of the earth, stirring the chi of the void-essence and, with both hands, carefully lift up a huge, expansive sphere of chi; at the same time, the internal chi should be consciously unified with the external chi. While transmitting chi into the navel, generate the ball of chi into the navel, thinking of The Door of Life; while one is imagining the lower Vital Center is filling with chi, chi will flow into the lower Vital Center through the navel like an endless stream. As the palms are turned down with the hands and arms spreading sideways, one now places oneself between heaven and earth, the hands pressing the earth chi and spreading out to the horizon; at the same time, chi is continuously being absorbed within. When the hands are at the back, transmitting chi into The Door of Life, again fill the lower Vital Center with the chi of the void-essence, visualizing the navel.

c. *Then lift both hands forward and upward, transmitting chi into the underarm points (Dabao), middle fingers pressing inward. Turn the fingers forward and stretch both hands out to the front within the width of the shoulders, transmitting chi into the mid-brow point (Yintang).*

Explanation: As the hands and forearms are raised to the underarm points, try to keep the palms face-up with the fingers pressing into the body; at the same time, open the chest and relax the shoulders, as shown in Figure 11. The *Dabao* is a key point in the collateral chi channel of the spleen. Pressing this point is helpful in opening this channel. The aim of this movement is to fill the middle (central body) Vital Center with chi. Then close the elbows backward, turning the tips of the fingers forward, stretching the hands forward. When the arms are stretched at the level and width of the shoulders, slightly withdraw the hands and arms, hollow the palms with the middle fingers pointing back into the Mid-brow Point, as shown in Figure 12. When transmitting chi into the Mid-brow Point, beginners may just hollow or withdraw the palms; skilled practitioners may slightly retract the tips of the middle fingers a little, transmitting the energy sphere in the palms back into the Mid-brow Point. The less movement there is the better the effect will be.

Imaginal Technique: When pressing the underarm point with the middle fingers, concentrate the attention deep within the points, imagining the tips of the two middle fingers nearly touching each other within the center of the body; thus the collateral chi channels can be easily pushed open. When stretching the hands and arms forward, consciously connect the two hands and arms with chi, forming a sensed unity, with the palms facing upward as if holding something (actually, holding the Hunyuan chi in the void-essence of heaven and earth). When transmitting chi into the Mid-brow Point while the tips of the middle fingers are pointing back, one feels as if two energy beams from the tips of the middle fingers are meeting within the Mid-brow Point. There may be various distinct sensations of chi. As more chi enters the head, the upper Vital Center can be opened, and vital points and paths within the head can be made more sensitive; this may lead eventually to the opening of the Eye of Heaven and the attainment of higher sensory abilities.

> d. *Spread out both arms sideways until they form a straight line with the shoulders. Rotate the palms first downward then upward, carry chi up above the head, pressing palms and fingers together.*

Explanation: Slightly rotate the wrists, with the fingers of one hand facing those of the other in a diagonal manner. Then, leading with the elbows, rotate and open them, leading the arms to spread sideways (Figure 13), and forming a straight line with the shoulders with the palms facing forward. Leading with the little fingers, continue to rotate the palms downward (Figure 14); then, as the arms rise, rotate the palms upward with the arms stretching straight, describing a wide arc, until they extend above the head (Figure 15). Press the palms and fingers together.

Skilled practitioners may wish to experience and observe three types of forces in the spreading of the arms. One is the resistance between the shoulder blades when the shoulders and upper back try to open as the arms spread sideways. Another is the attraction between the inner sides of the arms as the shoulders lead the elbows to open. The third is the expanding force between the arms as if a huge balloon is inflating between the arms. Imagining the hands spreading along the horizon may blend internal chi with external chi to form an entirety-field.

When the arms form a nearly but not completely straight line with the shoulders, start to rotate the palms and arms downward, leading with the little fingers; then, when the palms are nearly facing completely down, immediately rotate the palms upward. This is a continuous movement combining both the rotation and the rising of the hands and arms, thus maintaining a continuous flow of chi.

When lifting chi up along the edge of the heaven, the arms should be relaxed and straight, as if holding something in the palms. One may feel a heaviness and a strenuous sensation in the arms; this is a manifestation of supporting the chi of heaven and earth, in which the arms are filled with chi.

Imaginal Technique: When the arms are spreading sideways, one feels as if one's embrace is being filled with chi, which feels like a huge balloon expanding; the hands feel as if they are extending infinitely far away - all the way to the horizon, and spreading along the edge of heaven. At the same time, one is blending internal physical chi with external natural chi to form a unity. When rotating the hands and lifting chi up, consciously stir

200

the Hunyuan chi in the void-essence between heaven and earth, gathering chi upward along the edge of heaven. When the palms and fingers are pressed above the head, the attention continues to lead the gathered Hunyuan chi toward their convergence in the center of heaven above the head.

> e. *Slowly move the hands down along the central vertical axis of the body, then to the front of the chest, forming a praying-hands position.*

Explanation: Lower the pressed palms and fingers along the central vertical axis of the body until they are ten centimeters above the head, moving them forward and lowering them to the front of the chest to form a praying-hands position, about ten centimeters forward of the chest (Figure 16). The roots of the thumbs are at the level of the Mid-breast Point (*Tanzhong*), the fingers point straight up into the sky, and the upper arms form an angle of about forty-five degrees with the body, while the forearms form a level horizontal line. Led by the middle fingers, slightly rotate the pressed-together palms counter-clockwise.

Imaginal Technique: Pour the Hunyuan chi gathered in the void-essence down through the head into the middle Vital Center. As the palms rotate, gather chi into and mobilize chi in the middle Vital Center.

Benefits of the Beginning Posture: Though this beginning posture seems simple, it actually fills all of the three key energy centers within the human body with chi - the earth chi center (lower Vital Center), the human chi center (middle Vital Center), and the heaven chi center (upper Vital Center). The earth chi is cultivated through pressing chi down and pulling chi up and by transmitting chi into the navel and The Door of Life. Pressing the underarm point is for the purpose of filling the middle Vital Center with chi; transmitting chi into the Mid-brow Point is performed in order to fill the upper Vital Center with chi. The clasping of the hands above the head effects the pouring down of chi through the crown-point and The Gate of Heaven. The praying hands are placed into the middle Vital Center to govern both the lower and upper Vital Centers. Through the practice of the Beginning Posture, both the earth chi and the heaven chi, as well as the internal and external chi, are all mobilized and unified.

Most of the rotating movements of the palms are led by the little fingers; this is because the little finger is linked to the channel of the heart.

201

Moving the little finger first helps to retrieve the attention and aids it in becoming concentrated upon the practice.

The benefit of the praying-hands position is to connect the chi channels of the ten fingers and to promote a smooth circulation of chi; the coincided palm-center points can balance the chi in both the right and the left sides of the body. With the thumbs aiming at the Mid-Breast Point, the chi is unified with the blood; this will keep the mind concentrated and dispel distracting thoughts.

4. Posture One - Starting From the Front and Lifting Chi Up Laterally

> a. *Rotate and point the fingers to the front, stretch the clasped hands forward at the level of the shoulders. Separate the fingers and point the hands upward with the palms facing front. Separate the hands completely to keep them at shoulder width.*

Explanation: Resuming the praying hands position, rotate and stretch the tips of the fingers forward until the arms are straight out horizontally (Figure 17). While maintaining the contact of the forefingers and thumbs, separate the hands, starting from the little fingers, one pair of fingers after another, with the palms facing downward. Point the hands upward, with fingers pointing straight up as well; the thumbs and forefingers now form a triangle (Figure 18); push out the centers of the palms, with the palms forming a right angle with the forearms. Slowly separate the forefingers then the thumbs, with the arms at shoulder width; the palms are facing frontward with the center of the palms pushed out and The Door of Spirit (*Shenmen*) opened (Figure 19 - 20).

Skilled practitioners may wish to gaze into the triangle with narrowed eyelids; after a long period of practice, one may see chi or other visual phenomena.

Imaginal Technique: When the hands are stretched forward, visualize the internal physical chi as being connected with the fingers, stretching forward, far away into the void-nature; while separating the fingers, the attention moves from the parting of the little fingers to that of the other fingers until the open triangle is formed. Observe the chi phenomena within this triangle with a one-pointed mind. Experience and observe the resistance and attraction between the thumbs when slowly separating them.

202

b. *Push forward and pull backward: pull, push; pull, push; pull, push. Pull chi horizontally: open, close; open, close; open, close.*

Explanation: The overall requirement of pushing and pulling is to unify the shoulders, elbows, and the wrists, leading with the shoulders to rotate in a vertical circular motion: upward, backward, downward, and forward. At the start of the movement, before pulling back, extend the palms outward a little - connecting the chi in the palms with the universal chi. Then, lift the shoulders upward and backward, the elbows moving along with the shoulders, the wrists following the elbows, which remain slightly dropped. With the palms hollowed (withdrawn inward), naturally relax the fingers as if holding a ball of chi in the palms (Figure 21). During this process, the wrists should not be lower than the shoulders, and the hands should not be lower than the wrists, but rather raised slightly above them.

When pushing forward, use internal force in extending from the shoulders directly through to the wrists, at the same time using the roots of the hands (at the juncture of the wrists) to push the arms forward, endeavoring to make the hands form a right angle with the forearms in order to open the Door of Spirit. Flex back the tips of the fingers, pushing out the palms as the shoulders move downward and forward (Figure 22).

After three cycles of pushing forward and pulling backward, gently hold the palms erect and pull chi sideways along a horizontal plane: when opening, and leading with the palms, the arms are opened to an angle of fifteen degrees (Figure 23); then close them at shoulder width (Figure 24). This movement should be conducted slowly and smoothly.

The movements of pushing and pulling should not be made too expansive; rather, one feels as if one is kneading a small elastic ball deeply into the void-essence; the movements are slow and small, gentle and undulating. Through pushing and pulling, the internal physical chi is released and the external natural chi is absorbed. The horizontal open-close movements should not be too expansive, nor exceed an angle of fifteen degrees. The out-pushed palm-centers and back-bent fingertips can cause the released chi to flow back again into the body. Skilled practitioners may also wish to practice following an elliptical path of opening and closing. The principle involved is the same as in that of the chi-pulling of the Beginning Posture.

Imaginal Technique: When pushing forward, think of the depth of the void-nature; when pulling backward, think of the depth within the body.

Gather and collect the chi of the void-essence through the open-and-close pulling of chi.

> c. *Spread both arms out sideways until they form a straight line with the shoulders, push and pull sideways, pull inward, push outward; pull, push; pull, push. Pull chi vertically: rise up, pull down; up, down; up, down.*

Explanation: After three cycles of opening and closing, hold the palms erect and spread the arms sideways, forming a line level with the shoulders (Figure 25); then perform the sideways pushing and pulling movements. One also leads this movement with the shoulders, following the reverse circular rotation: upward, inward, downward and outward. When pulling back, lift the shoulders upward and inward, the elbows moving along with the shoulders, the wrists following the elbows, which remain slightly dropped. Hollow the palms and relax the fingers (Figure 26). When pushing out, as the shoulders move downward and outward, push the palms out, leading with the roots (base) of the palms, causing the palms to form right angles with the forearms; open The Door of Spirit and flex back the tips of the fingers (Figure 27). After three cycles of push-pulls, proceed to pull chi vertically for three cycles: leading with the middle fingers, raise the arms 15 degrees above the shoulders (Figure 28), and then lower them down to shoulder-level (Figure 29). The principle involved and practice requirements are similar to those of the front-facing push-pulls and open-closings; the only slight difference is that one should pay special attention to consciously absorb chi. In the vertical pulling of chi, an elliptical path is recommended for skilled practitioners.

Imaginal Technique: This is the same as that of the front-facing push-pulls and pulling of chi.

> d. *Relax the wrists and rotate both hands, with the palms facing upward, carrying chi up above the head; remain in this posture for a time-period of one cycle of breath, pouring chi down into the body through the top of the head. Relax the shoulders, allowing the elbows to descend, continuing to send chi into the body with the hands, moving further down along the face and down to the front of the chest. Rotate the hands, with the palms facing the chest, continuing to move them downwards*

*until they reach the navel; press the navel with the middle fin-
ger of each hand.*

Explanation: Relax the wrists, as the fingers slightly drop; leading with the little fingers, raise the hands and arms and at the same time rotate them until the palms are facing upward (Figure 30). Relaxing the shoulders, the hands and arms lift chi up above the head, with the wrists at shoulder-width; hollow the palms a little, aiming at the crown, and remain thus for the cycle of a natural breath (Figure 31). Relax the shoulders and lower the elbows, transmitting chi into the head as the hands move downward. The hands continue to move down just in front of the face, with the fingers facing the practitioner at a diagonal angle (Figure 32), until they arrive at the front of the chest; turn the hands so that the palms are facing the chest, with the finger tips pointing toward each other, nearly touching. With the palms nearly brushing the body, guide the chi within the body down to the navel. Press the navel, with the middle fingers touching one another (Figure 33).

One may experience certain special sensations when the chi sent into the navel meets the chi descending from the head. This meeting place is the lower central point of Zhineng Qigong. It is an indeterminate point where the flow of chi stops and beyond which it ceases to descend. One may carefully experience and observe, but should not desperately pursue such sensations.

Imaginal Technique: When relaxing the wrists, rotating the palms, and lifting chi up, one may imagine that the fingers are five huge columns of chi descending over the horizon. When they are nearly horizontal, scoop chi up from down deep within the earth and lift chi up along the edge of heaven. As it is carried upward, chi is also being sent into the body as if in an endless stream. When the hands are above the head, chi is being poured down into the body through the top of the head like a huge column of energy; at the same time, while maintaining a lifted perineum, one brings one's mind to the centers of the soles of the feet.

The intention here is to allow chi to pass through and to fill the whole body. During the interval of a natural cycle of breath, relax the body, letting chi pour down into the body with a long, deep, gentle, and even breath. When the shoulders are relaxed and the elbows are lowered, continue to absorb chi into the body. As chi is being guided down through the body, one may imagine the hands to be actually moving within the body, pulling chi down, suffusing the muscles and bones and even the bone-marrow, with chi. When pressing the navel, think of the Door of Life, filling the lower Vital Center with chi.

> e. *Slide along the waistline to the Door of Life, pressing it with the middle fingers. Slide both hands down along the back of thighs and calves, to the heels, then slide forward along the outer sides of the feet and place both palms upon the insteps.*

Explanation: All the fingers slide along the waistline to the back with the finger tips continually touching the body; with the middle fingers touching one another, press the Door of Life (Figure 34). Then move the hands down, along the back of the legs, at the same time lowering the body (Figure 35). The hands move from the hips to the thighs; separate the thumbs (at the side of the leg) from the other fingers (at the back of the leg) and slide them down over the calves, and finally to the heels. Along the outside of the feet, slide the fingertips forward, then rotate the palms, until they are facing downward. Place the palms upon the insteps, with the fingers pointing the same direction as the toes. (Attention: as the hands are sliding down the body, bend the knees and the whole body until the thighs are horizontal, with the hips slightly higher than the level of the chest, which touches the upper legs; relax and slightly drop the head down, Figure 36.)

Imaginal Technique: As the fingers slide along the waistline, the mind also rotates together with chi within the lower Vital Center; while pressing the Door of Life, think beyond to the navel. As the hands glide down, endeavor to cause chi to permeate through the marrow of the bones in the legs.

> f. *Press down, lift up; press down, lift up; press down, lift up. Separate the hands and pull chi up from the depths of the earth, sliding the hands to the inner sides of the feet, and then slide them up, with the palms facing the inner sides of the legs until they reach the navel. Press the navel with the middle fingers touching one another. Separate the hands and return them to the sides.*

Explanation: Perform the press-downs and lift-ups slowly and with good balance. When pressing down, close the two knees together and shift the center of gravity onto the hands and the front of the feet; do not lift up the heels, relax the centers of the palms and soles of the feet (Figure 37). When lifting up, leading with the Door of Life, rotate the hips backward and upward, shifting the center of gravity backward onto the feet, while withdrawing the centers of the palms and soles of the feet (Figure 38). This movement is very graceful if one does it correctly, as if a little boat is swaying on the sea. After three cycles of press-downs and lift-ups, raise the body a little bit, lifting the chest from the thighs, while at the same time the hands leave the insteps. Leading with the little fingers, pivot the palms outward, with the middle fingers at the outside of the little toes (Figure 39), while at the same time withdrawing the middle fingers upward and moving them above the insteps as if holding a chi ball in the palms, hollowing the centers in the soles of the feet. Then separate the hands, with the palms facing the inner sides of the legs, and guide chi up (Figure 40). Raise the body as the hands are guiding the chi up; when the hands are at the navel, the body is also completely upright. Press the navel with middle fingers touching (Figure 41); separate and return the hands to the sides (Figure 42).

Imaginal Technique: When pressing down, visualize the void-nature deep within the earth. When lifting up, think of the depths of the body, absorbing underground Hunyuan chi into the lower Vital Center, unifying there the chi absorbed through the head with the chi absorbed from the feet. As the hands pull chi up from the depths of the earth, try to imagine that chi is directed up from the void-essence under the earth, through the arches of the feet, along the central paths of the leg bones. When pressing the navel, absorb the up-guided earth chi into the lower Vital Center, unifying the human chi with the chi of nature within the navel. Then separate the hands and return to the original posture.

During this posture, the chi in the void-essence to the left and the void-essence to the right is lifted up and poured down through the body - mainly into the lower Vital Center, enhancing one's vital force.

5. Posture Two - Starting From Sides and Lifting Chi Up Anteriorly

    a. *Lift both arms up with the palms facing down until they form a straight line with the shoulders. Vertically lift the hands up, with palms facing outward. Push and pull sideways: pull inward, push outward; pull, push; pull, push. Pull chi horizontally: close, open; close, open; close, open. Close both hands and arms forward until they are at shoulder-width. Push forward and pull backward: pull, push; pull, push; pull, push. Pull chi vertically: lift up, pull down; up, down; up, down. Relax the wrists and rotate both palms facing upward, carrying chi up above the head; remain in this posture for the period of one complete breath in order to transmit chi into the body through the top of the head. Relax the shoulders and lower the elbows in order to transmit chi down into the body.*

Explanation: Relax both shoulders, allowing each shoulder to function as the axis of the following movements: lift the arms and hands, with the elbows following the shoulders, the wrists following the elbows, the fingers following the wrists and the palms facing down (Figure 43), until the arms form a straight line with the shoulders (Figure 44). Leading with the middle fingers, vertically lift up the palms - facing them outward (45). Push and pull while horizontally opening and closing for three cycles, respectively (Figure 46 - 49) (following the same instructions explained in Posture One - c.). Stretch out the arms with the palms lifted, slowly closing them forward at shoulder width (Figure 50 - 51). Push and pull as well as vertically pull chi frontward (Figure 52 - 56) (following the same requirements explained in Posture One - b., c.). Then relax the wrists, let down the palms, at the same time, leading with the little fingers, and rotate the hands with the palms facing one another in a diagonal manner. Hollow the palms a little bit and slightly withdraw the little fingers inward, lifting chi (Figure 57) above the head with the arms in the shape of an arc and held at shoulder width. Pause to pour chi down through the whole body for the cycle of one breath (Figure 58). Relax the shoulders and lower the elbows, continuing to pour chi down through the body as the hands arrive very near to the crown-point, and slide the hands forward and downward.

Imaginal Technique: As the hands and arms rise laterally, imagine that they are stretching out infinitely into the void-nature of the earth, like two huge wings pulling chi up from the depths of the planet. When lifting up the palms, leading with the middle fingers, flex the fingers backward, absorbing the chi of the earth into the body. During the sideways push-pulls and horizontal chi-pullings, use the same concentration technique as that described in Posture One. When closing the arms to the front, the palms are lifted, and merged with the universal chi in the void-nature; use the shoulders to close the elbows and arms, absorbing surrounding natural chi into the entire body. Use the same concentration technique as described in Posture One during the frontward push-pulls and vertical chi-pullings as well as in lifting chi up and pouring chi down.

   b. *Move both hands down until they reach the level of the Mid-eyebrow Point (Yintang); press it with both middle fingers, then slide the fingers along the eyebrows to the back of the head until they reach beneath the bone of the occiput (Yuzhen). Press there with the middle fingers, then move both hands along the back of the neck down to the third thoracic vertebra (as far as the hands can reach). Trace the hands back up over the shoulders, down under armpits, and then to the back, meeting the chi at the point where the hands stopped in their initial descent toward the third thoracic vertebra. Move both hands down to the Door of Life (Mingmen), and press the point with both middle fingers. Slide the fingers forward along the waistline to the navel, press it with the middle fingers.*

Explanation: As the hands reach the height of the Mid-eyebrow Point (*Yintang*), press the point with the middle fingers (Figure 59), issuing a stream of chi directed toward the occipital point. Then separate and slide the fingers along the eyebrows, passing over the tips of the ears, until they meet just under the occipital lobe, the bone of *Yuzhen*. Press the point with the middle fingers touching one another (Figure 60). Move the hands downward along the neck to the point just under the third thoracic vertebra, pressing there with the middle fingers meeting one another, the tips of the elbows pointing vertically up to the sky, the hands partially overlapped, the head upright and the *Mingmen* opened outward to the rear, (Figure 61). Move the hands upward and forward over the shoulders with the other four fingers leading the thumbs. When the thumbs reach the point

209

above the shoulders, open the elbows to the sides, and pull the thumbs across the underarms, backward toward the spine (Figure 62), with the middle fingers meeting and sliding up to the highest point they can reach (Figure 63). Guide chi down into the Door of Life and press the *Mingmen* with the middle fingers touching one another (Figure 64). Then slide the fingers forward along the waistline to the navel and press the navel with the middle fingers meeting one another (Figure 65), issuing a stream of chi directed toward the *Mingmen*.

Imaginal Technique: When pressing the *Yuzhen*, absorb the chi of the void-essence into the upper Vital Center while thinking of the *Yuzhen* (sensitive practitioners may experience certain special sensations when the chi coming within through the *Yintang* meets the chi coming down through the crown). This meeting point is the upper central point of Zhineng Qigong - an essential point called the "original aperture of the vital spirit" in traditional chigongs. As the fingers slide along the eyebrows to the *Yuzhen*, imagine that the hands are within the head, rotating around the center of the brain and back to the *Yuzhen*. With the attention penetrating within, think of the *Yintang* while pressing the *Yuzhen*.

As the hands move down along the neck to the point on the spine beneath the third thoracic vertebra, the *Shenzhu*, press it with middle fingers touching, allowing the attention to penetrate the body within, filling the body with chi through the *Shenzhu* point. When the hands trace beneath the shoulders returning to the back, try to reconnect with the chi in the *Shenzhu* point and guide it down to the *Mingmen*. Absorb chi into the *Mingmen* while pressing the *Mingmen*, with the middle fingers touching. As the fingers slide along the waistline to the navel, imagine the hands are rotating around the lower Vital Center further inside the body; transmit chi into the Vital Center while pressing the navel, visualizing the *Mingmen* beyond.

Use the same concentration technique as described in the corresponding parts of Posture One in the successive movements.

> c. *Move both hands down along the inner sides of the legs to the inner sides of the feet, then place both palms on the insteps. Press down, lift up; press down, lift up; press down, lift up. Separate the hands and pull chi up from the depths of the earth, slide the hands along the outer sides of the feet to the back sides, then move them up along the back sides of the legs until they reach the Mingmen. Press the Mingmen with the*

middle fingers touching one another. Slide the fingers along the waistline to the navel, pressing the navel with the middle fingers touching one another. Separate the hands and return them to the sides.

Explanation: With the hands nearly touching the body, move them along the inner sides of the legs, at the same time, bend both the knees and the body, slowly lowering the body (Figure 66). The requirements for the pressing-downs and lifting-ups are the same as those described in Posture One (Figures 67 - 68). After pulling chi up from the depths of the earth (Figure 69), slide the hands up along the back sides of the legs (Figure 70) to the *Mingmen*. When the hands reach the *Mingmen*, the body is again completely upright, pressing the *Mingmen* with middle fingers meeting (Figure 71). Then slide the fingers along the waistline to the navel, pressing the navel with the middle fingers touching one another (Figure 72). Separate the hands and return them to the sides (Figure 73).

Imaginal Technique: This is the same as that described in the corresponding movements in Posture One. In this posture, the chi in the void-essence before and behind one is lifted up and absorbed into the body - mainly into the upper Vital Center, but also, in passing, into the lower Vital Center.

Note: No matter where the hands may be, maintain at the same time awareness of the void-essence in the opposite direction. For example, when lifting chi up in a forward direction, visualize another two imaginary hands are also lifting chi up behind oneself. After four hands and arms can be successfully visualized, imagine that numerous hands stretching out of the body are lifting chi up at the same time in all directions. Thus, the chi of the void-nature can be absorbed into the body from all directions.

6. Posture Three - Lifting Chi Up Diagonally

a. *Carry chi up diagonally (at an angle of 45 degrees) to the top of the head with the palms aiming at the crown-point. Remain in this posture for a cycle of one breath, pouring chi down into the body through the top of the head. Then move both hands down along the sides of the ears to the front of the shoulders and rotate the palms forward.*

211

Explanation: While lifting chi up, relax the whole of the upper limbs, hollowing the palms, with the little fingers withdrawing inwardly slightly, as if holding something between the hands, keeping the arms at a 45 degree angle from front and sides (Figure 74). With the shoulders leading, the elbows follow the movement of the shoulders, the wrists following the elbows and the palms and fingers following the wrists. When the hands are at the level of the shoulders, the distance between the two hands is at its greatest. Gradually reduce this distance as the hands and arms rise until they are above the head, with the wrists at shoulder-width. Hollow the palms, aiming at the crown-point, pausing for a cycle of one natural breath, pouring chi down through the crown-point (Figure 75). Relax the shoulders and lower the elbows (Figure 76). When the hands reach the sides of the ears, rotate the palms forward as they are descending to a point in front of the shoulders. At this point, the palms are facing forward with the tips of the elbows hanging down, the upper arms touching the ribs, the fingertips slightly higher than the shoulders, the backs of the hands aligning with the pits of the shoulders (Figure 77).

The purpose of this movement is to lift chi up in a diagonal manner, with the hands describing big arcs in their paths of movement. A point to note is that the hands are closest at the two endpoints of the arcs, while they are farthest from one another when they are at shoulder level.

Imaginal Technique: When lifting chi up diagonally, imagine that the hands are first stretching into the void-essence of the earth, then pulling Hunyuan chi up from the depths of the earth, along the edge of the heaven, and directly overhead. When pausing above the head, pour the gathered heavenly chi down into the body, in harmony with the breathing and the turning of the mind within; the universal Hunyuan chi now fills the entire body like an endless stream. As the hands and arms are descending, continue to absorb Hunyuan chi with focused attention, allowing it to reach the perineum (while lifting it up), then proceeding down to the centers of the soles of the feet - causing chi to permeate the whole body.

> b. *Extend the right hand forward, with the palm forming a right angle with the forearm. When the arm is nearly straight, relax the wrist and rotate the hand, the palm facing left; leading the movement with the spinal column, turn the upper body to the left. When the arm reaches the left side (90 degrees from the front), press the Zhongkui finger point (the center of the middle*

212

joint of the middle finger) with the right thumb. Keep turning to the left, bending the right elbow and sliding the right hand across the left shoulder to the Door of Chi at the sub-clavicle point(Qihu). Press the Door of Chi with the right middle finger (the thumb still touching the Zhongkui). Push the left hand forward with the palm forming a right angle with the forearm. When the arm is nearly straight, relax the wrist and rotate the hand so that the palm is facing the right; leading with the spinal column (or trunk), turn the upper body to the right. When the arm reaches the right side (90 degrees from the front), press the Zhongkui point with the left thumb. Continue turning to the right, bending the left elbow and sliding the left hand across the right shoulder to the Door of Chi (Qihu). Press the Door of Chi with the left middle finger (the thumb still touching the Zhongkui). Inhale and exhale naturally for three cycles. Relax both thumbs and push both hands forward, rotating both hands like a blossoming lotus, and press the hands together to form a praying hands position in front of the chest.

Explanation: As the right hand pushes out, point the fingers upward with the right palm pushed out, forming a right angle with the forearm, and with the fingertips flexed back (Figure 78). When the arms are nearly straight, first relax the wrist and let down the palm; then, leading with the little finger, rotate the right hand so that the palm is facing left, with naturally stretched fingers and slightly hollowed palm. Finally, leading with the spinal column, turn the body, right arm and hand leftward - turning the spinal column (the trunk) first, then the shoulder, the elbow, the wrist, and finally the palm and the fingers - collecting Hunyuan chi in the left hemisphere of the void-essence. In actual practice, all of the above-described movements are conducted simultaneously.

As the right arm arrives on the left side (90 degrees from the front) with the body facing the left, press the *Zhongkui* finger-point (the center of the middle joint of the middle finger) with the right thumb, and gently close the other four fingers together (Figure 79). Continue to gather Hunyuan chi from the left until the right hand arrives at the back of the body, with bent elbow (approximate 180 degrees from the front). Slide the fingers over the left shoulder toward the front, with the right hand still pressing *Zhongkui* and the shoulders rotating back to the right (Figure 80). When the right hand arrives at the left Door of Chi point (*Qihu*) just under the mid-clavicle, the body is facing directly to the front. Press the left Door of Chi

213

(*Qihu*) with the right middle finger (Figure 81). Then perform the same movements with the left hand, following the same instructions on the opposite side in the reverse direction (Figures 82 - 83). (Attention: the movement of bending the elbow and sliding the hand over the shoulder emerges out of, and is continuous with, the initiating motion from the spinal column; thus, with the shoulder relaxed, the spine, shoulder, elbow, and wrist can be unified as a structural entirety.

At this point, the two forearms now form a crossed position, with the inner side of the left wrist touching the outer side of the right wrist. The upper arms are at a 45-degree angle to the body (Figure 84). Breathe naturally for three cycles - pressing the Door of Chi (*Qihu*) while inhaling, and gently relaxing the middle fingers (while still touching the body) while exhaling. Then relax the fingers, naturally stretching them out, keeping the upper arms fixed (still 45 degrees to the body), and the wrists touching one another (Figure 85). Leading with the forearms, push the wrists and palms forward until the forearms form a right angle with the upper arms. With the wrists still touching one another, allow the hands to descend, with the palms facing upward. Leading with the fingertips, fan the left hand out leftward on a horizontal plane simultaneously as the right hand fans out rightward, until the two hands form a straight horizontal line (turning the blossoming-lotus hands, Figure 86). Press the palms of the hands together upright and lower them to the correct praying-hands position (the same as that described in the Beginning Posture. Slightly rotate the palms to absorb more chi into the middle Vital Center. Then prepare to end the practice (Figure 87).

Imaginal Technique: When pushing the hand forward and turning leftward, let the attention travel to the horizon, gathering the distant Hunyuan chi in the hemisphere of the void-essence to the left side. Merge the spirit with the mind and absorb the gathered chi deep within while pressing the *Zhongkui* point. Continue to gather and absorb the Hunyuan chi in the rear of the left hemisphere of the void-essence. When pressing the Door of Chi (*Qihu*), fill the middle Vital Center with Hunyuan chi. Employ the same concentration technique for the movement of the left hand. While turning the blossoming-lotus hands, give attention to following the extension of the fingertips far beyond, to the horizon - rotating them along the edge of heaven; thus the Hunyuan chi is gathered and absorbed deep within the body from all regions of the cosmos. The forming and rotating of praying-hands unify the spirit, chi and body as an entirety - preparing us to conclude the practice.

Note: According to the Theory of the Main and Collateral Chi Channels, the thumb exists within the circuit of the lung channel (governing chi), and the middle finger exists within the circuit of the pericardium channel (governing blood); pressing the middle part of the middle finger with the thumb can integrate the chi with the blood.

According to Chinese medical theory, the inner side of the upper thumb is related to the spleen (governing consciousness), and the middle part of the middle finger is related to the pericardium (governing the spirit). Pressing the *Zhongkui* point with the thumb can help unify the consciousness with the spirit, stabilizing the heart and mind, as well as help in gathering, absorbing, and mobilizing chi.

7. Ending Posture

    a. *Bring the palms and fingers pressed together above the head, stretching them upward, rotating and separating the hands with the palms facing frontward. Slide both hands and arms down sideways as if gliding along the dome of heaven until they are almost level with the shoulders. Rotate the hands, with the palms turning to face upward, and close both arms to the front at shoulder width, transmitting chi into the Yintang while pointing the middle fingers backward.*

Explanation: When the hands, pressed together, complete their ascent above the head, endeavor to stretch up as high as possible. Starting from the little fingers, separate the fingers one pair after another. When the arms are at shoulder width in front, withdraw the palms and arms a little bit, pointing the middle fingers back, with the tips aiming at the *Yintang*. (Figures 88 - 91)

Imaginal Technique: Imagine the pressed-together hands rising from the middle Vital Center - guiding chi upward (along the central channel of the body) to the upper Vital Center and then out above the head. Use the internal chi to stretch the hands, arms, and body upward, mobilizing the physical chi in the lateral parts of the body as if the hands were nearly touching the distant dome of heaven (in doing this, do not use forceful effort, and take care to keep the feet touching the floor). When separating and rotating the palms, as well as lowering the arms, imagine that the hands are drawing two huge arcs along the edge of heaven, as if dividing the sky into two hemispheres. While closing the arms to the front with the palms facing upward, continue to gather and absorb Hunyuan chi while imagining that you are extending the arms to the distant horizon. With the middle fingers aiming at the *Yintang*, absorb chi into the upper Vital Center, visualizing it flowing beyond to the *Yuzhen*.

> b. *Lower and withdraw the elbows, pressing the Dabao with the middle fingers under the arms. Rotate and stretch the fingertips out backward, spread the hands and arms out to the sides, and gradually rotate both hands so that the palms are facing the front. Close the arms forward and transmit chi into the lower Vital Center. Place both palms onto the navel, nourishing chi there for awhile. Separate the hands and return them to the sides, and slowly open the eyes.*

Explanation: Follow the same instructions described in the Beginning Posture while pressing the *Dabao* (Figure 92) Stretch the hands out backward until the arms are straight, keeping the palms facing upward at the level of the Door of Life (*Mingmen*); then continue to spread them out to the sides. Leading with the little fingers, rotate the hands, with the palms facing front, during the process of forward-closing of the arms (Figures 93 - 94). Gather and absorb chi into the navel, placing both hands upon the navel (men placing the right palm over the left, women placing the left palm upon the right). Nourish the chi in the Vital Center for two or three minutes (Figure 95). Separate the hands and return them to the sides, and slowly open the eyes (Figure 96).

Skilled practitioners may wish to draw small circles first before pressing the *Dabao* points with the middle fingers (forward, upward, backward, and downward).

Imaginal Technique: While withdrawing the elbows, maintain the palms facing upward as if they were supporting something, unifying the two arms into a structural entirety with chi. When pressing the *Dabao*, fill the middle Vital Center with the gathered Hunyuan chi. As the hands stretch out backward and spread sideways, imagine the palms supporting the chi of the void-essence and stretching far behind one, then spreading the hands out along the horizon in a forward-moving direction. When closing the arms to the front and placing the hands upon the navel, gather chi from the horizon and absorb it within the navel.

216

Benefits: The Hunyuan chi in the natural world and the chi field which is formed during one's practice are once again gathered and absorbed within the body. In reverse order, the three key chi centers are filled with Hunyuan chi, coinciding with the Beginning Posture. Through the gathering, absorbing, and nourishing of Hunyuan chi, and through transmuting the absorbed chi of nature into one's own chi, one enhances one's own spiritual and physical health. The Ending Posture plays a role in unifying and consolidating the chi within the whole body; it is especially vital to remain concentrated and singleminded in this endeavor.

8. Summary

a. Through the practice of the Lift Chi Up and Pour Chi Down Method, the natural Hunyuan chi in the void-essence has been gathered, lifted up and absorbed into the body. This chi includes chi from the four cardinal directions - front and back, left and right (Posture One and Posture Two), chi from the four diagonal directions (Posture Three), chi from the heavens (absorbing chi through pouring chi down), and chi from the earth (absorbing chi through pressing down and lifting up). In a word, chi has been gathered and absorbed into the body from all points.

b. Through the practice of Posture One, the lower Vital Center is filled with chi; in Posture Two, the upper Vital Center (and also, in passing, the lower Vital Center) is filled with chi; in Posture Three, the middle Vital Center is filled with chi. Through the Beginning and Ending Postures, these three Vital Centers are repeatedly filled with chi. Before the practice, a chi field is consciously established; after the practice, the chi field is closed and gathered in, or harvested. Thus every part of the body is filled with chi, and the chi and blood within the body are abundant, plentiful, smooth, clear and unimpeded.

c. Through the practice of the Lift Chi Up and Pour Chi Down Method, not only can the Hunyuan chi within the body be increased, but its quality can be improved as well. Illness can be healed, vitality can be enhanced, and intelligence can be developed. The general practice of this form can play a role in balancing the chi within the body overall. Better and more rapid effects can be achieved upon a specific part of the body if one

217

consciously gathers and fills the part concerned with chi. The principle employed is to consciously fill the part with chi if the function of that part needs to be enhanced.

d. In order to practice this form well, one needs on one hand to perform the movements correctly, and on the other hand to conduct correct mental and spiritual cultivation - deepening one's understanding of the importance of this form, as well as the practice method of External Hunyuan, and employing correct techniques of sensory and supersensory concentration. During the practice of this form, one should give particular attention to making the movements fluent and elliptical, and to allowing the body to become soft and gentle, with the heightened extension and expansion of one's awareness far beyond oneself, and into the cosmos.

9. Words of Instruction (based upon Professor Pang's recorded tape)

Introduction: The Lift Chi Up and Pour Chi Down Method is the first practice level of Zhineng Donggong. It resides at the External Hunyuan stage of practice. The objective is to practice releasing the internal physical chi and absorbing the external chi of the natural world. Practicing this form can clear and open the vital points and channels connecting the human physical Hunyuan chi with the natural Hunyuan chi; thereby one can be benefited with restored and enhanced health, and one can experience the further subtleties of the gathering and absorbing of chi.

Let us now begin the practice of the Lift Chi Up and Pour Chi Down Method.

Preparatory Posture: Put the feet together, keeping the whole body upright, centered, and well balanced, naturally allowing both hands to hang down at the sides; gaze forward at eye level, withdrawing one's vision within oneself; gently close the eyes, and relax the entire body.

"Extend up into the sky and step down into the earth, relaxing the whole body and expand the awareness; be tranquil within and respectful without; clear the mind and maintain a reverent attitude; dispel all distracting thoughts and unify the attention; permeate the consciousness with the void-essence; introvert the awareness to observe the whole body, which is now warm, comfortable, and completely relaxed."

Beginning Posture: Rotate and point the hands forward, press down and pull the chi: push forward, pull back; push, pull; push, pull. Relax the wrists, rotate the palms, hold and carry chi up in both hands to the front at navel-level, transmitting chi back into the navel center. Rotate the palms downward and spread both arms sideways and to the back, transmitting chi into the *Mingmen*; then move both hands forward and upward, transmitting chi into the *Dabao*. Stretch both hands out to the front at shoulder level and width, transmitting chi back into the *Yintang*. Spread both elbows and arms out sideways until they form a straight line with the shoulders. Rotate the palms first downward then upward, lifting chi upward with the hands drawing big arcs to the point above the top of the head. Clasp both hands and slowly lower them to the front of the chest, forming a praying-hands position.

Posture One - Starting From the Front and Lifting Chi Up Laterally: Rotate and point the fingers to the front, stretching the clasped hands forward at shoulder level. Separate the fingers and lift the hands, pointing them upward with the palms facing front. Separate the hands completely, allowing them to come to shoulder width. Push forward and pull backward: pull, push; pull, push; pull, push. Pull chi horizontally: open, close; open, close; open, close. Spread both arms out sideways until they form a straight line with the shoulders, push and pull sideways: pull, push; pull, push; pull, push. Pull chi vertically: rise up, pull down; up, down; up, down. Relax the wrists and rotate both hands, with the palms facing upward, carrying chi up above the head; remain in this posture for a time period of one cycle of breath, pouring chi down into the body through the top of the head. Relax the shoulders, allowing the elbows to descend, continuing to transmit chi into the body with the hands, moving further down along the face and down to the front of the chest. Rotate the hands, with the palms facing the chest, continuing to move them downward until they reach the navel; press the navel with the middle finger of each hand. Slide the hands along the waistline to the *Mingmen*, pressing it with the middle fingers. Slide both hands down along the rear thighs to the heels, then slide forward along the outer sides of the feet and place both palms upon the insteps. Press down, lift up; press down, lift up; press down, lift up. Separate the hands and pull chi up from the depths of the earth, sliding the hands to the inner sides of the feet, and then slide them up along the inner sides of the legs until they reach the navel. Press the navel with the middle fingers. Separate the hands and return them to the sides.

Posture Two - Starting From Sides and Lifting Chi Up Toward the Front: Lift both arms up sideways with the palms facing down until they form a straight line with the shoulders. Lift the hands up to a 90 degree vertical position, with palms facing outward. Push and pull sideways: pull, push; pull, push; pull, push. Pull chi horizontally: close, open; close, open; close, open. Close both hands and arms forward, coming to within shoulder width of each other. Push forward and pull backward: pull, push; pull, push; pull, push. Pull chi vertically: rise up, pull down; up, down; up, down. Relax the wrists and rotate both palms, carrying chi up above the head, remaining in this posture for a time period of one cycle of breath, then pouring chi down into the body through the top of the head. Relax the shoulders, allowing the elbows to descend, continuing to transmit chi into the body with the hands, moving further down to the mid-eyebrow point (*Yintang*). Press the *Yintang* with both middle fingers, then slide the fingers along the eyebrows to the back of the head until they meet under the bone of the *Yuzhen*. Press this point (the occiput) with the middle fingers, then move both hands along the back of the neck down to the furthermost point that can be reached (the third thoracic vertebra). Trace the hands up over the shoulders, then down under the armpits and to the back, reconnecting with the chi at the point on the spinal column where the descending hands previously stopped. Move both hands down to the *Mingmen*, and press the *Mingmen* with both middle fingers. Slide the fingers forward along the waistline to the navel, pressing it with the middle fingers. Move both hands down along the inner sides of the legs to the inner sides of the feet, then place both palms on the insteps. Press down, lift up; press down, lift up; press down, lift up. Separate the hands and pull chi up from the depths of the earth; slide the hands along the outer sides of the feet to the rear, and move them up along the back sides of the legs until they reach the *Mingmen*. Press the *Mingmen* with the middle fingers. Slide the fingers along the waistline to the navel, pressing the navel with the middle fingers. Separate the hands and return them to the sides.

Posture Three - Lifting Chi Up Diagonally: Carry chi up diagonally (at a 45 degree angle from the front and sides) to the top of the head, with the palms aiming at the crown-point. Remain in this posture for one cycle of breath, pouring chi down into the body through the top of the head. Then move both hands down along the sides of the ears and down in front of the shoulders rotating the palms to face forward. Extend the right hand forward, with the palm forming a right angle to the forearm. When the arm is nearly straight, relax the wrist and rotate the hand so that the palm is facing left; leading with the spinal column (trunk), turn the upper body to the left. When the arm reaches the left side (90 degrees from the front), press the *Zhongkui* with the right thumb. While continuing to turn to the left, bend the right elbow and slide the right hand over the left shoulder to the Door of Chi (*Qihu*). Press the Door of Chi (*Qihu*) with the right middle finger (the thumb still touching the *Zhongkui*). Push the left hand forward, with the palm forming a right angle to the forearm. When the arm is nearly straight, relax the wrist and rotate the hand so that the palm is facing toward the right; leading with the spinal column, turn the upper body to the right. When the arm reaches the right side (90 degrees from the front), press the *Zhongkui* with the right thumb. Keep turning to the right, bend the left elbow and slide the left hand across the right shoulder to the Door of Chi (*Qihu*). Press the Door of Chi (*Qihu*) with the left middle finger (the thumb still touching the *Zhongkui*). Inhale and exhale naturally for three cycles. Relax both thumbs and extend both hands forward, rotating both hands like a blossoming lotus; then press the hands together to form a praying hands position in front of the chest. Slightly rotate the palms to absorb more chi into the middle Vital Center.

Concluding Posture: Move the clasped hands up above the head, stretching them upward, rotating and separating the hands with the palms facing front. Move both hands and arms down sideways, in a descending arc, until they nearly form a straight line with the shoulders. Rotate the hands with the palms facing upward and close both arms to the front at shoulder width, transmitting chi back into the *Yintang*. Lower and withdraw the elbows, pressing the *Dabao* point under the arms with the middle fingers. Rotate and stretch the fingertips out backwards, spreading the hands and arms to the sides, and gradually rotate both hands with the palms facing toward the front. Close the arms forward and transmit chi into the lower Vital Center. Place both palms upon the navel, nourishing chi there for a while. Separate the hands and return them to the sides, and slowly open the eyes.

10. The points involved

Crown-point (*Baihui*): Located one centimeter behind the center point on the line connecting the tips of the two ears, usually the center of the hair vortex on the scalp.

Door of Chi (*Qihu*): Beneath the midpoint of the clavicle.

Door of Life (*Mingmen*): On the spine, between the second and the third lumbar vertebrae.

Door of Spirit (*Shenmen*): At the ulnar extremity of the transverse crease of the wrist, in the depression of the radial tendon of the ulnar flexor muscle of the wrist.

Great Vital Point (*Dabao*): Under the arm, on the side central line, at the sixth intercostal space.

Mid-breast point (*Tanzhong*): On the midline of the sternum, level with the fourth intercostal space, between the breasts.

Mid-digit point (*Zhongkui*): The midpoint in the middle section of the middle finger.

Mid-eyebrow point (*Yintang*): The midpoint between the eyebrows, right above the bridge of the nose.

Mid-thorax point (*Shenzhu*): On the upper spine, between the third and fourth thoracic vertebrae.

Occiput (Jade Pillow) (*Yuzhen*): Opposite the **Mid-eyebrow point** (*Yintang*), the extruding bone at the base of the back of the head.

Palm center (*Laogong*): The point in the palm that the middle fingertip touches when making a fist.

Sole center (*Yongquan*): Approximately at the junction of the anterior and middle third of the sole of the foot (excluding toe).

B. THREE CENTERS MERGE STANDING FORM

1. Introduction

The Three Centers Merge Standing Form is a transitional practice bridging the practitioner's passage from the external Hunyuan practice (or the outer energy cultivation) of Lift Chi Up and Pour Chi Down to the Internal Hunyuan practice (or the inner energy cultivation) of the Body and Mind Form. Its purpose is to facilitate the absorbing of external chi within oneself. It is also a practice needed in making the transition from the Five One Form to the practice of Central Hunyuan - but with differing merging positions and concentration techniques. The characteristic features of the Three Centers Merge Standing Form reside in the fact that throughout most of it duration, it contains fewer movements within an unmoving practice position. It begins with simple movements, progressing through the readjustment of all parts of the body, followed by the mobilization of internal physical chi, at which point the body is maintained in a fixed posture while purely the activities of consciousness are employed in achieving the goals of practice.

The Three Centers Merge Standing Form consists of four postures: The Preparatory Posture, The Beginning Posture, The Standing Posture, and The Ending Posture.

2. The Preparatory Posture

> a. *Put the feet together, keeping the whole body upright, centered and well balanced, naturally allowing both hands to hang down at the sides; gaze forward at eye level, withdrawing one's vision within oneself; gently close the eyes, and relax the entire body.*

Explanation: The postural requirements and concentration technique of this phase are the same as those described in the Preparatory Posture of Lift Chi Up and Pour Chi Down Method (Figure 97).

> b. *Turn both vision and hearing within, into the center of the brain.*

Explanation: This requirement is actually an adjustment of one's awareness - in order to focus one's attention within, and to bind the eyes, ears, nose and mouth together by focusing their sensory activities upon one single locus - the center of the brain. One may do as follows: when withdrawing one's vision, retrieve the attention - together with the Hunyuan chi from the void-essence - into the center of the brain, the particular point of intersection of the line coming downward from the *Baihui* and inward from the *Yintang*. As the eyes gently close, gaze passively at any chi phenomena at this locus. Bring the attention of the hearing faculty within, in order to listen to the sound at the center of the brain. With the upper lips and teeth gently touching the lower, with the tongue, touch the point on the upper palate adjacent to the center of the brain. Move the attention from the tip of the nose down to the perineum, then back across to the tip of the tailbone, then up along the interior of the spinal column into the brain, merging the senses of vision, hearing and the stimulation delivered by the tongue all together at the center of the brain; then continue, sensing a dual-extension of energy upward, through the Heavenly Pass Point (*Tongtian*), as if two antennae or feelers are extending from out of the top of the head. Focus upon allowing the tips of these two "feelers" to

223

meet above the head, then withdraw this point of intersection back into the center of the brain. This imaginal technique plays a role in distributing both the attention and the chi within the head, in keeping the spirit and chi within, and in making spirit and chi within the head plentiful and abundant.

   c. *Step upon chi.*

Explanation: First shift the center of gravity backward to the heels, establishing the heels as axes of support, separating the front part of the feet to form an angle of 90 degrees with the inner sides of the feet (Figure 98). Then, establishing the pads of the feet as axes, rotate the heels 90 degrees outwards. Now the centers of the soles are at shoulder width, with the distance between the pads of the feet narrower and that of the heels wider than the width of the shoulders (Figure 99). Whether rotating the heels or rotating the front of the feet, the entire sole of the foot should touch the ground at all times - maintaining full contact with the floor (thus connected with the earth chi at all times).

Benefits: With the front of the feet pointing inward, the *yang* channels along the outer sides of the legs are filled with chi while the *yin* channels along the inner sides of the legs are naturally relaxed; thus, the functions of these channels can be enhanced. This movement distributes the attention and the chi within the feet and causes the chi within the limbs of power and support to be plentiful and abundant.

Note: In contrasting this practice with the Preparatory Posture of the Lift Chi Up and Pour Chi Down Method, we find the addition of a new imaginal technique - introverting the vision and hearing, and a new movement - stepping upon chi.

3. Beginning Posture

The movements and concentration techniques are the same as those described in the Beginning Posture of Lift Chi Up and Pour Chi Down Method (Figures 100 - 108)

4. Standing Posture (including postural requirements)

General requirements: *(Resuming the praying-hands position), separate the roots of the palms with the fingers touching or nearly touching in pairs, moving the palms down in front of the lower abdomen. Rest the edges of the thumbs and little fingers upon the lower abdomen (allowing the center-point of the circle formed by the thumbs and little fingers to be aligned with the navel). Endeavor to make the palms form a right angle with the forearms, hollowing the palms, and naturally stretching out the fingers. Bend the knees and lower the body, keeping the front joints connecting the thighs and hips empty. Relax and push out the Mingmen as if sitting upon something. Do not extrude the knees beyond the vertical line rising from the tips of the toes* (Figures 109-111).

Head: It is necessary to keep the head upright and suspended (extending upward from within as if a cord of chi were lifting one from above the *Baihui*). First, withdraw the Adam's apple; then tuck the chin, as if the chin were searching for the Adam's apple; while the attention continues probing further backward and upward to the occiput (*Yuzhen*), and finally to the crown-point (*Baihui*), holding it upright. In this manner the head assumes its correct position, as does the entire body. Focus the attention above the *Baihui* to lift it upright, at the same time remembering to smooth the eyebrows and drop the cheeks, with the corners of the mouth slightly lifted. Second, focus upon the tip of the nose, down to the chin, then further down to the perineum (*Huiyin*), backward across the perineum and upward along the inside of the spinal column, to the *Yuzhen*; then to the crown-point, holding it upright. Third, focus upon the mid-eyebrow point (*Yintang*), and inside (keeping the eyes still, with only the attention moving), to the center of the head, then up to crown-point, holding it upright.

In daily life, one may wish to form a good habit of keeping the head upright: place a small glass ball or any little ball upon the pit of *Baihui*; preventing this ball from falling may keep the head upright in the position required for chigong practice. After repeated practice, the head may come to always be held upright.

The correct position of the head is extremely essential in keeping the entire body upright, centered, and well-balanced. When the head is upright, chi can be mobilized and guided upward to nourish the brain and consciousness, enhancing the controlling ability of the spirit, while as a result the practitioner appears vigorous and energetic. If the head bends backward, chi in the Governor Vessel Channel (*Dumai*) cannot rise up,

225

which may cause the neck to feel tight and numb. If the chin points upward, chi in the Conception Vessel Channel (*Renmai*) is obstructed from descending, which may cause dizziness and high blood pressure. If the head is not lifted up, one appears dejected and dispirited, unbalanced, either bending forward or backward, or tilting to the right or to the left. Correct all these incorrect postures by maintaining the head upright.

Eyes: First, passively gaze forward at eye level for awhile, merging one's mind with one's vision (the focus of the mind and the vision may either be concentrated upon the distant horizon or an imagined space immediately surrounding oneself, occupying an area of one meter to the front). Gradually focus the attention and vision upon an imaginary point within this circumscribed area. Withdraw the vision and attention, gently closing the eyes: the vision follows the mind and withdraws within the mid-eyebrow point (*Yintang*); commencing at the outer corners of the eyes, gently and gradually allow the upper and the lower eyelids to close together. The eyes can be closed either completely or opened to narrow apertures; merging the attention with the vision, move the focal point of this spiritual vision out from the down-slanting space of the eyes and up across the center of the brain, finally returning it back to the *Yintang*. The former procedure is helpful in maintaining one's concentration upon the practice and in maintaining a peaceful and tranquil mind, while the latter is helpful in mobilizing and enhancing one's connection with, and absorption of, the chi of the natural world. As soon as the eyes are closed, try to maintain the eyeballs in the forward-looking position, neither moving them up nor down, to the left nor to the right.

Withdrawing one's spiritual vision is an important way of keeping the spirit within and concentrated. The eyes can direct chi, thus, when the vision is introverted, chi is also retained within. The spiritual vision can adjust moods such as joy, anger, worry, grief, and fear. If one is accidentally frightened during one's practice, the eyes are employed in recovering from shocks (shocks, especially after one becomes still and tranquil, may cause perturbation, irritation, sweating, and so forth, because chi is disturbed and in disorder). The proper response is neither to stop practicing nor to open the eyes; rather just turn the eyeballs to the far left (while not turning the head), then to the front, repeating the process twice more. Then look to the far right, back to the front, repeating the process three times more. In this way, the calm and tranquil state of the mind can be restored. Withdrawing the spiritual vision is a process of cultivating the spiritual vision (some chigong practitioners can heal illness with only a glance due to the fact that refined spiritual vision is more powerful than the external generation of chi).

There is also a way to heal diseases involving the use of the eyes: when gazing into the distant horizon, the attention and vision are not withdrawn, but completely concentrated far away into the void-field. Keep the vision at eye level without even batting an eyelid for several minutes, and have no concern if tears or other impurities flow from the eyes. Repeated practice can help heal various eye illnesses, and even internal diseases.

Note: If the eyes are not closed at an even speed, various distracting thoughts may emerge. The solution is to slowly open the eyes, gaze into the void-realm before oneself, and slowly close them again. The distracting thoughts can be dispelled through, at the most, three cycles of such slow opening and closing of the eyes.

Oral cavity: Relax the upper and lower lips, slightly withdraw the *Chengjiang* (the hollow part beneath the lower lip) and slightly tighten *Renzhong* (the point at the junction of the superior and middle third of the philtrum); then gently close the lips without leaking any chi. Without force, keep the upper front teeth aligned with and gently touching the lower front teeth, with the molar teeth in a position as if chewing something. Gently touch the upper palate with the tip of the tongue (for beginners, the position is at the juncture connecting the root of front teeth and the front gum). As the tongue becomes more flexible, the point touched can be moved backward to the junction of the soft and hard palates. If this can be easily performed, one may wish to stretch the tongue flat and cause the tip of the tongue to touch the juncture of the upper and lower front teeth, with the body of the tongue contacting the upper palate. There are two points under the tongue that relate to the kidneys, and that can generate saliva. If the tongue touches the lower palate and rotates a little while, more saliva can be generated. Those who need more saliva may touch the lower palate first, stirring it, swallowing the generated saliva, then touch the upper palate. The main purpose of the closed lips and teeth, as well as the tongue touching the upper palate, is to connect or unify the Governor Vessel Channel and the Conception Vessel Channel and to make chi smoothly circulate and flow along these two channels. With the tip of the tongue touching the juncture connecting the root of front teeth and the front gum, the chi flowing across the collateral channels and surface layers can be unified. When the tip of the tongue moves to the joint of the hard and soft palates, chi in the main channels can be unified. Through long-term practice, distorted teeth can be corrected. If plentiful saliva is generated, gently swallow it down into the lower Vital Center.

Note: If the tip of the tongue is touching the upper hard palate, one may feel sleepy - a way to help go to sleep quickly for those who suffer neurasthenia. After some period of practice, beginners may sense a pulsing at the mid-eyebrow point; just move the tip of the tongue backward and it will disappear.

Neck: It is necessary to keep the neck relaxed and straight by withdrawing the Adam's apple and tucking in the chin, giving one's attention to searching for the *Yuzhen*, then moving it up to the *Baihui* and holding the crown-point upright. A relaxed and straight neck can, on the one hand, reduce the physiological curve of the cervical vertebra, and, on the other hand, mobilize and direct clear *yang* chi up into the brain. If the neck falls too far forward, the head and neck may become numb and the *Yuzhen* cannot be easily opened. If the neck is pressed backward, chi is deadlocked, and the head and chest cannot be correctly relaxed.

Chest and back: It is necessary to keep the chest both hollowed and opened, the shoulders round and dropped, as well as relaxed, and the armpits empty. A hollowed chest refers to slightly hollowing the triangular area between and above the breasts. A hollowed and opened chest can keep the heart and lungs functioning peacefully within the chest - maintaining a smooth and unimpeded circulation and flow of chi and blood. A relaxed chest and back can help the connection and unification of the Governor Vessel Channel and Conception Vessel Channel, and also help connect the six *yin* channels together and enhance the functions of the internal organs. Various key vital points can also be cleared and opened. Relaxed shoulders can cause chi and blood to flow easily into the arms. Empty armpits create the conditions favorable for helping the chi to reach the elbows, the wrists and the Door of Spirit.

First, inhale deeply and at the same time lift the shoulders up (rounding them). Second, as one breathes out, lower the shoulders backward and downward (dropping them); then slightly close the shoulders in a forward direction (hollowing the chest) and immediately lift them upward and slightly outward (opening the chest). Finally relax the shoulders and lower them naturally (relaxing the shoulders and emptying the armpits).

Elbow: In order to relax the elbows and promote the unimpeded circulation of chi and blood around the elbows, it is necessary to both drop and suspend the elbows. Give gentle attention to dropping the lower tips of the elbows, and at the same time suspending the elbows from their upper tips using internal chi. In this manner chi and blood follow the attention to fill and flow smoothly through the entire elbow.

Wrist: It is necessary to form a dropped wrist. There is a slight down-pulling attention at the Door of Spirit that causes the wrist to drop down, at the same time, lifting itself up slightly from its outer side.

Palms and fingers: It is necessary to hollow (withdraw) the palm as if one were holding a chi ball. The fingers are naturally extended, with some space between the fingers, and with attention given to propping them out; the chi from the little finger and the chi from the thumb converge outside of the palm (about one hand's-breadth away). The fingertips are slightly withdrawn. The purpose of this position is to gather and absorb chi within, through the placement of the palms and fingers.

Lower abdomen: Withdraw the lower abdomen and do not allow it to protrude. Withdraw the navel inward toward the Door of Life (*Mingmen*), lift up the perineum and hold it firmly in place. Thus the acquired chi can be transmuted into original or innate chi; the vital chi in the lower Vital Center can be further absorbed deep within. The increased internal pressure will promote the chi in the Vital Center to circulate through and permeate the entire body.

Waist: Relax the second, third and fourth lumbar vertebrae (including lumbar ligaments and muscles) protruding them backward. Employ the following abdominal breathing method: withdraw attention to the Door of Life (*Mingmen*) while inhaling deeply, then slightly sit down and relax the lumbar region; three to five cycles of breath are recommended. Relaxing the tailbone as well as the waist and hips provides a short-cut to this end.

Hips: Relax both the front hip joints and the back sacroiliac joints in order to allow the lower limbs to become more agile, and to broaden the range of the lower Vital Center in order to accumulate more vital chi.

229

Tip of tailbone: It is necessary to drop and point the tip of the tailbone downward to the ground - making the heels form the apexes of an equilateral triangle, with the distance between the heels being the length of one side. Imagine that the tailbone is connected to a stick resting upon the center-point of this equilateral triangle. After long-term practice, the tailbone can be dropped down. Remember to lift the anus when dropping the tailbone. A relaxed tailbone can help generate and mobilize the *yang* chi throughout the body; thus chi can be easily gathered and absorbed into the Vital Center.

Crotch: It is necessary to hold up, adjust and round the crotch. Slightly contract both the anus and urethra as well as the muscles of the perineum region (including the inner parts of the thighs), and try to round the crotch, with relaxed hips, dropped tailbone, and inwardly bent knees. In Zhineng Qigong, the perineum is referred to as the opening of the ejaculatory ducts for men, and the opening of the cervix for women. For beginners, the chi from the perineum can be lifted to the center between the navel and the Door of Life (*Mingmen*).

Knees: Relax the knees and slightly bend them inward, with attention given to slightly - and without force - lifting the kneecaps. Thus the lower limbs can be unified into a structural whole.

Feet: Lay the feet flat upon the ground with the weight evenly distributed and in good balance. First, adjust the entire body to be upright and centered; then slightly contract the big toes to direct chi to descend, lowering the weight of the whole body from the crown-point along the ears, the shoulders, the sides, the outer sides of the legs, down to the arches, evenly distributing the weight upon the heels, soles and toes while consciously trying to lift the knees. After long-term practice, the arches can come to touch the ground - this is the so-called "feet laid flat upon the ground". It differs from a flat foot in that the flexibility of the arch is enhanced.

Concluding Posture: Leading with the crown-point (*Baihui*), slowly rise up and close the feet through "stepping upon chi" (in a closing rather than opening sequence, reversing the procedure from "stepping upon chi" in the Beginning Posture). Clasp and lift the hands to form the praying hands pose (Figure 112). The following movements and imaginal techniques are the same as those described in the Ending Posture of Lift Chi Up and Pour

Chi Down Method up to the point that the hands are placed, one upon the other, upon the navel (Figures 113 - 118). Massage chi as if the palms are pressing and twisting the lower abdomen, rotating in counterclockwise direction (left, up, right, down) nine times, then in a clockwise direction (left, down, right, up) nine times. Nourish chi there for a while. Separate the hands and return them to the sides, and slowly open the eyes.

Imaginal Technique: Gather and absorb chi into the Vital Center; transmute, condense, and accumulate chi throughout the body into the Vital Center.

5. Key Phrases

It is through these key phrases that the spiritual activities are controlled and the practitioner is helped to achieve a better energy-sensitive state (chigong-state). The adjustment of the body and mind are of equal importance and should be actively carried out throughout the entire process of practice.

The key phrases are:

    a. Close the seven apertures and, with the tip of the nose, stir up the Pass of Heaven.

    b. Step upon chi with the "bowl of the hands" upon the navel.

    c. When the three centers merge with the Vital Center, the center of the crown merges downward with the Vital Center, the centers of the hands merges inward with the Vital Center, and the centers of the soles of the feet merges upward with the Vital Center.

    d. The body is light, the chi is clear and bright, and a soft smile appears upon one's visage.

Explanations:

    a. *Close the seven apertures and, with the tip of the nose, stir up the Pass of Heaven.*

The seven apertures refer to the two eyes, two ears, two nostrils, and mouth. This is actually the "turning within of the vision and hearing" as described in the Preparatory Posture. This purpose is to withdraw the attention of the seven sensory apertures within, into the center of the brain - introverting the spirit and filling the head with chi and blood. It is necessary that one be consciously aware of this point throughout the entire practice.

b. *Step upon chi with the "bowl of the hands" upon the navel.*

Through "stepping upon chi", the feet and the entire lower part of the body are filled with chi. Thus both the head and the feet are connected with the chi, and the chi within the whole body is consolidated and balanced. The hands are resting over the navel like a bowl, to facilitate the gathering of the chi.

c. *When the three centers merge with the Vital Center, the center of the crown merges downward with the Vital Center, the centers of the hands merge inward with the Vital Center, and the centers of the soles of the feet merge upward with the Vital Center.*

The merging process usually starts from the center of the crown - the attention goes up to the crown (inside the body), then immediately down into the navel (Caution: do not try to consciously analyze the path and process involved, otherwise abnormal symptoms may occur). The same principle is applied to the centers of the hands and soles of the feet. Beginners may merge these centers within the Vital Center one after another. The method of merging in the practice of External Hunyuan is to merge the infinite extensions of the three centers in the cosmic void-essence with the Vital Center within. Always keep the merging attention within - first from the Vital Center to the three centers in the void-field, then from the three centers to the Vital Center; rather than forcing or pushing from the outside, conceive instead that the Vital Center is attracting or pulling the three centers inward. The purpose of this form is to enhance the ability to control the chi of the external world from within the Vital Center. Inhale when merging the three centers with the Vital Center, and exhale when opening out from the Vital Center to the three centers.

d. *The body is light, the chi is clear and bright, and a softly smiling visage appears within oneself.*

When the posture is proper and correct, one may experience and observe what are termed the "four ups and one down" - extending the crown-point upward, lifting the tongue to touch the upper palate, holding up the perineum, hollowing the arches of the soles, and dropping the tailbone down. Through the above-mentioned adjustments of posture and mind, the circulation of chi becomes smooth and unimpeded, the mind is concentrated and cleared of distracting thoughts, one continues being consciously or unconsciously aware of the Vital Center, and a comfortable and pleasant sensation emerges - with a feeling of inner joy, leading to a smiling appearance. On the other hand, it may sometimes be necessary to consciously adjust one's expression to present a smiling visage. In the long run, chi can be cultivated purely and clearly, and the practitioner may experience a lightness of body.

6. Benefits of the Three Centers Merge Standing Form

a In the bodily aspects: distorted parts of the body can be corrected, so that chi and blood can circulate and flow along the appropriate passages. As the physiological curve of the spine is corrected, the lumbar area, the hips and the tailbone can be relaxed. Correct posture will help the mind to remain peaceful and tranquil.

b In the spiritual aspects: one's inner activities are adjusted through key phrases, which help the practitioner to reach a deep state of energy-sensitivity and balance (chigong state), with a peaceful and tranquil mind as well as mobilized circulation of chi.

c In the aspect of chi: through the practice of this form, the true chi can easily and quickly be stimulated and mobilized. The health-enhancing effect is distinct. The sensations of chi, such as slight rocking or trembling of the body, warmth within the body, attraction and resistance between the hands, appear quickly. As the three centers merge with the Vital Center, the internal true chi is enhanced and consolidated.

7. Summary

a. The benefits of the healing of illness and progress in practice.

The essential conditions for the healing of illness and the making of progress are plentiful and abundant chi and blood and the smooth and unimpeded circulation of chi and blood. Many diseases are caused by the abnormal circulation of the chi and blood, due to incorrect physical postures. Through the practice of this standing form, every part of the body is adjusted to assume a correct posture, which further promotes the normal flow of chi and blood. Through the merging of the three centers, the chi in the Vital Center is further gathered within. In addition, the main aim of this form is to relax the lumbar area, the hips, and the tailbone, so that the range of the Vital Center is broadened, the chi throughout the entire body can be made plentiful and abundant, and the functions of the entire body can be enhanced.

b. The solution to distracting thoughts.

During the practice of this standing form, through the adjustment of the mind, vacillating, disorganized, and wandering thoughts can be dispelled; the attention is concentrated upon the sole thought of chigong practice.

However, in daily life, people are used to experiencing numerous and disorderly thoughts. Against the background of a tranquil mind, such distracting thoughts may re-emerge. When this occurs, it should be clear that this is the beginning of a tranquil chigong state, and the starting point for the eradication of the disorderly state of mind. It is not the result of chigong practice, but the manifestation of the underlying consciousness as it is experienced against the background of tranquillity. It is a reaction denoting the making of progress.

One should not become irritated or annoyed by distracting thoughts, but rather continue practicing until the scheduled period of time is fulfilled. Thus one may advance step by step. One is not to worry if one finds one's mind wandering away; just retrieve it and merge it with the Vital Center.

The following are various solutions to this problem:

1) Discard all worries. As soon as one senses the presence of distracting thoughts, allow thinking to cease - neither reasoning nor caring, but actively resuming one's practice in accord with the instructions.

2) Slowly open the eyes, then withdraw the spiritual vision and slowly close them, repeating twice more. The mind-field will ordinarily become peaceful and tranquil after three cycles of opening and closing the eyes.

3) Do not concern yourself at all about distracting thoughts.

c. Time of practice and height of posture

The time of practice depends mainly upon the physical condition and the level of the practitioner. For ordinary practitioners, it is required that this be practiced for at least 30 minutes, because the time period of the circulation of chi and blood is approximately 28 minutes. The time can be prolonged as the practitioner becomes stronger. Beginners may stand higher, while skilled practitioners may wish to stand as low as possible, as long as one correctly conforms to the requirements.

8. Words of Instruction (based upon Professor Pang's recorded tape)

Let us start the practice of Three Centers Merge Standing Form.

Preparatory posture: Put the feet together, keeping the whole body upright, centered, and well balanced, naturally allowing both hands to hang down at the sides; gaze forward at eye level, withdrawing one's vision within oneself; gently close the eyes, relax the entire body. Turn both vision and hearing within, into the center of the brain. Separate the two feet through stepping upon chi and stand in the required posture.

Beginning Posture: Rotate and point the hands upward, press down and pull the chi: push forward, pull back; push, pull; push, pull. Relax the wrists, rotate the palms, hold and carry chi up in both hands to the front at navel level, transmitting chi back into the navel center. Rotate the palms downward and spread both arms sideways to the back, transmitting chi into the *Mingmen*, then move both hands forward and upward, transmitting chi into the *Dabao*. Stretch both hands out to the front at shoulder width and level, transmitting chi back into the *Yintang*. Spread both the elbows and the arms sideways until they form a straight line with the shoulders. Rotate the palms first downward then upward, lifting chi upward with the hands drawing wide arcs to the point above the top of the head. Clasp both hands and slowly lower them to the front of the chest, forming a praying-hands position. Separate the hands from the roots of the palms with the fingers touching each other, lowering the hands down in front of the abdomen and forming a position in which the hands seem to be holding a semi-sphere, or bowl against the navel. Bend the knees and lower the body to a proper height.

Adjustments of physical parts: Suspend the head from the crown, smooth the eyebrows and loosen the cheeks, while creating a softly smiling expression. Touch the upper palate with the tongue and relax the neck. Hollow the chest and round the shoulders, relaxing the shoulders and emptying the armpits. Drop and suspend the elbows. Angle the wrists, hollow the palms and relax the fingers. Relax both the *Mingmen* and the hips in a sitting-yet-not-sitting posture. Drop the tip of the tailbone and hold up and tighten the perineum. Relax both knees and bend them inward. Round the crotch and place the feet flatly on the floor.

Imaginal Technique: Close the seven apertures and stir up the Pass of Heaven with the tip of the nose, Step upon chi with, the "bowl of the hands" upon the navel. When the three centers merge with the Vital Center, the body is light, the chi is clear and bright, and a soft smile appears upon one's inner visage. Merge the center of the crown downward with the Vital Center, the centers of the hands inward with the Vital Center, and the centers of the soles of the feet upward with the Vital Center; merge the three centers into the Vital Center. Relax and be singleminded.

Concluding posture: Now prepare to end the practice. Leading with the *Baihui*, lift the whole body slowly upward. Close the feet and put them together. Clasp the palms and lift them above the head, stretching them upward, rotating and separating the hands with the palms facing frontward. Allow both hands and arms to descend sideways until they are nearly level with the shoulders. Rotate the hands with the palms facing upward and close both arms to the front at shoulder width, transmitting chi back into the *Yintang*. Lower and withdraw the elbows, pressing the *Dabao*, under the arms, with the middle fingers. Rotate and stretch the fingertips out backwards, spreading the hands and arms to the sides, and gradually rotate both hands with the palms facing toward the front. Close the arms forward and transmit chi into the lower Vital Center. Place both palms upon to the navel, massage the abdomen: rotate counter clockwise in everwidening spirals: one, two, three, four, five, six, seven, eight, nine; rotate clockwise in diminishing spirals: nine, eight, seven, six, five, four, three, two, one. Nourish chi tranquilly for a while. Separate the hands and return them to the sides, and slowly open the eyes.

9. Energy points involved

In addition to the points introduced in the section of Lift Chi Up and Pour Chi Down Method, there exist several other points:

Chengjiang: The philtrum, or hollow area beneath the lower lip
Heavenly Pass Point (*Tongtian*): Double points on the top of the head: from the central point on the front hair edge, go right up 4 *cuns* (cun - the length of one's middle digit of the middle finger), then 1.5 cuns right and left.

236

Renzhong: The point at the junction of the superior and middle third of the philtrum

Note: For the following supplementary practice methods, one may employ the Beginning Posture and Ending Posture of the Lift Chi Up and Pour Chi Down Method before and after the practice of these extra forms. At the very least, simply adjust the body and mind in the beginning for awhile, and remember to gather, absorb, and nourish chi, as well as close the chi field, afterwards. (- X.J.)

C. WALL SQUATTING METHOD (*DUN QIANG FA*)

1. Introduction

Though it appears simple, the Wall Squatting Method had long been the best kept secret in the tradition of Immortal chigong and was strictly forbidden to reveal to the public. It is a basic practice for achieving the attainment of a weightless body, through the neutralization of the gravitational field, and it is also a shortcut to relaxing the spine, the lumbar region, and the tailbone.

At the Zhineng Qigong Recovering Center, the Wall Squatting Method is employed especially for the healing of deaf-mutes, atrophy and hypoplasia of the cerebellum, and other children's mental and nervous disorders. Professor Pang once said that there was nothing that could not be healed if one persevered in performing hundreds of wall squats every day over a considerable period of time.

In Zhineng Qigong, it is a basic supplementary practice by which to prevent and treat abnormal symptoms; it is also the best way to treat various practice reactions. The practitioner usually practices this form individually according to her own goal and level. (The time and difficulty of practice differ from person to person.)

2. Requirements

Stand in front of a wall with a flat surface, put the feet together flat on the floor with the toes touching the base of the wall. Keep the whole body upright, centered and well-balanced, leading the *Baihui* upward and keeping the chin tucked, pushing out the *Mingmen*, and trying to withdraw the lower abdomen a little bit. Drop the tailbone down and lift up the per-

237

ineum (maintaining this condition throughout the practice), as shown in Figure 119. Then slowly bend the knees and lower the body along the wall with the shoulders folding forward and inward, the tailbone tucking downward and forward as if the crown-point and the tailbone were stretching out the vertebrae, one by one, from both ends of the spinal column (Figure 120). When one has reached the lowest position, remain for a while (Figure 121), then lifting with the crown-point, slowly rise up with the tailbone still tucking forward. Try not to protrude the buttocks (Figures 122 -123). Then one may repeat this movement as many times as one can.

Notes: Diverse levels of practitioners may practice this form at various levels of difficulty. There are some tips that can make it either easier or even harder.

3. Tips for easier performance

   a. Do squatting without a wall.
The aim to doing squatting in front of a wall is to prevent the knees and the whole upper body from advancing beyond the vertical plane of the toes; thus the spine and the chi channels in and around the spine can be cleared and opened. However, if one cannot squat down at all directly adjacent to a wall, it is best either to keep a proper distance from it or to simply leave the wall. When doing squatting without a wall, also try to consciously follow the requirements mentioned above. As the spine becomes more relaxed, one may perform it in the required way, or at least in a better way.
Some may also choose to practice with a tree replacing the wall, because the chi of a tree is much greater than that of a wall, thereby making the squatting much easier. However, a wall is the rule for objectively evaluating what level one has reached.
   b. To help initially, the feet may be left apart.
In fact, this was the manner in which wall squatting was first taught. But it is better to close them if one can, in order to nourish and replenish the kidney chi.
   c. Keep the crown-point lifted and the chin tucked at all times. Fold the shoulders inward and forward, with the arms and hands placed in front of the body rather than at sides to keep the body balanced. Try to consciously grasp the earth with the toes, with the weight shifted slightly to the front of the soles.

d. If this is still too difficult, one may hold onto something in front of oneself to aid in practicing.

4. Increased difficulty

If one can easily do perfect wall squatting, one may wish to increase the difficulty by seeking to further relax the spine. One way is to do wall squatting with the side-stretching of the arms and the up-pointing of the palms. Another is to do wall squatting with the arms and hands bent back behind one.

D. THE PULLING-CHI (*LA-QI*) AND FILLING-CHI (*GUAN-QI*) THERAPY

1. Introduction

This therapy is an external-chi healing method derived from the Lift Chi Up and Pour Chi Down Method. It directly employs the essences of the latter to treat either others or oneself. It is also the basis of external-chi therapy. It is the fundamental skill of Zhineng Qigong and should be mastered by every practitioner. Through pulling chi, one can easily experience and observe the existence of external chi (chi in the natural world and around one's own physical body); it is also an effective way to gather or accumulate chi. Through filling the body with the gathered chi, the sick can be restored to health, the weak can become strong, and the old can appear young again.

2. Explanation

This form can be done in any posture (sitting, standing, and lying on one's back). First, adjust the body and mind according to the postural and spiritual requirements as described in the previous sections. Then naturally place the two hands in front of the abdomen with the palms facing one another, with a distance of approximately ten centimeters between them, fingers pointing to the front. Relax the whole body, slowly close the eyes, clear the mind and concentrate the attention on the space between the two palms (Figure 124). Now push them together, the closer the better, but do not let them touch each other (Figure 125); then pull them apart within the above-mentioned distance (Figure 126). Repeat this opening and closing movement until one feels that there is attraction and resistance between the palms - something preventing the hands from closing and opening. That is chi - a fusion of the chi in the natural world and one's own chi, distributed around one's physical body. When one personally experiences and observes the existence of chi, one should actively and consciously gather and accumulate the chi from nature into the palms - employing the concentration techniques introduced in the Lift Chi Up and Pour Chi Down Method while pushing-pulling and opening-closing.

What is the use of this chi? It is a healing chi with which to bring about the cure of illness. When enough chi is gathered between the palms, transmit it into the physical part in which it is needed in order to relieve anyone from suffering and to bring about a cure. This is called filling the body with chi (the *Guan-qi* Method). This filling of chi is the same as that employed in the Lift Chi Up and Pour Chi Down Method. The key concept is to bring the external original Hunyuan chi which has already been gathered between the palms into the body, filling the body, causing chi to penetrate into the locus of the illness, and then blending it with one's own chi and restoring the abnormal chi or condition to normal.

Beginners may not know how to transmit chi within. Simply use thought direction and, with one's own mind, transmit chi wherever one wishes - with the chi following the attention. The deeper one's attention probes, the deeper chi penetrates. For example, if one wants a suffering part to be normal, just imagine that one is able to actively transmit the ball of chi gathered between one's palms into the ailing part, penetrating it and filling it with healthy chi and "commanding" it become normal. Do not try to analyze how chi enters the body and how it functions. If one tries to reason out the details, one's attention may be distracted, and because of this, one may fail to bring about any change in the condition. The movement of the attention, merged with chi, should be sharp, quick, and concentrated. Repeated attacks upon and into the sick part are all right, but do not linger too long. The effectiveness of the healing depends upon the penetrating and radiating power of the spirit (mind).

After becoming skilled in the Pulling-Chi Method, it is better to place that part of the body needing attention between the palms while performing pulling-chi and filling-chi upon it. For example, if one of the knees hurts, place it between the hands, pulling chi through the knee from one hand to another, filling it with healthy chi and "ordering" it to stop hurting and to return to normal.

There is no time limitation for the open-close pulling-chi. One may practice it as long as one enjoys, anytime and anywhere. After a given period of practice, the opening-closing movement of the hands will result in the opening-and-closing of the whole body; actually it is the opening and closing of the mind-field that leads to the opening and closing of the chi and the body. The mind is concentrated upon the conscious thought itself and upon the sensations of the body. With the opening of the hands, the whole body and mind also open into the vastness of the blue sky, the Milky Way, and the depths of the cosmic void-nature; when closing, all these return deep within oneself - bringing the purest universal Hunyuan chi back into the place where it is most needed in order to restore normalcy.

Some skilled practitioners perform their opening and closing practice in their minds throughout the whole day. It is essential, not only for the sick but also for the healthy, to be more aware of chi and to enhance the ability to make use of it.

E. STRETCHING-CHI METHOD (*CHEN-QI FA*)

1. Introduction

The Stretching-Chi Method is one of the Eight Methods of Chi-Cultivation, which are taught after the Five One Form (*Wu Yuan Zhuang*). However, the Stretching-Chi Method itself is taught everywhere and to everyone in China, because it is a very effective way to stimulate and mobilize the internal physical chi and to unify the chi within the entire body as a whole. It is also a shortcut to the developing of superintelligence.

2. Explanation

The Preparatory Posture is the same as that of the Lift Chi Up and Pour Chi Down Method (Figure 127). Following this, raise the arms sideways, forming a downward angle of approximately 45 degrees from the level line of the shoulders (Figure 128). Point the hands up with the roots of the hands forming right angles with the wrists and forearms, the fingers flexing back towards the arm as much as possible, the palms pushed out with the arms staying straight (Figure 129). Leading with the shoulders (in an inward-upward movement of the shoulder blades), the arms and hands move diagonally up (with the consequent relaxing of the palms, Figure 130) and then down (in an outward-downward movement, with the pressing down and out of the centers of the palms and the places between the roots of the fingers, Figure 131). Repeat the up-down movements for a considerable length of time

Make sure that the hands form a right angle with the forearms and that the fingers flex backward to their limit. The arms should be straight at all times, in this way, the in-and-out flow of chi through the hands can be increased, and the sensation of flowing chi becomes stronger. This sensation of the flowing of the internal physical chi may move from the fingers up along the arms, to the shoulders and to the head as, one by one, channels and vital points are cleared and opened.

Follow the postural requirements in the Preparatory Posture throughout the practice (excluding the moving parts). The minimum time for the practice of this form is approximately 14 minutes, in order to stretch the chi out throughout the entire body; the longer the better. When the practice ends, place the palms upon the navel, nourishing chi as introduced in the Lift Chi Up and Pour Chi Down Method (Figure 132).

In the beginning there will be pain and soreness in the shoulders, neck, palms and fingers. When the chi channels and vital points are cleared and opened, any pain will be gone and a feeling of joy and comfort will be experienced. Once one starts this form, it is necessary to do it every day; otherwise, if one resumes the practice after a period of not practicing, the pain will reappear.

F. METHOD OF ESTABLISHING A CHI FIELD (*ZUCHANG FA*)

1. Introduction

The Method of Establishing a Chi Field for the practice and application of Zhineng Qigong is one of the greatest of Professor Pang's innovations. This method is based upon the Hunyuan Entirety Theory founded by him. The Method of Establishing a Chi Field is applied to group healing, group teaching and scientific experiments, as well as to practical production in both agriculture and industry. Although there are many ways to establish a chi field, the basic principle is identical throughout.

2. Explanation

Because most Western practitioners practice alone, a simple method of establishing a chi field for oneself is introduced here.

a. Adjust each part of the body to conform to the requirements of chigong practice as introduced in the Preparatory Posture of the Lift Chi Up and Pour Chi Down Method. Consciously relax the entire body, from crown to toe.

b. One may either use Professor Pang's Eight Key Phrases to adjust the mind, or one may reflect upon the following suggestions in adjusting both the mental and spiritual activities in order to reach a deep chigong state.

c. Think of, or imagine, the vast expanse of outer space deep into the six directions, with oneself extended upward into the blue sky, stepping downward, into and through the earth and into the blue sky upon the opposite side of the planet. The body infinitely expands into the deepest recesses of the Milky Way, to the front and to the back, and to the left and to the right. Endeavor to sense or imagine the finest and most subtle original Hunyuan chi in the cosmic void-realm, blending one's attention with that chi, gathering and accumulating the chi in the depths of the void-essence, and then bringing back as much of it as one can to fill the space around oneself. One now exists at the center of this chi field.

d. Repeat step c. several times, then think of the huge chi field in China, at the Center, while connecting one's own chi field with that field, thinking of Professor Pang and all one's fellow practitioners with respect, and bringing chi back into one's own chi field again. Leading with the crown-point, slightly rock or rotate one's entire body, sensing one's own chi field and the chi field surrounding oneself. Then one is both filled with chi and surrounded by chi. The sensation is not unlike that of swimming in water. One may start one's practice now, in this warm, peaceful, comfortable, and tranquil chigong state.

Remember to close the chi field once one ends one's practice. Give attention to "harvesting" within oneself the chi gathered from the distant chi field as well as that around one's physical body, gathering in or absorbing the chi into the lower Vital Center, or wherever one most needs it, adding positive chi-filled affirmations to oneself - "I am better than I was yesterday, and I will be even better tomorrow!" Deepen your belief in *Hunyuan Ling Tong!* Finally, nourish chi for a few minutes.

Last Word: Of the forms introduced, it is recommended that one practice the Method of Stretching-Chi first (however, if they comprise part of a scheduled practice, several dozen wall squats may be practiced before Stretching-Chi; if the number exceeds one hundred, it is better to practice wall squatting separately). Then practice the Lift Chi Up and Pour Chi Down Method, and finally the Three Centers Merge Standing Form. However, this suggestion is not in any sense an absolute requirement, and one may arrange the forms according to one's own needs.

Due to the technical limitations of photographic illustrations, if there are any perceived differences between the postures illustrated in the following sections and those described in the preceding texts, it is recommended that the student take the literal explanations as the most accurate description of the poses or movements concerned, particularly the latter. (-X.J.)

FINAL INNER REFLECTIONS

"How should a novice begin his or her training in chi? One should relax completely. The aim is to throw every bone and muscle of the body wide open so that the chi may travel unobstructed

. . .A tornado is but the massed movement of air and a tidal wave that of water. As a whiff, nothing is more pliable than air' as a drop, nothing more yielding than water. But as tornadoes and tidal waves, air and water carry everything before them.

. . .Your head is held as if suspended by the scalp from the ceiling of the room. . .This strengthens the spine, the vital inner organs, and the brain itself. Make a habit of concentrating on the chi. This can be done at work or play, walking or riding.

. . .During the exercise, limbs and other body components are moved not so much by localized exertions as by the force of the chi.

. . .Observe a child. Note how he breathes – not hight in the chest but low in the abdomen. See too, how he meets an accident – relaxed and with no apprehension in his mind. You may charge this to ignorance, but, this notwithstanding, the child more often than not emerges from accidents unscathed. Perhaps the experience and intelligence clogging the adult's mind and causing his body to stiffen is really not such an asset after all.

We can truly learn from children. . .progress can be made only if one becomes like a child."

Cheng Man-ch'ing

G. PHOTOGRAPHIC ILLUSTRATIONS

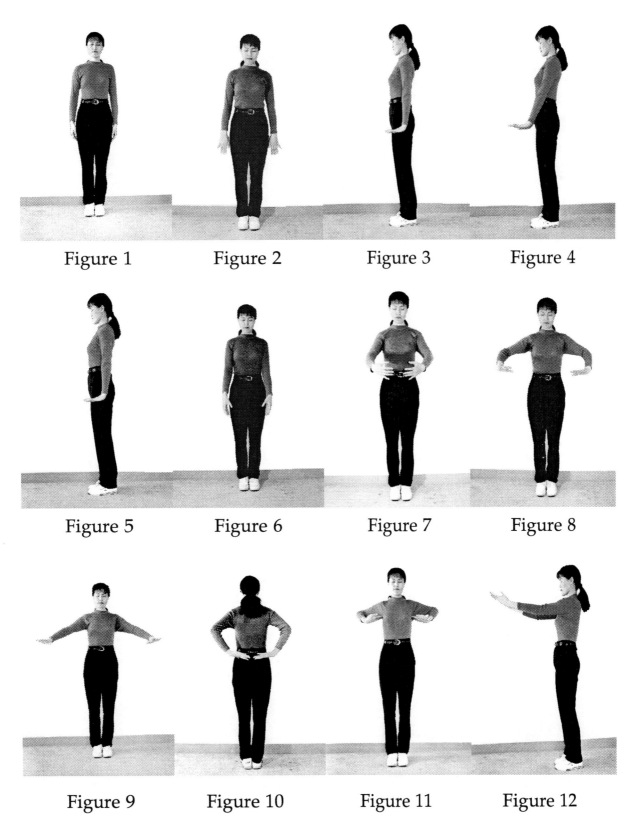

Figure 1   Figure 2   Figure 3   Figure 4

Figure 5   Figure 6   Figure 7   Figure 8

Figure 9   Figure 10   Figure 11   Figure 12

Lift Chi Up Pour Chi Down Method (Figures 13 - 24)

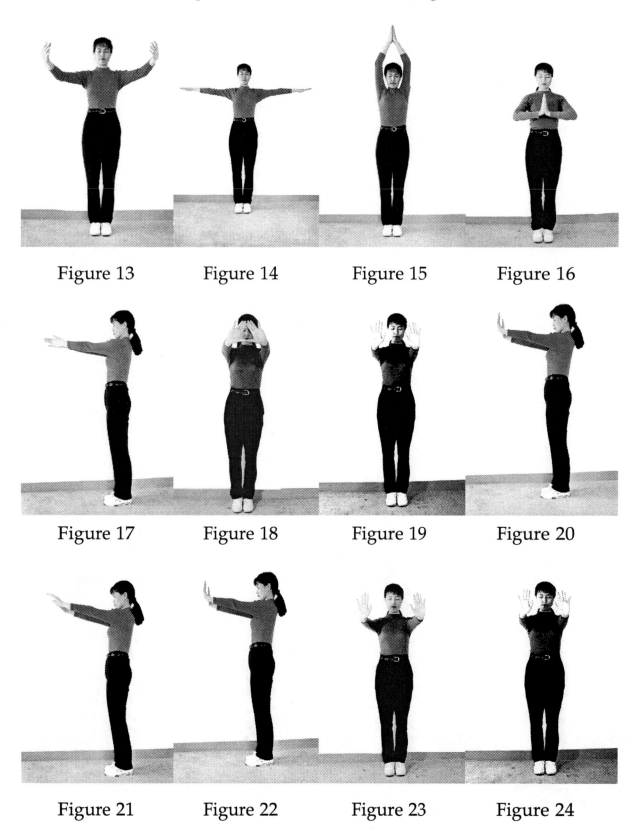

Figure 13　　Figure 14　　Figure 15　　Figure 16

Figure 17　　Figure 18　　Figure 19　　Figure 20

Figure 21　　Figure 22　　Figure 23　　Figure 24

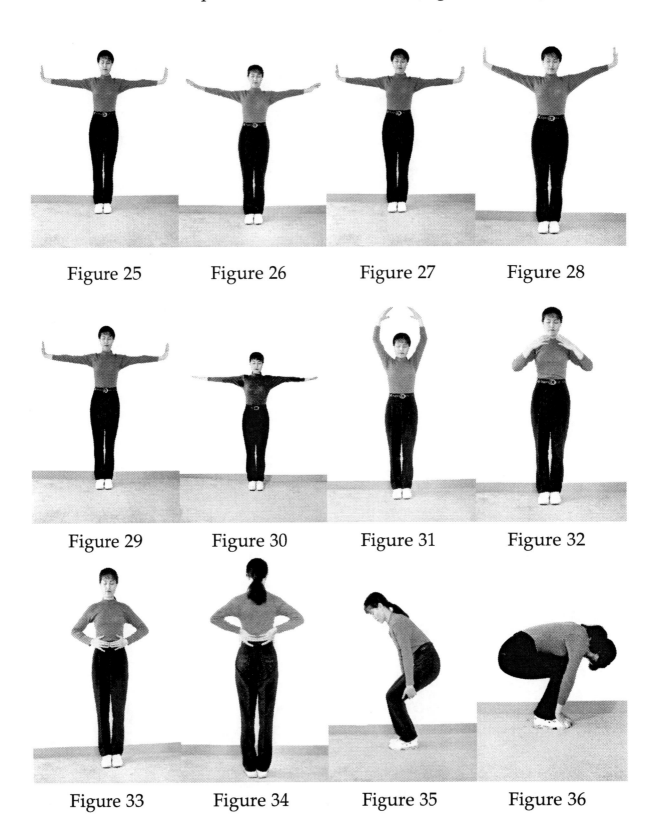

Figure 25   Figure 26   Figure 27   Figure 28

Figure 29   Figure 30   Figure 31   Figure 32

Figure 33   Figure 34   Figure 35   Figure 36

Lift Chi Up Pour Chi Down Method (Figures 37 - 48)

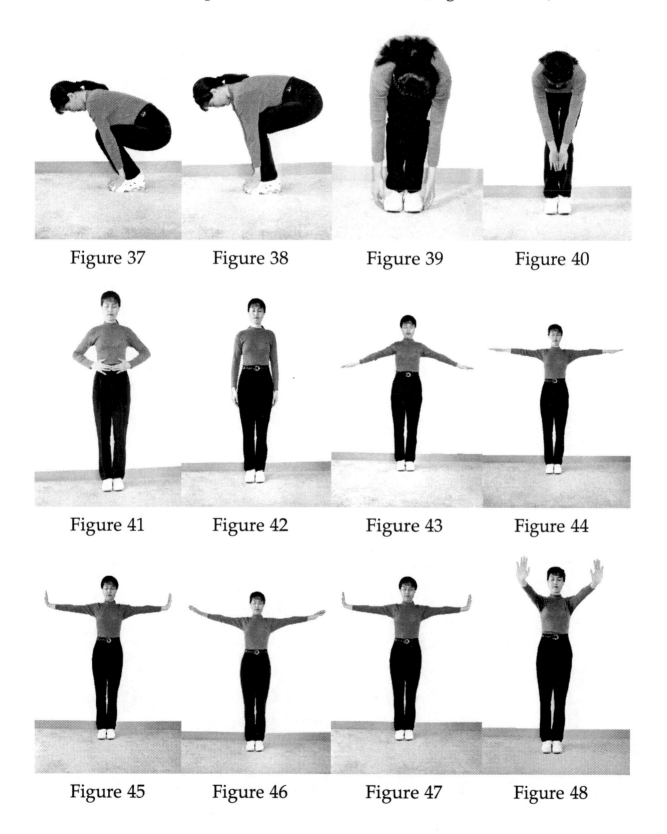

Figure 37   Figure 38   Figure 39   Figure 40

Figure 41   Figure 42   Figure 43   Figure 44

Figure 45   Figure 46   Figure 47   Figure 48

Lift Chi Up Pour Chi Down Method (Figures 49 - 60)

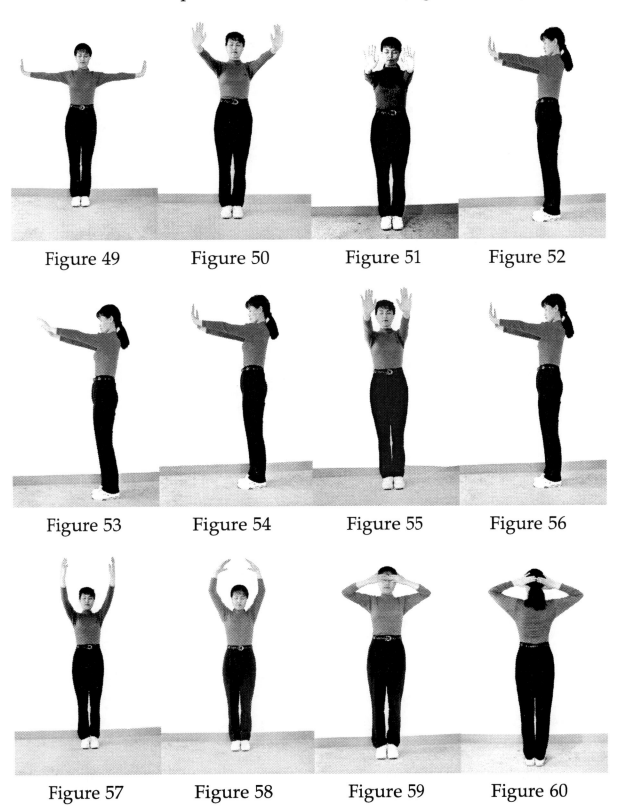

Figure 49

Figure 50

Figure 51

Figure 52

Figure 53

Figure 54

Figure 55

Figure 56

Figure 57

Figure 58

Figure 59

Figure 60

Lift Chi Up Pour Chi Down Method (Figures 61 - 72)

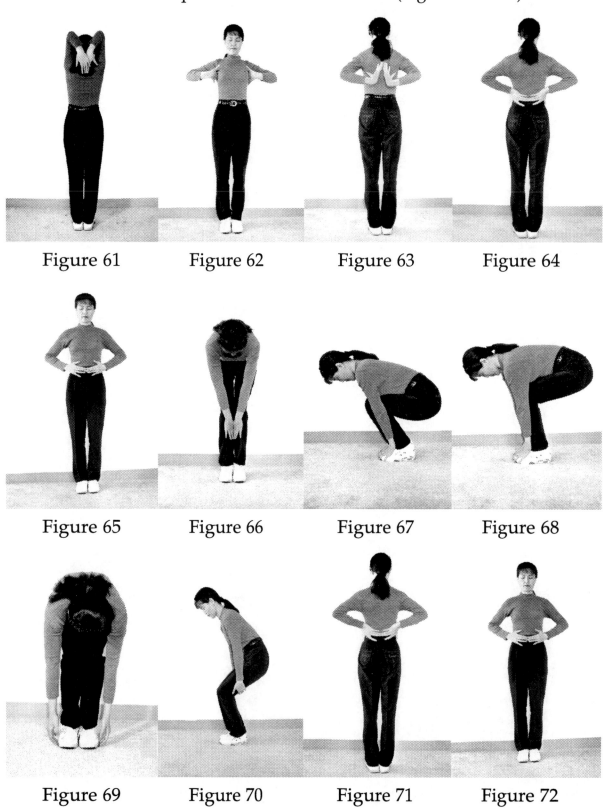

Figure 61　　　Figure 62　　　Figure 63　　　Figure 64

Figure 65　　　Figure 66　　　Figure 67　　　Figure 68

Figure 69　　　Figure 70　　　Figure 71　　　Figure 72

Lift Chi Up Pour Chi Down Method (Figures 73- 84)

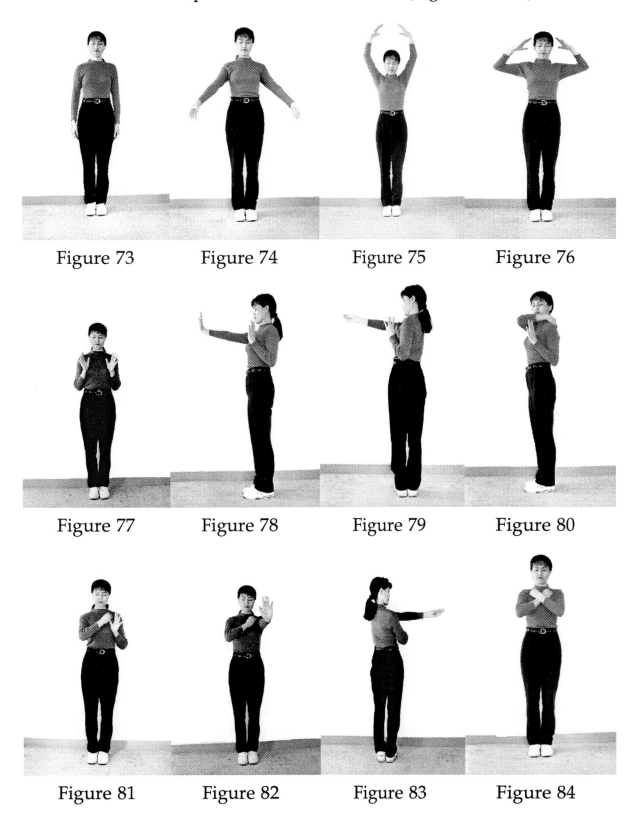

Figure 73

Figure 74

Figure 75

Figure 76

Figure 77

Figure 78

Figure 79

Figure 80

Figure 81

Figure 82

Figure 83

Figure 84

Lift Chi Up Pour Chi Down Method (Figures 85 - 96)

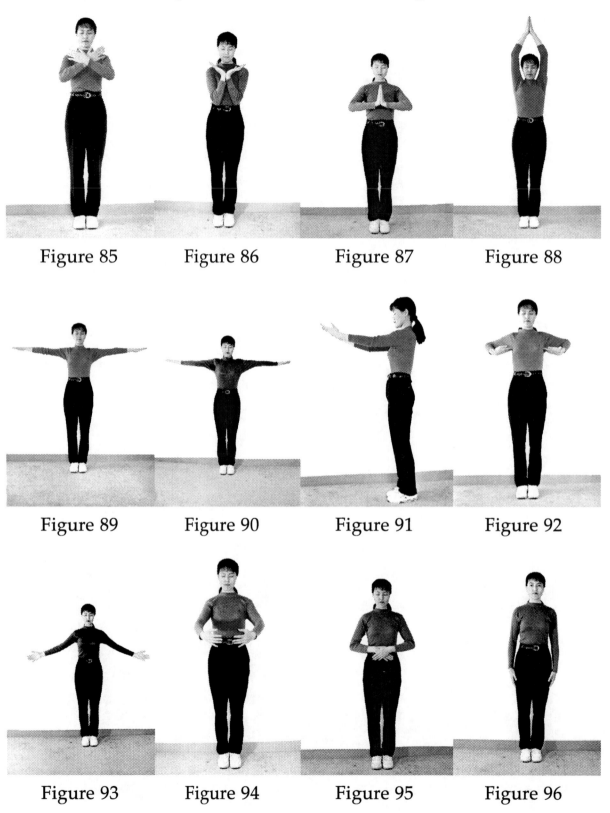

Figure 85   Figure 86   Figure 87   Figure 88

Figure 89   Figure 90   Figure 91   Figure 92

Figure 93   Figure 94   Figure 95   Figure 96

Three Centers Merge Standing Form (Figures 97 - 108)

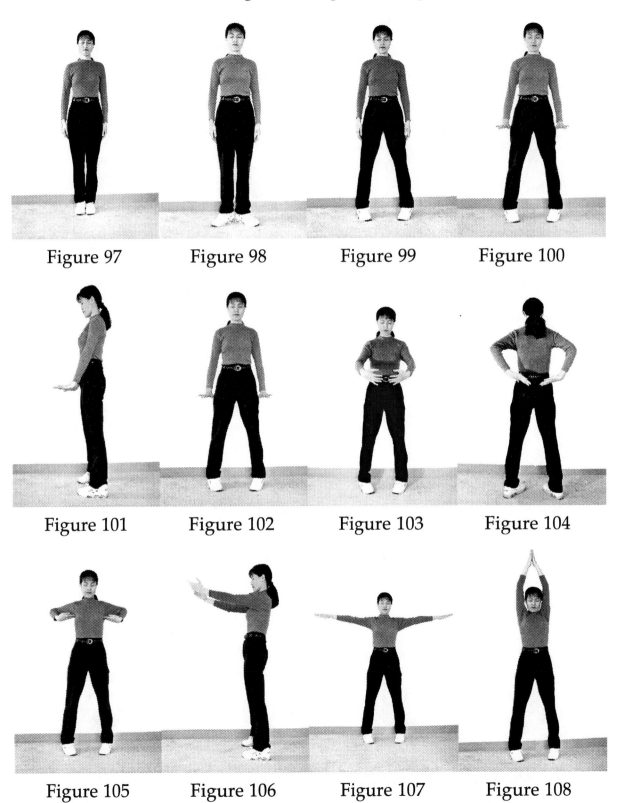

Figure 97   Figure 98   Figure 99   Figure 100

Figure 101   Figure 102   Figure 103   Figure 104

Figure 105   Figure 106   Figure 107   Figure 108

Three Centers Merge Standing Form (Figures 109 - 118)
Wall Squatting (Figures 119-120)

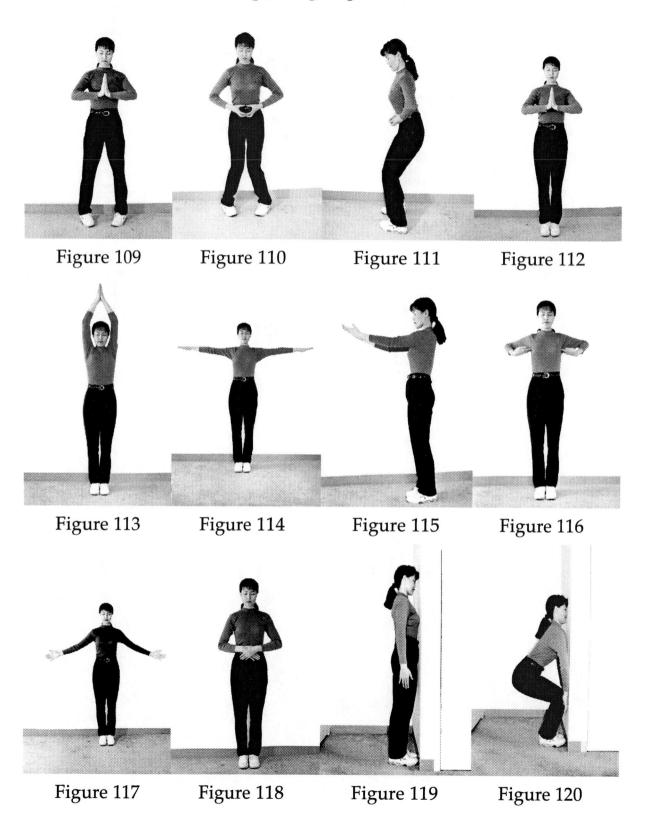

Figure 109   Figure 110   Figure 111   Figure 112

Figure 113   Figure 114   Figure 115   Figure 116

Figure 117   Figure 118   Figure 119   Figure 120

Wall Squatting (Figures 121 - 123), Pulling Chi Therapy (Figures 124 -126)
Stretching Chi Method (Figures 127 - 132)

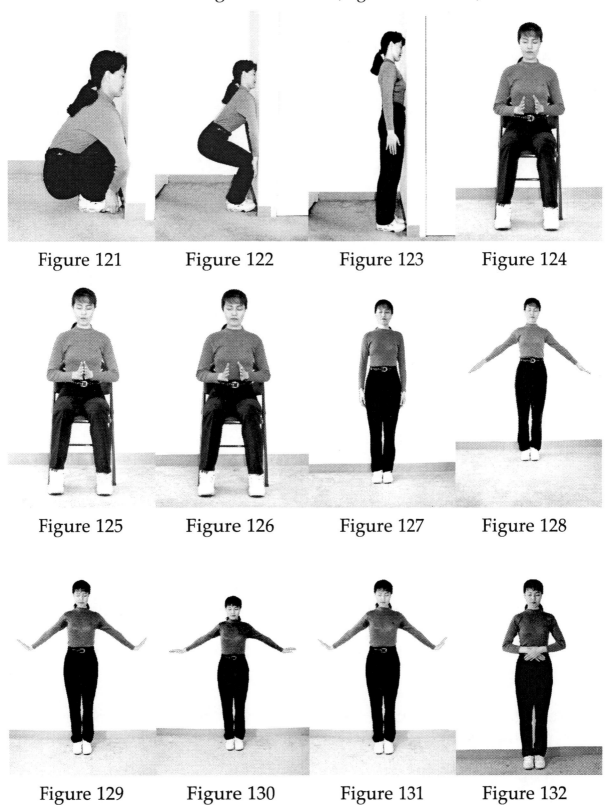

| Figure 121 | Figure 122 | Figure 123 | Figure 124 |

| Figure 125 | Figure 126 | Figure 127 | Figure 128 |

| Figure 129 | Figure 130 | Figure 131 | Figure 132 |

H. THE ART OF TRUE PRACTICE

Note: While not drawn directly from the writings of Ming Pang, this section embodies forms and extensions of his teachings emerging from the personal understanding, experience, thoughts, and insights of the authors. (-J. M. and X. J.)

1. Reflections Before Practice

* Zhineng Qigong practice may be considered a primary form of self-respect, or going further, of self-love - in the best sense of the term - an ongoing, committed and caring process by which and through which one orders, balances and enhances the substance of his or her existence - the chi, or life-energy, and by extension, impacts the greater world of mankind and society. It is helpful to gently remind oneself of this in those inevitable moments when one's practice has, unawares, fallen into the nature of a neutral routine.

* In one of his speeches, Professor Pang has shared five key principles with Zhineng Qigong practitioners:

    1) Purity of purpose - to be sincere, honest, open-minded, fully embracing Zhineng Qigong – the cultivation of energy-intelligence.
    2) Strong faith - to believe, trust, and have great confidence in Zhineng Qigong.
    3) True commitment - to practice deeply no matter what one may experience; to be fearless in hardship, pain, discomfort or fatigue.
    4) Wholeheartedness - devotion to, concentration upon, and absorption in Zhineng Qigong, without external distractions or the dangers of other chigong practice involvements.
    5) When imbued with the above-mentioned essential virtues, Zhineng Qigong works very surely!

* Reflect on the intriguing and consoling fact that, simultaneous with one's own seemingly solitary efforts, there exists a population of more than ten million men, women and children - young, mature and elderly, sick, in transition and well - who are performing Zhineng

Qigong faithfully, silently, stoically and uncomplainingly, in China and throughout the world. Take courage from this thought and, going within, connect from the heart with the truly awesome body of humankind who are walking the path that you now walk - some haltingly, some stumbling, some dragging themselves, some running.

* Contemplate the implications of the China Sports Bureau survey and evaluation of the major publicly taught qigong methods in China, which recognized Zhineng Qigong as the most effective qigong method for health and wellness, and that the government now promotes the value of Zhineng Qigong to its citizens to increase their well-being and for the reduction of their health care costs.

* Absorb the impact of the impressive statistics that, over the years, the Center in China has treated more than 200,000 patients with more than 450 disease conditions, and has achieved an overall healing effectiveness rate of 95 per cent, and realize that, as a consistent practitioner, these parameters of success include you as well.

* Agree that, rather than a perfunctory mechanical performance of prescribed movements, your practice can be a creative and ever-deepening exploration into dimensions yet to be revealed, carrying you beyond the narrow limits of the predictable human life-patterns; thus, approach your practice with care, humility and a certain natural reverence - as one would an ancient Redwood or a magnificent sunset. This will insure that it retains a quality of specialness and purity.

* Remember that the quality of the movements, and of your consciousness, is crucial to transformation. Mindless repetition and mechanical run-throughs can never replace sensitive practice and deepening awareness.

* Endlessly endeavor to refine your movements. While they may already be soft and smooth without, realize that, ultimately, one must be soft and smooth within one's own self, within each nerve and fiber, each cell and sinew.

* Always seek the dynamic over the static; when one's awareness unknowingly fixes itself into crystallized structures, such as habitual

tensions, repetitive thoughts or routine postures or positions, thaw the consciousness into movement again and allow the body to resume its subtle flow through space, for it is at these times, and not the static, fixed moments, that the true processes of transformation of matter and energy are enabled to occur.

* Realize that, at its best, Zhineng Qigong is a palpable way of - in a phrase - 'making love' with the universe, a tangible means of extending oneself into the Cosmos and of inviting the Cosmos within one's very self, in an ever-deepening rhythm.

* Reflect upon the truth that, to whatever extent you are effective in your practice - your 'rendezvous with infinity' - you are creating - or re-creating - a better, deeper, richer self with which to impact all whom you encounter, and with whom you live and work, throughout the rest of your life activities beyond the practice of Zhineng Qigong.

* Reorder your life priorities so that there is time available to consistently undertake your practice, no matter what. This may mean relegating the television to weekends, rising earlier, or saying no to habitual diversions, temptations and indulgences.

* Whenever possible, seek for and practice in the company of like-minded others, be they friends, family or simply companions on the path. When this is not possible bear vividly in your mind and heart the vision and feeling of your participation in and belonging to an extended community of fellow seekers throughout the world.

* Frequently read the stories of the healing journeys of others, as published in Luke Chan's *101 Miracles of Healing*, the *Chi-Lel™ Qigong News* quarterly, and, if literate in Chinese, in the publications available by the China Center, realizing that what one has done, all can do. Likewise, study and reflect upon the deeply seminal words of Professor Pang, who has not written a work of abstract theory, but rather one of dynamic principle. Continuously deepen your understanding of Zhineng Qigong through repeated immersion in the teachings shared in this book, and seek to view the diverse levels of life through the consciousness which those writings inspire.

* Look upon the healing phenomena of history and of other cultures in the light of chigong, seeking to perceive the essential principles and parallel modes of operation involved - whether these be from other chigong practices, Western energy-healing traditions, or, for that matter, traditional religious sources.

* In time, personalize your Zhineng Qigong practice, creating a regimen which is tailored to your particular nature, needs and inclinations, and which yet respects the integrity of the teachings. For example, one might wish to begin the day with a series of Soft Chi-Gatherings (*la chi*) followed by some quiet minutes of the Three Centers Merge Standing meditation, or perhaps conversely, end the day this way. One inclined to vigorous early morning activity might be inspired to perform a substantial series of wall squats after arising and before breakfast, choosing to perform Lift Chi Up and Pour Chi Down in the evening.

2. Sensitizing the Body and Mind for Transformation

While mechanical in their expression, the instructions for practice actually describe an exceedingly elegant and poetic process involving nothing less than the dissolution of self-limiting boundaries, both physical and psychospiritual. These are comprised of long-held behavioral patterns generated by personal, cultural and archetypal conditionings undergirding the functional grid of human life-energy. Once these are released - and this may take some time - there follows the beginning of the dilation of one's individualized being into the dimensionless matrix of the void-essence, which turns out not to be void at all, but rather formless, unconditioned energy-intelligence.

It is of crucial importance that one always bear this in mind, lest one be distracted and ultimately derailed by a myriad of formal directives and details: the essence of practice is one of self-softening, opening, expansion, merging and harmonizing, receiving, gathering, and consolidation, proceeding in a ceaseless cyclic rhythm.

Thus, once the movements are properly learned and capable of being accurately executed, one should take the opportunity of proceeding to the next level of subtlety. If the movements are now proper in form and sequence, begin to bring the awareness to bear upon their softness, smoothness and openness. If these are all present, proceed further to sense the extension of this softness, smoothness and openness into the atmospheric depth of the greater field of chi beyond the body. If this is achieved, one may then begin to develop a sensitivity towards cultivating the omni-directional expansion and contraction of self-boundaries simultaneously upward, downward, forward, backward and bilaterally, or more accurately, spherically.

In the course of alternately expanding one's attention beyond - and then contracting or condensing it within - the physical body, it is important to do so without the focus of the attention becoming either totally possessed by or exclusionary of either the body or the cosmos; instead, one's awareness should maintain, as it were, a dual hold on these two polarities - fully condensed form and totally expanded formlessness. True, as awareness flows between them, it will be more filled with first one and then the other of these two focal points, but, if properly done, there will still be an intuitive background awareness of the dynamic dual polarity.

The more one feels oneself to exist as a being of solidity and substance, the less will one be able to feel chi. The lighter and emptier one renders the sense of oneself in practice, the fuller and more obvious will be one's experience of atmospheric chi. These two perceptions exist in an almost direct inverse proportion to each other. As one's movements become smoother, softer and lighter, to a greater or lesser extent one's sense of physicality will gradually diminish and dissolve, until there comes a shift in the perceptual differential between self and environment, due to the increasing sensitivity of one's energy field. At this crucial point, that which has always been assumed to be empty - three-dimensional space - is experienced as full, and that which has long been thought to be static - the inner body and the outer world - is now perceived as dynamic and flowing.

Here the journey into Zhineng Qigong - the cultivation of energy-intelligence - only begins.

At this stage, one has moved beyond the mere mechanical performance of a required regimen of physical movements and postures, reinforced and held in place by willpower, faith and commitment; and one has passed into the realm of true exploration and empirical research. One is no longer practicing merely to 'get through' the various practices, or to log them onto an ever growing list of achievements – or 'gongs'.

Instead, one is practicing as part of living itself, immersing oneself completely in the stream of chigong without hurry or inertia, and with no rigid time constraints. In this way one can practice in such a manner as to insure the acquisition of true stillness and softness, while inviting spontaneous discovery which does not appear through force or manipulation. In so doing one may retain the qualities of mystery and innocence which will enhance one's desire to daily penetrate further into the depths of practice.

Without these, any practice - even one designed to benefit humankind - soon becomes jaded and lifeless, and ends up by being dogmatic and harsh. Above all, one should seek to preserve the sense of poetry and humanity which rightfully belong to all truly worthwhile endeavors, those given to healing most of all.

If you find yourself inadvertently caught up in a strenuously effortful practice which gives birth to a subtle, if unadmitted, sense of resistance or even loathing, it is safe to conclude that you have undertaken your practice in the wrong spirit and need to reframe your approach. These misguided efforts may easily weary the body and exhaust the spirit, undermining everything that one may have been striving for.

The wrong kind of effort comes from the subconscious belief in separateness and isolation. In such an instance, the practitioner deeply feels herself to exist apart and against her frame of reference - her world. This approach emerges from and reinforces the quality of hardness and tends to further isolate one, until all of one's actions take on the quality of struggle, strain and resistance.

The right kind of effort is, in a very real sense, effortless; it springs from an intuitive conviction of the interconnectedness of all things and the unity of life. In this case, the practitioner senses herself to be part of an underlying continuum which supports and nurtures her, and her efforts will have the qualities of softness, surrender and acceptance.

3. Carriage, Posture and Tone

The fulfillment of the human form emerges only when and if the practitioner comes to experience her own body as an extension and a completion of the body of the universe, and not merely an isolated fragment. One who has rediscovered her natural heritage as a child of the cosmos no longer roams the world as a disconnected entity confronting an alien landscape. Instead she enjoys a living unity with heaven and earth - as well as the realm of humanity - which supports and nurtures her.

On the physical level, this manifests as a spontaneously balanced and upright posture deeply rooted in the earth, but lifting freely towards heaven, almost as if one were the connecting rod between the two. The horizontal body axis is likewise expansive, suggesting an open embrace of the whole of life, from horizon to horizon, without rigidity or affectedness.

The properly rooted human being draws upon the stabilizing power of the earth while simultaneously lifting into the limitlessness of heaven, like a freely soaring kite launching upwards from its home tether. It is, in fact, this rooting itself which endows man with the stability and courage to explore the infinite depths beyond his earthly moorings.

Thus, in Zhineng Qigong, one's physical attitude should be founded upon a relaxed, yet profound rootedness in the earth and its gravitational field. To the extent that one is able to relax, one will feel its strength and consolidating power, and to the extent one attempts to exercise purely personal or ego-centered control and effort, one will be deprived of any transpersonal or deeper sense of support and empowerment, and will experience life as if one were existing purely by one's own efforts and struggle.

Although one may be firmly rooted and balanced in the earth-field, this in no way implies a sunken or hunched posture, enfolded upon itself in a false imitation of humility, and manifesting a denial of the upward-lifting dynamic which is the natural counterpart of the centripetal force bonding one with the earth. Rather, one who is truly rooted in the earth will tend to more fully give expression to the complementary counter force thrusting heavenward and expanding outward as the selfsame centripetal earth force flows through its centrifugal (or earth-transcending) phase.

In the illusion of fostering 'softness and relaxation', many various traditional chi practices - such as Tai Chi and chigong disciplines - have fallen into the regrettable extreme of stressing only the downward flow of force, thereby distorting both the physical form and attitude into a sunken-chested, bottom-heavy parody of nature's original design for mankind.

As ever, trees reveal the ideal dynamic balance to be emulated: profoundly rooted in the earth, yet flexibly expanding outward and upward toward the light of the heavens. The lower body represents the trunk, the upper body the branches and leaves. One should feel one's entire lower extremities, including hips, pelvis and abdomen to be powerful extensions plunging into and emerging out of the depths of the earth.

The spinal column is fully extended as if being lifted from within and above, so that there is the natural elongation of the neck in conjunction with a forward-upward thrusting of the posterior crown, with a consequent lowering of the chin. As the upper body blossoms upward, the base of the spinal column releases itself downward, creating a powerful thrust through the legs and soles of the feet, penetrating into the earth.

The shoulders release themselves downward and outward, easing their grip on the chest and the upper body, which then assume their appropriate openness. In natural succession there follows the release of the arms, hands, fingers and palms, through which energy will be felt to flow.

A special sensitivity of the palms and fingers should be cultivated, whereby one gradually comes to sense what has previously believed to be only 'empty space' as full. By constantly seeking to empty oneself and one's limbs - particularly the palms - of tension and fixity, a transparency of form begins to be experienced which enables one to palpably sense the ambient surrounding atmosphere and its various inherent conditions, such as pressure, warmth, density and flow.

Little by little, one will develop this sensitivity to the point where one experiences all space and atmospheres in a fashion very similar to the way a swimmer experiences water - as environments full of substance of varying densities, currents of flowing force, and fluctuating polarities.

Further, with the freeing of the thoracic, intercostal and abdominal cavities and their consequent relaxation, the breath will be experienced as spontaneously emerging from the depths of the umbilical diaphragm (the hara), which flexibly expands and contracts, generating only minor referred movement to the areas above; more expansive upper-body movement should only become noticeable in situations of extreme respiratory activity.

One's breathing should be soft, smooth and soundless - almost superfine, always through the nose and without the slightest strain or struggle.

One's state of mind should be alert, yet without tension, and tranquil, but without lethargy, as if one were in a waking dream.

One's inner state should become increasingly fathomless and free, as if, in that moment, one had been born out of eternity - mindless, unblemished and without care, a spirit moving ahead freely on the Great Way.

4. The Unbroken Stream

The continuity of practice

In their private moments, some practitioners and would-be practitioners have wondered if the rather stringent injunctions against missing even a single day's practice are not perhaps just a little extreme in their dogmatism. They have encountered the formidable concept of 'gongs' and further 'gongs', and sensed the perilous implications of ever lapsing in these critical endeavors, lest all be lost. Professor Pang provides further cause for concern in reaffirming in fairly incisive terms the importance of sustained and uninterrupted practice, especially for those who are experiencing positive recovery from serious illness, suggesting the possibility of relapse and retrogression.

Are these admonitions purely doctrinal or gratuitously disciplinarian? Or do they contain some genuine insight?

The momentum and power of a river is in direct proportion to the depth and the width of the riverbed through which it flows, as well as to the period of time over which it has been flowing. This is true of the practice of Zhineng Qigong as well. The parameters of the riverbed itself are shaped, altered and expanded by the coursing of the river through it; with more rain and fuller, more numerous tributaries, the floor of the riverbed will erode and deepen correspondingly and even the very banks will widen to accommodate the increased current,

If, perchance, after a drought, we were in need of restoring such a waterway and we had limited flow, we would have to proceed very carefully, confining our conduit to a fairly narrow framework so that a continuous, unbroken flow of water could be created, however slight. This would insure that at least limited amounts of the life-giving substance was arriving at its destination.

However, if our vigilance lagged and we permitted the source-flow to drop, then there would come a drop in the current, and very possibly a complete break or interruption in the flow, leaving bare, dry ground in various places, interspersed with pools of motionless water. This picture embodies the dynamics involved when we are involved in stimulating and harnessing a flow of chi throughout the bodily pathways during the practice of Zhineng Qigong. While such practice does gather and generate chi, an inconsistent, interrupted or fragmentary practice compromises or completely disrupts the steady and even flow of chi, as well as effectively sabotaging its chances of increasing in amplitude and momentum.

While it is possible to re-establish the flowing current, it will require much time and energy merely to arrive at the same point and level that was initially lost. The full restoration of the flow can not be achieved until all discreet, interrupted pools have been irrigated, augmented and re-united by new externally generated currents of water.

Thus, one's time and energies have, to a greater or lesser extent, been squandered, consumed in the process of re-stimulating and restoring what was lapsed and lost.

This is why it becomes crucial to view the exercise of Zhineng Qigong as a life-practice, an integral part of one's intimate existence, interfacing and impacting all dimensions of one's being: physical, mental, emotional and spiritual. In this way there will be no conflict in trying to somehow integrate a peripheral or appendage-like practice into one's way of living.

5. Opening the Body/Mind-Field

Clearing the paths

While Zhineng Qigong is a complete system addressing all areas and levels of the body and mind, until one comes to learn the second level, which concerns itself with the loosening and clearing of joints, ligaments, tendons and fascia so that chi may flow more fully and freely, it would be valuable for the student to undertake a series of simple breath-coordinated bendings and stretchings prior to practice for this purpose.

These may be drawn from traditional chigong warm-ups, hatha yoga exercises, Aikido workouts, the Five Tibetan Rites of Rejuvenation or modern dance calisthenics, all of which, in their respective ways, work the joints, ligaments, muscles and spinal vertebrae, loosening, lengthening and toning them, and to some extent stimulating and opening the energy channels within them.

Some of the obvious areas to focus such exercises upon are: the neck, spine, shoulders, wrists and hands, hips, deep abdomen, thighs, knees, ankles and toes.

6. Aids and Precautions for Practice

* Weather-permitting, it is always preferable to practice in as close contact as possible with the energies of nature, barefoot or thinly slippered, lightly clad, as near as possible to mature trees and running water. These will add freshness and vitality to your practice. During practice, direct sunlight should be avoided after 11 a.m. and before 3 p.m., as it can easily sap one's energy and create weariness and fatigue; so likewise should one avoid extreme cold, heat, chill winds and dampness, especially where active perspiration is experienced as a result of practice.

* It is of great value to take one half to one glass of tepid or slightly cool spring water - the fresher the better - before and after practice, to hydrate and lubricate the entire system, and to offset any internal metabolic and energetic activities, which consume a great deal of moisture.

* It is advisable to allow from thirty minutes to one hour to elapse after eating before undertaking the practice of Zhineng Qigong, as a great deal of one's circulation and energy are involved with the processes of digestion and assimilation of nutrients.

* It is to one's advantage to undertake one's practice following evacuation of the bowels.

* Following practice one should avoid immersion in or exposure to cold water for at least one hour, taking care to maintain a moderate temperature if one does choose to bathe or shower.

7. Designing a Practice

If one is undertaking extended practice and experiences fatigue, it is perfectly all right to take periodic respites and then resume one's practice.

If one wishes to perform greatly extended periods of practice, it would be wise to create an interesting and varied sequence of practices; this provides contrast and refreshment. Such a sequence, lasting one, one and a half, and two hours, respectively, might be:

One-Hour plan (A):
1) Lift Chi Up and Pour Chi Down Method - 30 minutes
2) Three Centers Merge Standing Form - 15 minutes
3) Gathering Chi - 15 minutes

One-Hour plan (B):
1) Lift Chi Up and Pour Chi Down Method - 30 minutes
2) Three Centers Merge Standing Form - 30 minutes

One and a Half Hour Plan (A):
1) Lift Chi Up and Pour Chi Down Method - 45 minutes
2) Three Centers Merge Standing Form - 30 minutes
3) Gathering Chi - 15 minutes

One and a Half Hour Plan (B):
1) Wall Squatting - 15 minutes
2) Lift Chi Up and Pour Chi Down Method - 45 minutes
3) Three Centers Merge Standing Form - 30 minutes

One and a Half Hours Plan (C):
1) Stretching Chi - 15 minutes
2) Lift Chi Up and Pour Chi Down Method - 45 minutes
3) Three Centers Merge Standing Form - 30 minutes

Two-Hour Plan (A):
1) Wall Squatting - 15 minutes
2) Forward Push-Pulls - 15 minutes
3) Lift Chi Up and Pour Chi Down Method - 45 minutes
4) Three Centers Merge Standing Form - 30 minutes
5) Gathering Chi - 15 minutes

Two-Hour Plan (B):
1) Wall Squatting - 15 minutes
2) Stretching Chi - 15 minutes
3) Lift Chi Up and Pour Chi Down Method - 45 minutes
4) Three Centers Merge Standing Form - 30 minutes
5) Gathering Chi - 15 minutes

Note: Wall Squatting and Stretching Chi perform the function of warming-up the system, by initially mobilizing and stimulating physical chi. The practice of The Lift Chi Up and Pour Chi Down Method promotes the absorption and flow of the chi within the membranes and collateral chi channels. The practice of the Three Centers Merge Standing Form further merges the chi from the three centers within the Vital Center. Finally, chi is gathered to fill the whole body and to bring about healing and the enhancement of health.

8. Breathing in Harmony

While Professor Pang explained various breathing techniques in another book - *Essences of Zhineng Qigong Science*, which we included little of in this edition, to the seasoned practitioner, it soon becomes obvious that there is a natural, almost inevitable movement and rhythm of one's respiration which enhances one's practice of Zhineng Qigong. Frequently, it is the case that the outgoing chi will travel upon an exhalation, and the incoming chi upon an inhalation - but not always. In some instances, the sense of internal energetic opening and closing will override this, dictating the appropriate breathing which best accords with the parallel movements made by the body at the moment.

In all instances, however, the ideal remains to maintain a soft, silent, long, deep, even and superfine breathing, emerging from and returning to the lower belly, which continues gently expanding and contracting circumferentially (omni-directionally), as one proceeds through one's movements.

- The Deeper Dimensions of Wall Squatting

While a seemingly simple – almost mechanical - exercise, the sustained and sensitive exploration of wall squatting will begin to manifest a power out of all proportion to its perceived simplicity; the deepening practice of this ancient temple-secret will bring the student through levels of chi development which might otherwise have long remained inaccessible.

Due to its ability to consolidate both the physical form and the forces within that form into a powerfully unified totality, wall squatting places a major impetus upon the heaven and earth energy gates – particularly the crown and the soles of the feet. This practice produces a highly concentrated stimulation upon and delivers a potent cyclic charge to the chi receptor sites at the base and summit of the spinal column, the soles of the feet, and ultimately, the whole body. When done correctly the practice of wall squatting also opens and clears the ascending energy channels throughout the complete length of the spinal column, as well as the descending channels along the front of the body, culminating in a heightening of chi flow throughout the microcosmic orbit, as well as a concentration and condensation of chi within the lower Vital Center.

As in the other practice forms, the optimal benefits of wall squatting will increasingly manifest themselves as the consciousness of the practitioner succeeds in alternately extending and expanding itself from the surface to both the depths of the body and progressively throughout the regional and remote dimensions of the cosmos.

Its very simplicity enables the one to achieve a deep concentration of spirit relatively quickly, and to sustain and extend this singlemindedness over a considerable span of time. Highly committed practitioners may find themselves sensing that they are in possession of a benign and immensely powerful weapon with which they may ultimately penetrate and dissolve the barriers of chronic, acute or even normally terminal conditions – provided they possess the power of will that emerges from boundless faith.

268

BOOK IV

LIVING WITH LIFE-ENERGY

RESOURCES

COMPILED BY
JOSEPH MARCELLO

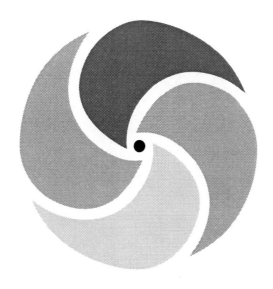

LIFE-ENERGY ENHANCEMENTS –

THE CHIGONG LIFESTYLE

Complementary Practices

Until and unless one commences the study of the Body and Mind Form - Level Two of Zhineng Qigong, it would be helpful and advisable to undertake a regimen of exercises which open and loosen the joints, vertebrae, ligaments and tendons, in order to maximize the flow of the chi created by the practice of Level One, Lift Chi Up and Pour Chi Down. Several excellent choices are given below.

Tai Chi Chuan (*Tai Ji Quan* - Supreme Ultimate Fist)

Originally developed as a martial art, with its founding credited to the famed Taoist adept Chang San-feng (1279-1368), Tai Chi bears some striking similarities to Zhineng Qigong in both its movements and its inner qualities. Handed down from teacher to student in great secrecy, it remained a zealously guarded private practice discipline throughout the following centuries. Employing long forms of sequential elliptical movements of a subtle and flowing nature, the main intent of Tai Chi practice was the distribution of chi for purposes of enhancing one's ability to deal with external physical challenges, as opposed to self-healing per se. Even so, the successful practitioner would likely experience certain inner benefits as a result of such heightened chi flow.

Employing deep diaphragmatic breathing, with the center of gravity maintained in the lower abdomen, the Tai Chi adept practices the deflection or delivery of blows through the redirection of chi in a fluid and dynamically responsive manner. Through deep, focused relaxation in movement, the chi is invited, gathered, concentrated and mobilized as needed.

These obvious differences in intent lead the energy to work in distinct ways within and around the body, with the chi field phenomenon most greatly in evidence during the practice of Zhineng Qigong, where no mutually antagonistic (even if spiritually harmonious) relationship exists within one's practice partners. Yet these two highly affinitized practices mutually enhance each other and pose no essential conflict of interest, as both are based upon the same principle: chi follows mind, body follows chi.

Tai Chi falls under the umbrella of subsidiary chigong practices, and is among the many disciplines which were practiced and explored by Professor Pang, and from whose essence the practice of Zhineng Qigong was distilled.

Further reading:

Chia, Mantak Chia, *The Inner Structure of Tai Chi - Tai Chi Kung I*, Healing Tao, Huntington, NY, 1998.

Dang,Tri Thong, *Beginning T'ai Chi*, Charles E. Tuttle, Rutland, VT, 1994.

Man-ch'ing, Cheng, and Robert Smith, *T'ai-Chi* ,Charles E. Tuttle, Rutland, VT, 1976.

Hatha Yoga - Harmonizing the Human Forces

Hatha yoga provides another such choice, rendering the body, particularly the spinal column and deep connective tissues, firm and flexible. In addition, it places great emphasis on postures and exercises which insure the integrity of the vital internal organs, including the heart, the lungs and the brain, the efficiency of the abdomino-thoracic structure, and the endocrine glands, with the purpose of rendering the physical body as perfect a vehicle as possible for the pursuit of spiritual awakening.

The original meaning of hatha yoga is the yoga of force, for the physical and vital control of the body by physiological means for purposes of higher concentration. Later on, the word hatha came also to symbolize the two biomotor processes of the body, the energy-consuming and the energy-acquitting, which are called respectively the sun (ha) and the moon (tha).

The hatha yoga techniques are collectively knows as *nadi suddhi* processes, that is, processes for purifying the nerves and vitalizing the body. There are four broad divisions of techniques: 1) postures (*asana* and *mudra*), 2) breath - or more accurately - life-force control (*pranayama*), 3) dynamic contraction exercises (*charana*), 4) cleansing, special control and locking exercises (*shatkarma, bandha* and *mudra*).

Many excellent texts exist delineating these techniques. As with any other practice, optimal results are obtained when the disciplines are undertaken in a spirit of gentle exploration, with singleminedness and persistence, and without rigidity or unnecessary force.

Further reading:

Iyengar, B. K. S., *Light on Yoga*, Schocken Books, NY, 1974.

van Lysebeth, Andre, *Yoga Self-Taught*, Harper & Row, Pub., NY, 1971.

Vishnudevananda, Swami, *The Complete Illustrated Book of Yoga*, The Julian Press, Inc., NY, 1964.

The Eight Pieces of Brocade (Pa Tuan Chin - *Ba Duan Jin*)

Emerging from twelfth-century China, this series of chigong exercises was said to have evolved from Yueh Fei, a military leader, for the specific purposes of strengthening the various parts of the body, eliminating disease, and enhancing immunity and vitality. It is one of the most widely practiced sets of exercises throughout China, being practiced either in isolated sets or complete sequence.

Each exercise targets a specific area, organ system or energy network, and while comprising part of the set, may be performed on its own or in conjunction with others as desired.

Further reading:
Cohen, Kenneth S., *The Way of Qigong*, Ballantine Books, NY, 1997.
Reid, Daniel P., *The Tao of Health, Sex & Longevity*, Simon & Schuster, 1989.

The Five Tibetan Rites of Rejuvenation

A superb series of rejuvenatory total body and spinal exercises, the Five Tibetan Rites of Rejuvenation, sometimes known as the Five Tibetans or the Five Rites of Rejuvenation, provide a profound re-structuring and overhauling of the entire musculo-skeletal framework, with deep beneficial effects on the nervous, respiratory and circulatory systems, the endocrine glands and the brain.

Originally couched in highly dramatic, mysterious and - to some - even inspiring narrative extolling its youth-restoring powers, the practice of the Five Rites may be profitably practiced on its own merits, quite apart from the mythology - or history - surrounding it. It represents a highly concentrated, palpably energizing regimen which may be easily learned by almost anyone and performed, according to desire, in anywhere from 10 to 20 minutes.

The practice of the Five Tibetan Rites is to be highly recommended, both for its simplicity, comprehensiveness and its immediate rewards.

Further reading:
Kelder, Peter, *The Ancient Secret of the Fountain of Youth*, Doubleday, NY, 1998.

Lynn, Harry R. et al, *The Ancient Secret of the Fountain of Youth, Book II,* Harbor Press, Gig Harbor, WA, 1999.

Kilham, Christopher S., *The Five Tibetans,* Healing Arts Press, Rochester, VT, 1994.

Swimming - Experiencing the Ultimate Flow

One of the profoundest means of enhancing overall health, swimming in fresh - and particularly salt - water is second to none in purifying, strengthening and energizing the energy field. The total polymorphous stimulation of the water, rich in the broken-bonded negative ions which thrive wherever water breaks over itself, such as seashores, running brooks and streams, and heavily rained upon areas, provides maximum cleansing effect to the human system, mobilizing total lymphatic circulation, intense peripheral blood flow, and spontaneous, sustained deep breathing. Both physiological and energetic stagnation are completely dissolved, with resultant penetration of chi into the deepest recesses and the furthermost extremities of the body, particularly as the alternating currents of air, wind and water rhythmically play over the body.

A British study has established that of all the exercises, swimming distributes the blood most evenly throughout the entire body. Due to the equilateral support of the body in the water through submergence and flotation, all unbalanced stresses - such as those imposed by gravity - are removed, and joints and vertebrae are relieved of any disproportionate burden of weight. With the greater part of the bio-energy devoted to dynamic movement rather than anti-gravitational effort, the liabilities of jogging, tennis and other earth-bound aerobic endeavors are removed.

Employing simultaneous, sequential and symmetrical motions such as stretching, stroking, flexing, kicking, turning and gliding, the body experiences a freedom of movement unparalleled by any comparable land activity with the possible exception of rebounding.

In addition, the ocean provides both aqueous and atmospheric trace mineral nourishment, absorbed directly through the skin, as well as the benefits of sunlight, which, if taken before 11 a.m. and after 3 p.m. is highly beneficial and free of the dangers of ultraviolet exposure.

The author, a lifetime long-distance outdoor swimmer, has repeatedly experienced a distinct and profound purification and expansion of the physical, psychic and spiritual life-fields during and following sustained immersion and movement through natural waters. This is followed by a highly enhanced sensation of internal and external magnetic flow and conductivity lasting for some hours, at times, the entire day. This heightened energy-sensitive - or chigong - state is one of the most pleasurable paradoxes that can be imagined, in that it simultaneously imparts an exhilarating sensation of supercharged power while bequeathing an inner state of deepest calm and peace.

Barbara Brennan, well known healer and author of *Hands of Light* and *Light Emerging,* two encyclopedic texts on energy healing, considers ocean environments and ocean swimming among the highest regenerative energy sources for mankind.

Further reading:
Thomas, David G., *Advanced Swimming, Steps to Success*, Human
  Kinetics, 1990.
Counsilman, James E., *Complete Book of Swimming*, Macmillan, 1979.
Counsilman, James E. and Brian E., *The New Science of Swimming*,
  Prentice Hall College Div., 1994.

The Alexander Technique

A graceful and effortless means of enhancing one's conscious awareness of physical and psychophysical poise and balance, the Alexander Technique is a highly subtle, deeply elegant practicum which stands in contradistinction to almost all prior and present approaches to implementing the integrity of the human body. The catalyst which has enabled many professionals - including many famous musicians and actors - to free their bodies and psyches from unconscious stresses and misguided efforts, the Alexander Technique is dearly prized for the gentility with which it imparts its benefits, and with which it enables its practitioners to live their daily lives. It is particularly welcome to those who have, consciously or unconsciously, become enmeshed in overly effortful modes of living.

Virtually impossible to learn second-hand, from books or audio and video tapes, it is absolutely essential that the Alexander Technique be experienced at the hands of a qualified teacher to be truly appreciated.

Further reading:
Jones, Frank Pierce, *Body Awareness in Action*, Schocken Books, NY, 1976.
Gelb, Michael J., *Body Learning, An Introduction to the Alexander
  Technique*, Henry Holt, 1996.
Stransky, Judith and Stone, Robert B., Ph.D., *The Alexander Technique*,
  Beauport Books, NY, 1981.

ENERGY-RICH LIVING

The Chi in Air, Water and Food

Whatever enhances health nurtures chi, and whatever weakens health dissipates chi - even though these processes and behaviors may seem only remotely related to traditional chigong practices. At every moment of our lives, whatever we are doing is either actively augmenting or diminishing our energy field, be it what we are eating, breathing, reading, thinking, feeling or doing (or what we are not eating, breathing, reading, thinking, feeling or doing). Some of these activities are obvious and need no pointing out; others are subtle and require keen perceptiveness. A number of each has been included as a means of encouraging students to undertake a review of the full spectrum of their daily lives, with an eye toward bringing them into alignment with an energy-enhancing lifestyle. Only in this way can we even begin to set foot upon the path of cultivating a chi-sensitivity beyond that slender fraction of the day in which we may perform our formal Zhineng Qigong practice.

This may come to comprise a sustained practice in itself: the dynamic moment-to-moment sensitivity to - and search for - purity, energy and balance in one's individual journey. How we stand, how we breathe, whether there is poise or agitation in our movement, a soft smile or a tight grimace on our visage, a sense of care or impatience in our spirit, a spontaneous affection for our fellows, or a defensive mistrust, a deep-running reverence for life, or a profound cynicism - all these may well be as crucial and indispensable to our well-being, our internal energy-flow, the openness of our channels - physiological and psychospiritual - as any chigong practice we may ever encounter.

We have all seen dedicated, even slavish devotees of various esoteric disciplines whose humanity has been severely compromised by the extremity and imbalance of their immersion in various refuges of self-development. In the presence of such people - full of heroic ascetic agendas, and complex transcendental transmutational theories, we cannot escape the poignant impression of sacrificed selfhood which characterizes those who have mistaken obsessive discipline for true living.

We wish to point out that, among the myriad of energy-enhancing modalities discussed here, there has been no attempt to censor or otherwise adulterate valuable and time-proven practices or substances in order to make them conform to the protocols of this or that particular system, be it Western or Eastern in origin. While the reader will doubtless recognize modalities drawn from various healing traditions, such as hydrotherapy, enzyme nutrition or macrobiotics, few of which take advantage of the revelations and considerable benefits of the best in systems outside their own traditions, we feel that it would be tragic to omit genuinely life-renewing resources purely because of the provincialism endemic to such conceptually exclusive philosophies of practice.

Likewise, despite the national dietary and therapeutic traditions - and at times, prejudices - of Zhineng Qigong's country of origin, no attempt has been made to limit this overview to the traditional health practices native to that land. Indeed, when an empirical examination of the benefits or weaknesses of any given practice was ultimately made, irrespective of which country or tradition it happened to emerge from, the only criterion which was applied was a particular modality's relevance and effectiveness in freeing the body of stagnation, toxicity and blockage and re-establishing the free flow of energy and vitality throughout the system.

A simple example of how common practice can inadvertently dictate tradition - which then comes to assume the position of authority and dogma - is the widespread third world dependence upon grains as the basic staple food. While relatively healthful from one viewpoint, and cleansing when taken in balanced proportion with vegetable foods, a deep study of the anthropological evidence from numerous cultures over many centuries does not confirm that grains, as such, constitute either the ideal staple food for mankind then or now.

It is true that a grain-based diet can and does relieve many of the dietary sufferings of particularly those who have been conditioned into the denatured Western diet of processed, chemicalized foods, hormonalized meats and sugar addictions. It achieves this effect primarily through the cessation of the ingestion of the offending disease-producing substances such as dairy foods, meats, canned, processed and denatured foods, junk foods and white sugar products). which allows the body to gradually discharge its collected toxins, replacing them with the relative cleanliness of such substances as organic grains, vegetables and sea vegetables. The diet cannot, however, be said to provide a truly superior set of building with which to reconstruct new tissue, nor to provide optimal energy for the various life-processes. An objective exploration of the Weston Price's stunning anthropological survey, *Nutrition and Physical Degeneration* will more than bear this out.

Yet, it remains the unspoken caveat that, seemingly from time immemorial, rice and vegetables, with perhaps some occasional fish or meat, is the truly balanced archetypal meal, when in reality, it is only what millions of Asians have habitually had recourse to, given their populations, economic situations, and available resources

An equally unfortunate example of such enshrined misinformation has been the macrobiotic bio-philosophy's denial of and deprivation of water as an aliment needed in great abundance by all living creatures, a clearly vital fact as proven by many empirical scientific studies, but conveniently theorized away by esoteric conceptual legerdemain.

However, it is not a phenomenon alone limited to the macrobiotic diet, and it can be seen amidst those who cling narrowly to any dietary "ism", including raw foodism, vegetarianism, veganism, and many other similar approaches; each carries its own perils. One risks not only one's health but one's inner balance. In becoming so psychospiritually invested in any protocol of eating, a person may become incapable of developing and trusting their own intuitive wisdom, thus sacrificing the ability to flexibly adjust and be creative with regard to diet and nutrition, and in all areas of life.

Further reading:
Colbin, Annemarie, *Food and Healing*, Ballantine Books, NY, 1986.
Kushi, Aveline and Monte, Tom, *Thirty Days* (Macrobiotic regimen),
    Japan Pub., Inc., 1991.
Schmid, Ronald F., N.D. *Native Nutrition*, Healing Arts Press, Rochester, VT, 1994.

The Vital Elixir of Life

No other activity or practice bears as immediate and intimate a relationship to the processes of life as does breathing. Throughout the millennia, the culture of the breath has been the pre-eminent physical and psychospiritual practice of self-development of mankind; in forms crude and esoteric, strenuous and subtle, conscious or unconscious, it provides the keynote - the unspoken mantra – of all earthly human life. With a little insight, it is not difficult to gauge the physical and psychospiritual condition of a person purely through keen study of his or her breathing patterns, habits and attitudes.

A perfect metaphor for the rhythm of existence, with its cyclic rise and fall, inflow and outflow, creation and dissolution, the breath is a lifetime companion, reflecting and responding to every moment in dynamic flexibility. Eloquent in its revelation of our openness to or defendedness against life, the breath flows between the polarities of our existence with quicksilver sensitivity: tension - relaxation, explosion - quiescence, anxiety - relief, never reflecting us amiss, never lying about who and what we have become, and how we have become it, and never failing to offer us an ever-present avenue leading toward our aliveness and wholeness.

At any and every given moment, the tide of the breath presents us with a ceaseless opportunity to deepen, broaden and in every way enhance our awareness, presence and balance. Protean in nature, the breath will respond readily to our desire to work physically, psychologically or spiritually, as we intend.

Conscious breathing may constitute a periodic practice or a continuous discipline, depending upon our needs, and while we, in our distractedness, may find ourselves unconsciously abandoning it, it will never abandon us.

While many breathing practices exist in fulfillment of the various purposes and pursuits of mankind, their common bond is the conscious participation of the practitioner in his or her own greater being through the deepening and focusing of her breath awareness.

As stated earlier, the qualities to be desired are not very different than those found in the young child or in unspoiled tribal and traditional cultures - a tranquil respiration that emerges from deep within the lower belly, softly expanding and contracting concentrically from a source-point behind and just below the navel, generating a gentle, almost imperceptible lift and ebb to the ribcage and chest. In dynamic activity this diaphragmatic breathing naturally augmented by the expansion of the ribcage and intercostal areas for maximal output; however, of themselves, the lower lobes of the lungs account for more than 60% of the airspace in the respiratory system and contain neural receptors which trigger a relaxation response.

The arsenal of complex breathing techniques aside, this practice alone would ensure the free influx of energy into and out of the earth center - an indispensible prerequisite for effective energy practice.

Further recommended reading:
Bragg, Paul & Patricia, *Super Power Breathing*, Health Science, Santa Barbara, CA, 1998.
von Durckheim, Karlfried Graf, *Hara, The Vital Centre of Man*, Allen & Unwin Ltd., 1962.
Reid, Daniel P., *Harnessing the Power of the Universe*, Shambhala, Boston and London, 1998.

Reid, Daniel P., *The Tao of Health, Sex & Longevity*, Simon & Schuster, 1989.

Sky, Michael, *Breathing*, Bear & Co., Santa Fe, NM, 1990.

The Fountain of Life

After oxygen, nothing else consumed by man approaches the crucial importance of water in providing the foundations for health and vitality. All physiological systems, without exception, have a primal dependence upon adequate hydration for their optimal assimilation of nutrients, purification of toxins and proper functioning.

Dr. F. Batmanghelidj, a Western-schooled physician born in Tehran, Iran, has written several books concerning the astonishing therapeutic powers of water. He made his discoveries after being sentenced to death by the government of Iran, which commuted his sentence to life imprisonment, forcing him to treat the illnesses of thousands of suffering inmates with nothing but plain water. Amazingly, the conditions that were ameliorated by adequate hydration ranged from the chronic to the life-threatening, from ulcers and hypertension to Alzheimer's Disease. To enumerate but a few of the myriad interactions which are crucially water-dependent:

> The flow of water through the cell membrane can generate "hydroelectric" energy (voltage) that is converted and stored in the energy pools in the form of ATP and GTP - two vital cell battery systems. ATP and GTP are chemical sources of energy in the body. The energy generated by water is used in the manufacture of ATP and GTP. These particles are used as "cash flow" in elemental exchanges, particularly in neurotransmission.
>
> Proteins and enzymes of the body function more efficiently in solutions of lower viscosity. . ."*Water, the solvent of the body, regulates all functions . . . .*" (Author's italics, J.M.)
>
> The adequate hydration of the human body in itself constitutes a profoundly health-enhancing act, through which literally thousands of complex biological systems are catalyzed and balanced.
>
> Most human beings and disease conditions present a picture of minor or major systemic dehydration.

An abundance of water throughout the day will enable the channels of elimination in the human ecosystem to continually cleanse themselves of their accumulated wastes it will also provide optimal tone to all the immune-enhancing mucous membranes in the body. It is particularly important to take sufficient water before and after meals, where it will insure the most favorable interactions between foods taken and the forces of assimilation. By creating an easily flowing fluid interchange and access between all the organs and their paths of elimination, an equilibrium is established amongst them which prevents any single system from being overtaxed and subject to dysfunction or breakdown.

Stress of any kind immediately and dramatically draws upon and consumes the available level of water in the tissues, thereby reducing the fluidity and the optimal functioning of all the systems of circulation, including the circulatory, the respiratory and the lymphatic. Therefore, under moderate or severe stress, one should take care to immediately and substantially increase one's intake.

As a flexible rule of thumb, one should consume at least six to eight full glasses daily, or approximately two to two and a half quarts. While pure, unchemicalized water is always preferable, if this is not readily available, rather than reducing one's intake, one should avail oneself of the best that one can find. A good habit is to drink from one half to two glasses of mildly tepid water upon waking. Likewise, one should take a glass prior to retiring, to insure the optimal tissue repair and organic interchange while sleeping.

It is important to note that no beverages can successfully substitute for pure water in their hydration effect and catalyst potential; only unadulterated water will achieve the best results. The first rule of any distress or discomfort, whether physical or psychic: When in doubt, drink more water.

Further reading:
Ballard, Juliet Brooke, *The Hidden Laws of Earth*, A.R.E. Press, Virginia Beach, VA, 1979.
Batmanghelidj, F., M.D., *Your Body's Many Cries for Water*, Global Health Solutions, Inc., Falls Church, VA, 1995.
Bragg, Paul & Patricia, *Water - The Shocking Truth*, Health Science, Santa Barbara, CA.
Frejer, B. Ernest (compiled by), *The Edgar Cayce Companion*, A.R.E. Press, Virginia Beach, VA, 1995.

Living Food

Dr. Edward Howell, biochemist, clinician at the Lindlahr Sanitarium and life-long researcher in the field of enzymes has written extensively and eloquently on the subject of living foods, with their rich store of enzymes intact, and their profound relationship to optimal human health. His *Food Enzymes for Health & Longevity* distills the research from over 435 medical and nutritional journals on the subject in a compelling manner.

Secreted by the pancreas, enzymes are considered biochemical catalysts which assist and are in fact indispensable to virtually every phase of life-function thus far explored by medical science - from the lubrication of the eyes to the breakdown of all nutriments within the body.

Howell takes care to delineate the fact that, "Catalysts are only inert substances. They possess none of the life energy we find in enzymes. For instance, enzymes give off a kind of radiation when they work. This is not true of catalysts." (*Healthview Newsletter*, 1979)

Elsewhere, he states this in a slightly different manner: "The enzyme complex is a biological entity composed of corporeal (material) and incorporeal (energetic) fraction . . . " It is clear from these extracts that the enzyme complex may be regarded as a minute quantum of energy-carrying matter.

Howell demonstrates the dramatic difference in an enzyme-sacrificing dysfunction and an enzyme-sparing one: "Loss of pancreatic enzymes by experimental or human pancreatic fistula (opening) is rapidly fatal, invalidating the supposition that extensive fecal excretion of enzymes is tolerable. On the contrary, death is not inevitable in experimental or human biliary fistula where no enzymes are sacrificed . . . "

A direct relationship exists between tissue enzyme levels and vitality, being highest in the young and the healthy, and almost nonexistent in the sick and the aged, so much so that Howell has written: "When it gets to the point that you cannot make certain enzymes, then your life ends."

When foods deprived of their natural enzymes through cooking arrive in the digestive tract, the body immediately signals a release of the appropriate endogenous enzymes from its own organs and tissues for the breakdown and assimilation of those foods, engendering an expenditure of its own precious resources to replace the missing enzymes. Over the course of three meals a day, 1,195 meals a year, throughout the span of many years, this represents an immense expenditure on the part of one's own energy resources. Eventually, this loss of capital registers as lowered vitality, compromised health and impaired ability to facilitate tissue repair.

Through the extensions of enzymatic processes, all life-maintaining bodily fluids and activities are catalyzed: from hormones to every manner of internal and external secretion upon which life depends. Thus, when these heat-labile entities are exposed to temperatures beyond their capacity to endure - such as intensively high fevers - life effectively ceases.

Immense medical anthropological evidence exists confirming the supremacy and power of those diets in which the native enzyme complements have been preserved, the extensive studies of Drs. Robert McCarrison, Frances Pottenger, and Weston Price being pre-eminent in the annals of this field of science.

As one example among many, the Pottenger experiments, conducted at the Pottenger Sanitarium, demonstrated both the epidemic proportions of diseases generated by the cooked-food regimen, and the virtual immunity from degenerative disease afforded by the adoption of a raw-food diet: "The experiment was conducted over a period of ten years on approximately nine hundred cats. All cats were fed alike, except that one group was fed cooked meat while the other was kept exclusively on raw meat. Both groups were fed two-thirds meat, one-third raw milk, plus cod-liver oil." According to Dr. Pottenger, the results were dramatic:

> The cats receiving raw meat and raw milk reproduced in homogeneity from one generation to the next. Abortion was uncommon . . . and the mother cats nursed their young in a normal manner. The cats in these pens had good resistance to vermin, infections, and parasites.
>
> They possessed excellent equilibrium; they behaved in a predictable manner. Their organic development was complete and functioned normally.
>
> Cats receiving the cooked meat scraps presented an entirely different picture: (They) reproduced a heterogeneous strain of kittens, each kitten of the litter being different in skeletal pattern. Abortion in these cats was common, running about 25 per cent in the first generation to about 70 per cent in the second generation. Deliveries were in general difficult, many cats dying in labor. Mortality rates of the kittens were high, frequently due to the failure of the mother to lactate. The kittens were often too frail to nurse. At times the mother would steadily decline in health following the birth of the kittens, dying from some obscure tissue exhaustion about three months after deliv-

ery. Others experienced increasing difficulty with subsequent pregnancies. Some failed to become pregnant.

Cooked-meat-fed cats were irritable. The females were dangerous to handle, occasionally viciously biting the keeper. The males were more docile, often to the point of being inaggressive. Sex interest was slack or perverted. Vermin and intestinal parasites abounded. Skin lesions and allergies were frequent, being progressively worse from one generation to the next.

Pneumonia, emphysema, diarrhea, osteomyletis, cardiac lesions, hyperopia and myopia (eye diseases), thyroid diseases, nephritis, orchitis, oophoritis, hepatitis (liver inflammation), paralysis, meningitis, cystitis (bladder inflammation), arthritis, and many other degenerative diseases "familiar in human medicine", took a heavy toll among these cats.

Unhealthy conditions of mouth and teeth, degenerative skeletal changes, and malalignment of teeth were found in most of them.

In autopsy, cooked-meat-fed females frequently presented the picture of ovarian atrophy and uterine congestion, whereas the males often showed failure in the development of active spermatogenesis. The bones of these cats showed "evidence of less calcium" and they generally showed signs of shriveling or wasting or became overly fat with distended abdomens. Dr. Pottenger reported:

> In the third generation of cooked-meat-fed animals, some of the bones became as soft as rubber and a true condition of osteogenesis imperfecta (imperfect bone structure from birth) was present . . . Of the cats maintained entirely on the cooked meat diet, with raw milk, the kittens of the third generation were so degenerated that none of them survived the sixth month of life, thereby terminating the strain.

An interesting sidelight is that it is virtually impossible to gain weight on a raw food diet, whereas the same quantity of food, when cooked, will result in a weight gain. Due to the premature breakdown of tissues and fiber, an over-absorption of nutriment is encouraged where there is no remaining roughage to sweep the substances through the gastrointestinal tract as rapidly as nature intended, resulting in weight gain.

Beyond the preservation of the all-important enzymes, an uncooked or lightly heated diet encourages the retention of various vitamins and minerals often destroyed and leeched out through various cooking techniques.

While far from a complete treatment on this complex subject, a general guide might include the increasing of the ratio of raw to cooked food in one's diet until raw food approaches 30% - 50% of one's diet in colder seasons, and at least 70% of the diet in more temperate seasons The inclusion of such healthful, high enzyme foods as miso, tofu, tempeh, fermented foods, sprouted grains, seeds and nuts (whose vitamin and enzyme potential and digestibility increase markedly after several days of sprouting) is very beneficial.

Additionally, enzymes, vitamins, minerals and other live-food factors may be largely preserved by preparing foods through marination, brief blanching, light sauteing, and steaming just to the point of tender firmness and crispness. Sun or air-dehydrated foods also retain a considerable measure of their nutrients, and may be rehydrated for later use. Fresh pressed fruit and vegetable juices provide rich amounts of enzymes.

Finally, a whole new food science has evolved which offers encapsulated enzymes of many varying kinds, singly and in combination, for consumption just prior to meals as an infusion of exogenous support for the work of digestion and assimilation previously borne by the body. This has led to an entirely unique mode of holistic medical treatment: enzyme therapy, which specifically targets various disease conditions through the use of specific enzyme formulas. Its results are highly effective while having the virtues of being supremely non-toxic and non-invasive.

As dicussed earlier, the macrobiotic diet, almost entirely heat-treated, can provide a highly valuable transition program which has demonstrated its ability to reverse many degenerative diseases and even terminal conditons; but over a period of some years on a strict macrobiotic regimen, deficiencies of various kinds - usually explained away as 'cravings' - tend to manifest, resulting in lowered energy levels, poor growth in children, compromised immunity and psychophysical stress disorders. Despite heroic and stoical adherence to the regimen, these symptoms will not disappear until such deficiencies are adequately addressed.

To be sure, these diets represent a generally healthful way of eating, resulting in low incidence of heart disease, cancer and other illnesses, and certainly provide a far superior choice to the common American diet, but this does not engrave them in stone as the optimal nutritional profile for all mankind at all times and places.

Further reading:

Cousens, Gabriel M.D., *Conscious Eating,* Vision Books International, Santa Rosa, CA, 1992.

Howell, Edward, M.D., *Food Enzymes for Health & Longevity,* Omangod Press, Woodstock Valley, CT, 1980.

Howell, Edward, M.D., *Enzyme Nutrition,* Avery Publishing Group, Wayne, NJ, 1985.

Jensen, Bernard, Ph.D., *A Hunza Trip,* (also *The Wheel of Health* by G.T. Wrench, M.D.), Bernard Jensen International, 24360 Old Wagon Road, Escondido, CA, 92027.

Santillo, Humbart, *Food Enzymes, The Missing Link to Radiant Health,* Hohm Press, Prescott Valley, AZ, 1987.

Santillo, Humbart, *Intuitive Eating,* Hohm Press, Prescott Valley, AZ, 1998.

ENERGY-ENHANCING FOOD COMBINATIONS

Creating Internal Harmony

Approximately 35% of all the bio-energy produced in a single day is given over to the tasks of breaking down, assimilating and eliminating that which we consume. Foods are generally classed into three large categories: proteins, carbohydrates and fats. Within these categories one may enumerate further subdivisions, but that is the subject of another study. A great deal of evidence exists to show that the congenial combination of these categories will substantially reduce the burden placed upon the body, so much so that proper combining will spell the difference between lethargy or a comfortable lightness after a meal.

Seen another way, the lethargy would imply a heavy energy expenditure, with much blood flow re-directed toward the organs of assimilation - and later, elimination - in order to deal with the challenge of the food consumed, while the lightness after meals would imply a minimal energy expenditure, with modest circulatory demands on the internal organs as a result of good food combining.

While no one will perish on the spot for lack of proper food combining, it will, over time, take a heavy toll on one's organic vitality and reduce one's general level of energy.

The principle involved, then, is fairly simple, requiring respect of the differing digestive scenarios of proteins and complex carbohydrates with regard to their differing enzymatic needs during digestion and their differing digestive time frames. In short, they should be eaten at different meals, and accompanied by foods which will facilitate their assimilation. The clinical proof and elaboration of these principles may be found in the works listed below; for now, we shall concern ourselves with the practicalities of implementing the harmony of foods.

Proteins are the most concentrated of nutriments, the richest in physiological building blocks, and yet the most difficult for the human body to break down and the source of the most potentially toxic by-products. Requiring the longest time to process, they galvanize an intensive internal effort on the body's part which may last many hours; therefore, proteins should ideally be eaten between the morning and mid-afternoon, after which they should be avoided. Otherwise the body will be denied the opportunity for complete physiological rest during the hours of sleep, as it continues to labor on an organic and cellular level. If the proteins are taken early enough, this period will see completion prior to the sleep-cycle.

Even so, there are proteins which are stressful for the body to metabolize in any great quantity, and other proteins which are easy for the body to deal with in a relatively short period of time.

Low-stress proteins (proteins which provide more energy than they consume):

Sprouted beans, cooked without boiling
Chicken, organically grown, range-fed
Coconut, green and young
Conch
Cottage cheese, raw milk, low or nonfat
Eggs, free-range organic, briefly poached just until whites solidify
Miso
Nuts (a medium to high-stress protein whose value is improved
    when used as nut milk (nuts soaked in water and blended for
    liquid form) and especially when sprouted
Ocean fish
Octopus
Scallops
Soy ferments
Sprouts, especially sunflower
Squid
Tahini
Tofu
Wild rice, cooked without boiling

Medium-stress proteins:

Avocado, game birds (cornish hens, quail, pheasant, doves), feta cheese, soaked nuts, turkey

High-stress proteins (proteins that consume more energy metabolizing than they provide)

Beef muscle, brewer's yeast (except in small amounts), cow's milk, lamb, raw nuts in large quantities, peanuts, pork, protein powder, sardines, non-fermented soybean products (soy milk, soy flour), veal.

In short, one must eat proteins:

1) Without carbohydrates/sugars
2) With a variety of vegetables (which enhance rapid digestion and absorption)
3) In complete protein groups (that is, with the addition of several spoonfuls of mixed nut-seed sprouts, such as sunflower, sesame, almond and pumpkin, to insure complete amino acid chains, thus preventing the body from borrowing its own to complete the incomplete chains of protein itself)
4) Early in the day
5) With a small amount of good quality oil (in salad)
6) Without liquid beverages.

These steps will insure the optimal assimilation of proteins.

One may then have a carbohydrate meal (grains, breads, etc.) at a different time of the day, and combined similarly with vegetable components as catalysts for optimal breakdown and absorption. However, the difference in quality between complex and simple carbohydrates is crucial. Such complex carbohydrates as rice or spaghetti have inordinately rapid absorption rates, ranking high on what is known as the glycemic index, which monitors the rapidity with which sugars in a food register in the bloodstream; yet the simple carbohydrates of such substances as fruits and vegetables for the most part maintain a very low rating on the glycemic index, indicating a moderate to low impact on the blood sugar level, and a consequent benign insulin reaction.

Therefore, it is well to remember that the simpler, more visibly vegetable carbohydrates are much more beneficial for the body than the complex, and one should seek to have them in a ratio of at least two to one with complex carbohydrates or starches.

This accords well with a by now almost traditional wisdom with regard to the optimal balance of acid-alkaline food for the maintenance of health. Edgar Cayce, a deeply gifted psychic seer, in his extensive discourses on diet and health, indicated that it would be almost impossible for illness or colds to manifest in a bloodstream which was balanced toward the alkaline, and further stipulated that, to achieve this balance, the most ideal intake of alkaline to acid foods was in the ratio of 80%-20%.

The chart below delineates these categories:

Alkaline Forming Foods:

> All fruits, fresh and dried (exceptions: cranberries, large prunes and
>   plums.)
> All vegetables, fresh and dehydrated except legumes (dried peas,
>   beans and lentils)
> All forms of milk (buttermilk, yogurts, cottage cheese)
> Apple cider vinegar
> Fresh, raw juice
> Honey
> Lima Beans
> Millet
> Molasses
> Potatoes
> Sea vegetables
> Sprouts

Acid-Forming Foods:

> Meat
> Poultry
> Fish
> All cereal grains (except millet; brown rice is less acid forming)
> All high-starch and protein foods (pasta ,white sugar, syrups)
> Alcohol and soft drinks

Animal fats and vegetable oils
Canned and frozen food
Black Pepper
Chocolate
Coffee
Distilled Vinegar
Egg whites (yolks are not acid-forming)
Foods cooked with oils
Fruits that have been glazed or sulphured
Nuts & Seeds
Legumes
Popcorn
Processed cereals
Salt
Sugar
Tea (except caffeine-free tea)
Tofu and soy products
Wheat products

Good general guidelines:

*   Drink a glass of water 30 minutes before and two hours after meals.
*   Fruits, being rapidly digested and largely juice, should be eaten alone early in the day, and prior to any other food with which they may cause fermentation; the same is true of freshly pressed fruit juices.
*   A large vegetable salad should be eaten daily, either with a protein or a carbohydrate.
*   Lightly steamed, sautéed or blanched vegetables should accompany the second meal if further raw vegetables are not desired.
*   Foods should be consumed directly after preparation, as they will begin to lose their values to oxidation from the moment they are cut, shredded or otherwise prepared.
*   Chewing well aids the body in its task and relieves it of extra work, requiring the secretion of fewer enzymes, as does eating modest quantities of food, which gives the internal organs rest.
*   Eating in peaceful settings, undistracted by other activities or focal points such as television, radio or intense intellectual or emotional discussions helps harmonize the energies while taking one's meals.
*   A brief period of stillness is a wonderful prelude to a meal, an invitation for the energy to gather and settle.

Another study could be made of special foods which are highly beneficial to human well-being, among these being almonds, grapes, beets and many others; for these, the reader may consult those source-works listed below.

A recently studied phenomenon known as 'The French Paradox' has contributed some remarkable insights to the practice of enlightened eating; the term comes from the observation that, as a culture, the French have traditionally eaten ample meals quite high in many of the 'offending substances' decried in the American diet: fats, oils, wine and pastries and yet have less than half the incidence of cardiovascular disease as Americans.

John Douillard, a chiropractic and Ayurvedic physician presently writing a work on the subject, has explained that the major reasons for this enviable immunity lie in two long overlooked factors: the time of day such meals are consumed and the traditional midday interval built into Mediterranean cultures which affords the body the opportunity to fully metabolize what it consumes. He points out that organ systems possess biorhythms with distinct energy peaks and troughs, and that the powers of the digestive system function most optimally from late morning to early afternoon. A substantial meal taken at the optimal functional period for the organs of the digestive system – between 11 a.m. and 2 p.m. – will be easily broken down, absorbed and assimilated, even if it contains considerable quantities of fats and protein, (particularly if one rests for 10 to 20 minutes after eating), whereas, by contrast, the same meal consumed in the evening will encounter a quiescent digestive system capable only of functioning at a much lower level, eventually overtaxing the body and burdening the body with harbored fats, proteins and carbohydrates.

This crucial insight enables us to shift from our often obsessive focus upon the "what" of nutrition to the "when" and "how" of the art of eating.

Further reading:

Dispenza, Joseph, *Live Better Longer*, (The Parcells' Plan), Harper San Francisco, 1997.

Price, Weston, *Nutrition and Physical Degeneration*, Keats Publishing, New Canaan, CT, 1989.

Reid, Daniel P., *The Tao of Health, Sex & Longevity*, Simon & Schuster.

Reilly, Harold J., Ph. D., D.S., and Ruth Hagy Brod, *The Edgar Cayce Handbook for Health Through Drugless Therapy*, MacMillan Pub. Co. Inc., NY, 1975.

Shelton, Herbert, *Food Combining Made Easy*, Willow Pub., Inc., San Antonio, TX, 1962.

Tips, Jack, N.D., Ph.D., *The Pro Vita Plan*, Apple-a-Day Press, 1996.

Cleansing Foods of Toxic Residues:

It goes without saying that organic food contains the highest nutritional value, but if one cannot procure or afford it, one can still insure removal of pesticides and herbicides by immersing the produce in a sink full of water to which one capful of original Clorox bleach has been added. This has the effect of stripping all external chemicals from the surface of the food without leaving any residue, provided one is careful to spray the foods with running water for a few minutes, or to resoak the food in a sink full of fresh water for from five to ten minutes.

Further reading:
Dispenza, Joseph, *Live Better Longer*, (The Parcells Plan), Harper San Francisco, 1997.

THE GIFTS OF EARTH

Nature's Miraculous Botanical Pharmacy

There exists a category of extremely potent natural substances called superfoods, whose effect on the body is profoundly beneficial in relatively small amounts. Their ability to energize, rejuvenate and renew the structures of the body is marked, and their track record spans millions of people over the course of many decades. Several of the most potent and effective are listed below; it is highly recommended that the reader approach their usage with an open mind and a spirit of exploration and experimentation, allowing sufficient time for the more subtle aspects of the various substances to achieve their effect - sometimes a matter of several months.

It is a now a well known tenet of nutrition that one is nourished not by the bulk of what one consumes, but by the specific elements which one absorbs and efficiently metabolizes. While the Western mind has been browbeaten by innumerable commercial health pitches promising bigger and better delivery of mega-supplements of every kind, each purporting to be the result of a proprietary process which renders it unique and supreme amongst its competitors (not to mention prohibitively expensive), the fact remains that the body may safely utilize only what it can easily absorb and incorporate into itself, and the key to both of these processes is the recognition on the body's part of the bio-compatibility of the substance in question.

In fact, a relatively modest amount of the right substance, when benignly received by the body, can go a surprisingly long way towards achieving dramatic benefit. It is in this light that the superfoods serve a decidedly superior role; they are not perceived as aliens, products of the laboratory created by the current and ever-transient vogue regarding what is best for the body. Rather, they are natural substances which have existed and coexisted with man on planet earth for millennia. Created by natural processes and harvested by man, they find ready recognition and relatively easy acceptance by the human organism, often resulting in dramatic energy enhancement.

Bee Pollen

"As far back as 2735 B.C., the Chinese emperor Shen Nung compiled a vast medical encyclopedia, still authoritative today, that features the gifts of the bees. As recently as A.D. 1991, Columbia University published a study on the cancer-fighting properties of one bee-made product, propolis." (*The Bee Pollen Bible* by Royden Brown)

"Bee pollen is a complete food. The optimum of vigor and resistance to poor health and disease was obtained by adding twenty percent bee pollen to food. Bee pollen is rich in rare and precious nutritive compounds. It works in a deep and lasting fashion." (Royal Society of Naturalists of Belgium and France)

Olympic coaches routinely report a 10 - 20% increase in the optimal performance of their athletes following the adoption of bee pollen in their program.

Demonstrated to contain every nutrient known to man, bee pollen alone has been shown to sustain generation after generation of life without the least compromise of health and vitality. The German publication *Naturheilpraxis* describes bee pollen's ability to normalize cholesterol and triglyceride levels in the blood: "Upon the regular ingestion of bee pollen, a reduction of cholesterol and triglycerides was observed. High density lipoproteins (HDL) increased, while low-density lipoproteins (LDL) decreased. A normalization of blood serum cholesterol levels was observed in forty patients."

Among its impressive array of benefits are included immune-strengthening effects, delay of onset of laboratory induced tumors in experimental mice, prevention of radiation aftereffects in cancer patients, increase in blood lymphocytes, gamma globulins and blood proteins, the restoration of sexual potency in both males and females due to the micro-hormonal constituents, normalization of prostatitis (inflammation and enlargement of the prostate gland), the stimulation of ovarian function, improvement of the ovum's ability to withstand the incubation period, and the amelioration of a wide range of menstrual problems categorized under the heading of Dysmenorrhea, as delineated below:

> Following the ingestion of the compound during two full menstrual cycles, symptoms improved in almost all patients. Symptoms persisted in only five cases out of the sixty girls given the compound . . .
>
> The positive effects of this preparation are due to the effects of the herbal hormones contained in the bee pollen and royal jelly. The compound may be administered for a long time. It is easily tolerated and does not give rise to undesired side effects. (*The Bee Pollen Bible by* Royden Brown)

Likewise, bee pollen has rescued many women from the vagaries of menopause, or prematurely induced menopause as a result of surgical removal of the reproductive organs due to cancer, or destruction by radiation:

> We proved that the compound exerts a beneficial effect throughout the whole system affected by radiation. Thanks to the therapeutic action of the compound, these women have experienced a general improvement in their condition. They feel fresher, more dynamic, open to every activity, and mentally calmer. The compound is easily taken and rarefy causes side effects. The beneficial effects of the preparation are noticeable after only 14 days of treatment. (*The Bee Pollen Bible by* Royden Brown)

Pollen is profoundly effective in treating allergies. The following is by Leo Conway, M.D. of Denver, Colorado, who treated his patients with bee pollen:

> All patients who had taken the antigen (pollen) for three years remained free from all allergy symptoms, no matter where they lived and regardless of diet. Control has been achieved in 100 percent of my earlier cases and the field is ever-expanding.

Since oral feeding of pollen for this use was first perfected in my laboratory, astounding results have been obtained. No ill consequences have resulted. Ninety-four percent of all my patients were completely free from allergy symptoms. Of the other six percent, not one followed directions, but even this small percentage were nonetheless partially relieved.

Relief of hay fever, pollen-induced asthma, with ever-increasing control of bronchitis, ulcers of the digestive tract, colitis, migraine headaches, and urinary disorders were all totally successful.

British author and nutritionist Dr. Maurice Hanssen says,

I look on pollen as being part of the athlete's ideal diet. I define the ideal athlete's diet as that diet which produces maximum performance when it is required, with no long-term harmful side effects. Your body is continually being renewed in the average half-life, which is the time taken for half your cells to be replaced. Protein, for example, is in the body for 80 days, but the time differs in different tissues. Blood serum, heart, liver, and kidneys are all 10 days, while bone, skin, and muscle are 158 days.

The extraordinary richness of pollen in micro-elements cannot be stressed too much. We just cannot be sure that a normal diet produces enough in available forms, but the absorption properties of pollen allow the trace elements to be incorporated into the body structure without excessive loss.

The British Sports Council recorded increases in strength as high as 40 to 50 percent in those taking bee pollen regularly. Even more astounding, the British Royal Society has reported height increases in adults who take pollen.

Antii Lananaki, coach of the Finnish track team that swept the Olympics in 1972, revealed, "Most of our athletes take pollen food supplements. Our studies show it significantly improves their performance . . . ."

Alex Woodly, past director of the prestigious Education Athletic Club in Philadelphia, said, "Bee pollen works, and it works perfectly. Pollen allows superstars to increase their strength and stamina up to 25 percent. This increase in strength and endurance may be the key to the secret regenerative power of bee pollen. Bee pollen causes a definite decrease in pulse rate.

The whole beauty of bee pollen is that it's as natural as you can get. No chemicals. No steroids."

The list of bee pollen's miracles is virtually limitless; the main concern with regard to supplementing one's diet with this superfood is the absolute assurance that the pollen in question is fresh, and soft to the touch, as opposed to brittle and crunchy (stale), in which case many of its properties may not be active.

In response to a possible note of concern regarding possible allergic reactions to bee pollen, it should be understood that there exist two types of pollens - anemophile pollens and entomophile pollens. Anemophile pollens are those carried by the wind. As breezes blow, they are scattered into wind; it is these pollens which cause allergic distress to individuals who suffer from such conditions as hay fever and rose fever, irritating the mucous membranes, and causing swelling and watering of the eyes.

Entomophile pollens are borne aloft by insects, primarily honeybees foraging among blossoms. These are heavier pollens and of a different variety than wind-borne pollens. Entomophile pollens never become airborne and are not those responsible for allergic reactions. Rather, it is the case that pollen is an effective treatment for seasonal pollen-induced allergies as well as allergies of other origin. The American statesman Senator Tom Hankin, at one time almost incapacitated by allergies, recovered totally through the sustained use of bee pollen.

A minimum of three teaspoons a day is highly recommended, and greater amounts in situations where substantial physiological renewal or support is required. It is likewise important that the pollen not be encapsulated, a process which requires its pulverization, resulting in premature oxidation of its nutrients.

Further reading:
Brown, Royden, *Bee Hive Product Bible*, Avery Pub., 1993.
Brown, Royden, *The World's Only Perfect Food*, Hohm Press, Prescott, AZ, 1993.
Johnson, Noel, *The Living Proof*, Britic (USA), Inc., N.Y., 1989.
Wade, Carlson, *Bee Pollen and Your Health*, Keats Publishing, 1978.

Fresh raw pollen sosurce: C.C. Pollen Co., Phoneix Arizona 85018 (800) 975-0096.

Green food concentrates

These are cold-processed cereal grasses harvested at their richest chlorophyll-producing stage, just prior to jointing; the most commonly used are barley grass, rye grass and wheat grass. Usually found in powder form, they may be added to drinks or taken as is, providing a boost to the hemoglobin-producing capacity of the bloodstream and maintaining an overall alkalinity of the blood. Such concentrates are of immense value for those with lifestyles which routinely default on the need to consume fresh, chlorophyll-rich vegetables on a daily basis.

Further reading:
Jensen, Bernard, D.O., *The Healing Power of Chlorophyll*, Bernard Jensen Publications, Escondido, California, 1973.
Seibold, Ronald L., *Cereal Grass—What's In It For You?*, Wilderness Community Education Foundation, Lawrence, Kansas, 1990.
Swope, Mary Ruth, Ph.D., *The Green Leaves of Barley*, Swope Enterprises, Inc., Phoenix, AZ, 1990.
Wigmore, Ann, N.D., *The Wheatgrass Book*, Hippocrates Health Institute, 1986.

Spirulina

A rich and nutritious concentration of ocean-harvested algae, considered the first plant life to appear on the planet, the blue-green varieties being the most primitive. Spirulina is about sixty percent protein, and that protein is complete, containing all essential amino acids, existing in a form very easily assimilated, due to the high digestibility of its cell walls. Higher in beta-carotene than all other foods, in a form assimilated ten times more easily than synthetic beta carotene, spirulina is rich in B vitamins, minerals and enzymes.

However, the reality of spirulina is not in its clinical nutrient portrait, which may be considered modest by some standards; only a course of supplementation with a fresh and organically harvested product will yield its subtle energy-enhancing capabilities, its absolute affinity for the human system, its ready absorption, and its benign and broad systemic effect.

Those products which are grown and harvested in purified sea water pools are to be preferred.

Further reading:

Henrikson, Robert, *Earth Food Spirulina*, Ronore Enterprises, Inc., 1997.

Hills, Christopher, Dr., *The Whole Truth About Spirulina*, Dr. Hills Technologies, 1982.

Morgan, Helen C., & Moorhead, Kelly J., *Spirulina*, Nutrex, Inc., 1993.

Vitamin E (alpha tochopherol)

(Natural- source vitamins are always to be used)

A potent antioxidant, which was first pioneered into clinical use and public awareness by two Canadian cardiologists, Evan and Wilfrid Shute, M.D.'s has been the subject of literally thousands of research papers confirming its effectiveness in treating and reversing such conditions as coronary thrombosis, angina pectoris due to coronary artery narrowing, thrombophlebitis, the dissolving of arterial thrombii, Buerger's Disease, peripheral vascular arteriosclerosis and insufficiency, intermittent claudication, diabetic and arteriosclerotic early gangrene, diabetic and arteriosclerotic retinitis, acute rheumatic fever, indolent leg ulcers, kidney disease, infertility, menstrual problems, first, second and third degree burns and scar tissue removal, and in many other conditions. It has also been found to enhance aerobic metabolism and delivery of cellular oxygen when given to athletes and racehorses, maximizing the usage of endogenous oxygen by as much as 25%.

A staple of contemporary holistic supplementation regimens as well as enlightened allopathic practices, Vitamin E has entered the domain of generic acceptance as a broad-spectrum health-enhancement substance.

Further reading:

Bailey, Herbert, *Vitamin E - For a Healthy Heart and a Longer Life*, Mass Market Paperback, 1993.

Challem, Jack, *All About Vitamin E*, Avery Publishing Group, 1999.

Shite, Wilfrid E. M.D., and Harold J. Taub, *Vitamin E for Ailing and Healthy Hearts*, Pyramid House, 1969.

Sinatra, Stephen T. M.D., *Heartbreak and Heart Disease: A Mind/Body Prescription for Healing the Heart*, Keats Publishing, 1999.

CoQ10

An enzyme found in every body cell, but in highest concentrations in the heart, CoQ10 has a profoundly beneficial effect on the energy-producing potential of the cardiac muscle, so much so that it is considered the most effective holistic treatment for hypertension; this effect derives from its enhancement of cell metabolism within the heart muscle, restoring functional efficiency to the entire organ.

In addition, CoQ10 neutralizes free radicals, enhances Vitamin E's antioxidant abilities, and improves the body's immune system by supercharging the cell metabolism of the entire body; a boost in the energy level is among the first perceived fruits.

CoQ10 is routinely prescribed by a majority of physicians in Japan. One should commonly allow six to ten weeks in order to experience its benefits. Maintenance doses range from 100 - 200 milligrams daily, while therapeutic doses for cardiac conditions and hypertension generally run from 300 to 500 milligrams, with gel forms better absorbed than capsules, and capsules better than tablets. Cardiologist Stephen Sinatra, M.D., founder of and director of the New England Heart Center considers CoQ10 the greatest health discovery in decades.

More than 15 million Japanese take CoQ10 daily, and in Western Europe doctors regularly recommend CoQ10 as nutritional support for healthy hearts. Ten times more CoQ10 is found in the heart than in any other organ. When CoQ10 levels fall to 25% or less than normal, organs may become energy deficient; when levels fall to 75% less than normal, serious health problems may occur. Levels of CoQ10 production decrease with age.

Further reading:
Sinatra, Stephen, M.D., *The CoQ10 Phenomenon*, Keats Publishing, 1998.

Hawthorn extract

As an adjunct to CoQ10, fresh herbal tincture of hawthorn provides an invaluable cardio-tonic, enhancing the propelling power of the heart muscle, as well as the stroke-volume, without raising blood pressure. It is the classic herbal treatment for enlarged or otherwise impaired hearts, with many cases of virtual resurrection from cardiac invalidism to its credit. Daily maintenance doses are two droppers full twice a day, and more if one's purposes are therapeutic in nature.

Further reading:

Lucas, Richard, *Secrets of the Chinese Herbalists*, Parker Publishing, West Nyack, NY, 1987.

Murray, Michael T. N.D., *The Healing Power of Herbs*, Prima Publishing, Rocklin, CA, 1995.

Siberian Ginseng (Eleuthero)

A time-honored, multi-faceted adaptagen thoroughly studied and tested by the Russian government, Siberian Ginseng has a full-spectrum effect upon the human body, enhancing its ability to work harder and longer, endure stress better, resist illness and organic breakdown, and sustain overall physiological and psychological balance in the face of life's demands. With none of the stimulatory and sometimes stressful effects of its generic cousins, Panax and American ginseng, eleuthero's effect on the body is gentle and benign, achieving its effects quietly and over a gradual time-frame. A trial in which it was secretly (and perhaps somewhat un-ethically) administered over a period of months to thousands of Russian factory workers via their lunch meals resulted in a dramatic decrease in worker illness and absence.

Further reading:

Lucas, Richard, *Secrets of the Chinese Herbalists*, Parker Publishing, West Nyack, NY, 1987.

Murray, Michael T., N.D., *The Healing Power of Herbs*, Prima Publishing, Rocklin, CA, 1995.

Ginger (Zingiber officinale)

Herbalist Paul Schulick, author of an exhaustive treatise on ginger's remarkable healing powers, *Ginger - Common Spice & Wonder Drug*, cites among its medicinal properties: the prevention and amelioration of such conditions as heart attacks, arthritis and ulcers; it is a potent aid to improved digestion, and is a powerful anti-inflammatory. Ginger contains a substance known as zingibain, a potent protein-digesting enzyme, one gram of which is capable of tenderizing 20 pounds of meat. More effective than all non-steroidal anti-inflammatory drugs on the market today, ginger is capable of counteracting arthritic and rheumatoid inflammation. Extremely potent in its antioxidant properties (having more than 12 constituents superior to Vitamin E), enzymatic properties (it is considered the premier digestive aid, and Confucius is recorded to have said he never dined without it) and a profound modulator of eicosanoid (precursory micro-hormonal) balances, preventing the development of cardiovascular disease in a manner far superior to the present usage of aspirin for the same purpose, ginger ranks as one of - if not *the* - premier herbal healer of all time. Found in more than half of all traditional Chinese herbal medical formulas, ginger's broad and profound biological effects have been noted for centuries throughout many cultures around the world.

Further benefits of ginger: analgesic, anti-diabetic, antihelmintic, anti-thrombic, anti-ulcer, immune supportive, anti-bacterial, anti-emetic, anti-inflammatory, anti-tumor, anti-viral, thermoregulatory, anti-cathartic, anti-fungal, anti-mutagenic, antitussive and hypocholesteremic.

One may easily supplement one's diet with ginger in many forms: grated raw, juiced with fruits or vegetables, crystallized and powdered. Encapsulated ginger is available for convenience when traveling.

Further reading:
Schulick, Paul, *Ginger, Common Spice & Wonder Drug*, Herbal Free Press, Ltd., 1994.
Lucas, Richard, *Secrets of the Chinese Herbalists*, Parker Publishing, West Nyack, NY, 1987.
Murray, Michael T. N.D., *The Healing Power of Herbs*, Prima Publishing, Rocklin, CA, 1995.

Other Herbs of Great Value:

Aloe vera (skin and tissue healing), cayenne (prime emergency herb for quickly arresting strokes and heart attacks), echinacea (immune-sytem enhancer), garlic (potent full-spectrum antibiotic), ginkgo biloba (cerebral circulatory enhancer), goldenseal (antibiotic, immunostimulatory), grape seed extract (antioxidant, cardiotonic), kava (relaxant), licorice (adrenal-support), lobelia (anti-spasmodic, anti-seizure), milk thistle (liver-protective), *Panax ginseng*, peppermint (digestive tonic), St. John's Wort (anti-depressive), tea tree oil (fungicidal), turmeric (cancer preventative, antioxidant), valerian (relaxant, sleep-inducer).

High quality organic & wildcrafted herb supplier: Pacific Botanicals, 4350 Fish Hatchery Rd., Grants Pass, OR 97527 (541) 479-7777

High quality herbal formulas by Dr. Richard Schulze: American Botanical Pharmacy, P.O. Box 3027, Santa Monica, CA 90408 (800) 437 2362.

Other Superfoods of Great Value:

Almonds, aloe vera, amaranth, avocado, bee propolis, beets, blackstrap molasses, Bragg's Amino Acids, Brewer's Yeast (or nutritional yeast), cabbage, carrots, cauliflower, chlorella, corn, dulse, eggs (softly poached), flax seed, garlic, grapes, kelp, onions, papaya, peaches, peppers, pineapple, quinoa, raisins, brown rice, sardines, salmon, tuna and mackerel, soybeans, spouts, strawberries, sunflower seeds, tomatoes, walnuts, wheat germ, yogurt (best among dairy foods).

Other Vitamins and Nutrients of Great Value:

(Seek first in the diet, then supplement. Avoid all synthetic vitamins.)
Vitamin A, Vitamins B1, B2, B3, B5, B6, B8, B9, B12, Vitamin C, Vitamin D, choline, inositol (the preceding two substances are found in lecithin) PABA, Vitamin F, Vitamin K, Vitamin P (citrin, rutin hesperidin).

Minerals of Great Value:

(Seek chiefly in the diet, then supplement with superfoods if needed.)
Boron, calcium, chlorine, chromium, copper, iodine, iron, magnesium, manganese, molybdenum, phosphorus, potassium, selenium, silicon, sodium, sulfur, vanadium, zinc.

FREEING THE CHI-FLOW THROUGH BODY-CLEANSING

The critical importance of inner cleansing in relation to healing cannot be overestimated, especially in the late-twentieth-century technological-industrial environment. It is no accident that, far from the early-century cancer incidence of one person out of a hundred, we now find that, by the new millennium, one out of two human beings in the contemporary industrial society will be dealing with cancer. Since the advent of the post World War II era, humanity has been both subtly and relentlessly exposed to massive quantities of non-biodegradable substances, breathed, consumed and absorbed at virtually every moment of life since birth.

The body, never designed to process these alien deluges of petrochemical, pesticidal and other biological poisons, immediately seeks to sequester them from participation in the systemic circulation, and thereby creates internal toxic storage sites which eventually mutate cell metabolism into

302

the anaerobic, fermentative process specific to cancerous growths. Unless or until the bio-energy or chi attains a level sufficient not only to fully implement the body's immediate biological imperatives - those maintaining metabolism and vital functions - it will not and cannot begin to access and eliminate the deeper intracellular waste and deposits of toxins for mobilization and excretion.

Because of this impasse, it becomes crucial to take a consistent and aggressive approach to internal detoxification if we are ever to even or better the odds with relation to environmental health, internal and external.

While a diligent study of contemporary holistic medicine will yield a host of invaluable aids in ridding the system of such stored carcinogens - including everything from therapeutic enzymes to chelation therapies of dramatic effectiveness - there are a number of other simple and equally potent means at our disposal.

World-renowned medical herbalist Dr. Richard Schulze, who insists upon an initial bowel and blood-cleansing regimen for every new patient who comes under his care, has repeatedly stated that, throughout decades of treating over 12,000 patients in his clinic, no matter what condition or pathology the incoming patient has suffered from, after the initial four-, six-, or eight-week cleansing regimen, over 85% of all such patients discovered that their disease conditions had disappeared.

This is a very dramatic yet very accurate depiction of the indivisible nature of the relationship between disease, detoxification and healing.

Fasting and Juice Fasting

A perusal of the collected medical and therapeutic documents from numerous ancient and modern cultures routinely reveals innumerable testimonies of dramatic reversal of almost every known disease condition through some variety of fasting; whether complete or partial, of brief or long duration, or of religious or secular in nature, the indisputable proof of fasting's power to heal becomes undeniable.

However, due to the fear of relinquishing a lifetime habit of consuming two to three meals a day, and due also to the association of abstinence from food with starvation, doubts and reservations usually arise in the minds of most human beings when the prospect of fasting is encountered. Subconsciously, people know that this will entail some major shifts in priorities, as well as considerable self-restraint, and it is usually not until someone has arrived at a nearly desperate stage that he or she will actively entertain the idea of undergoing a fast.

303

The ordinary - never mind the obese - individual has reserves enabling him or her to sustain at least six to ten weeks of fasting before the process of autolysis, or living from one's own stored substance, and the complete consumption of these reserves crosses over into the metabolizing of lean tissue and what is called starvation.

For the most part, despite the overwhelming historical evidence from healers and physicians of every era and culture, the technology-oriented practitioners of North American twentieth century allopathic medicine constitute almost a blind spot with regard to fasting's merits; this, despite the fact that fasting has been extensively studied and ardently approved for life-threatening conditions ranging from schizophrenia to heart disease by leagues of highly experienced Russian, European and mainstream and holistic American physicians.

In short, fasting itself does nothing to heal the body, except to liberate the body's innate self-healing powers. By removing the constant influx of food, and thereby relieving it of the immense labor of breaking down, assimilating and eliminating a constant stream of nutriments - many of which cannot be properly utilized due to organic stagnation and dysfunction - fasting provides a deep physiological rest to the body, during which time its energies are redirected toward the purpose of unburdening the system of much of its collected toxins.

Fasting facilitates the absorption of non-essential organic structures, dead or diseased tissues, chemical and organic deposits such as drugs, pesticides, lipids and cholesterol, metabolizing and eliminating them through a process of self-consumption. In this process, many if not most metabolic processes tend to undergo normalization: heartbeat, blood pressure, digestive ability, assimilatory and eliminatory ability, sight, hearing, respiration, sleep, and vitality and endurance. Chronic conditions tend to abate, even those which have persisted for decades, and severe conditions rapidly reverse themselves.

It is common knowledge by all those involved in the study of life extension that rat populations routinely underfed tend to live from 30 to 50 percent longer than their freely fed cousins; this tallies well with the aforementioned principle of the enzyme theory, in which it is stated that all foods taken in make a demand upon the body's endogenous enzyme reserve, which becomes increasingly depleted throughout the course of life unless actively replenished, and that, when enzyme capacity is exhausted, life effectively ends.

Some valuable, little known facts about fasting:

* Fasting does not deprive the body of any essential nutrients, whose levels remain remarkably constant throughout even a long fast.
* Fasting can eliminate smoking and drug addictions.
* Fasting slows the aging process.
* Fasting frequently restores lost fertility.
* In the animal kingdom, fasting is a routine practice, both seasonally and in times of illness.
* Fasting is a rite in all religions, and is mentioned 74 times in the Bible.

Brief fasts are relatively easy, make no excessive demands upon the lifestyle, and have the effect of renewing and resting the physiological organism and preventing the buildup of fatigue and the internal accumulation of toxins. They may involve as little time as a single day or three to seven day periods, such as long weekends and vacations.

These may be done on pure water alone or taking freshly pressed juices, with much bed rest and relaxation and a minimal amount of emotional or intellectual stimulation, such as interpersonal encounters, family and social activities, or exposure to media stimulation.

While juice fasting cannot strictly be called fasting, as one is still taking a form of nourishment, it constitutes such a radical abstinence from the burdens of treadmill food consumption and it effects such dramatic physical renewal that, in one sense, it is entitled to be called a fast in its own right. The process of inner cleansing and renewal goes on in a slightly less dramatic fashion, yet without a number of the physical and psychological challenges that can accompany pure water fasting, such as the heightened sensitivity and spiritual openness accompanying prolonged abstinence from food. Likewise one is more likely to experience some periods of weakness as the body readjusts to pure water over a period of days and enters a more hibernatory metabolic pattern, whereas in juice fasting, one's energy level is often experienced to be highly dynamic, and one's mood at times euphoric.

A reasonable plan might be to experiment with a day or two of fresh juice fasting to experience its comfort and exhilaration, repeating this periodically until it becomes natural, and then, when one feels comfortable, to proceed to explore a day or two of pure water fasting and experience its relative effects on the body and mind.

Unless one's family or companions are completely supportive, it is often best to take oneself elsewhere, where one can be at peace while pursuing one's exploration of fasting. Well intentioned intimates often constitute the most stressful of adversaries in this simple process, frequently voicing their reservations out of a private fund of their own fears regarding the matter.

A day or two are required before the habitual gastric reactions signaling hunger subside and the faster is left in relative peace; usually, by the third day, a genuine sense of enjoyment is experienced, along with a long-forgotten sensation of physiological lightness and comfort. Abundant water should be taken, or juice, if a juice fast, and one's exercise should be light and natural. If one feels the inclination to sleep, one should indulge the need for as long as desired. The theme of fasting is physical and physiological renewal through organic rest and tissue repair, which often proceed at a faster rate than when eating.

Upon resuming normal eating after a brief fast, one should make the first meal a juice if one has water fasted, or a dish of fresh fruit if one has juice fasted. Proceed to the next meal from juice to fruit, then from fruit to fresh salad, from salad to lightly steamed vegetables with a low-stress protein or carbohydrate, until one has resumed one's normal eating patterns by the end of twenty four to thirty six hours.

Fasting is neither complicated nor dangerous, and it should not be demonized or mysticalized; it is merely the optimization of the processes which are already and always at work within the body, whether eating, sleeping or fasting.

Further reading:
Bragg, Paul, *The Miracle of Fasting*, Health Science, 1966.
Carrington, Hereward, Ph.D., *Fasting for Health and Long Life*, Health Research, Mokelumne Hill, CA, 1963.
Cott, Alan, M.D., *Fasting, the Ultimate Diet*, Bantam Books, 1975.
Fuhrman, Joel, M.D., *Fasting and Eating For Health*, Griffin Trade Paperback, 1998.
Shelton, Herbert M., *Fasting Can Save Your Life*, Natural Hygiene Press, 1967.

CLEANSING THE CHANNELS

Internal Purification

The United States now has the distinction of having the highest rate of colo-rectal cancer in the world. It is the highest occurring form of cancer

306

amongst the total population of men and women. This information, coupled with the fact that this same population possesses the slowest bowel
transit times leads to an inescapable conclusion: the congested colon is the
genesis of unprecedented disease.

A periodic cleansing of the lower gastrointestinal tract can perform
near wonders in ridding the body of its backlog of uneliminated elements,
providing a lighter, purer chi. While it would be comforting to believe that
the natural eliminatory process would fully perform this cleansing, due to
the decades of dietary and chemical insult that it has sustained, the bowel
harbors a large and growing reservoir of breakdown products and fecal
residues, mucous deposits and encrustations which seriously threaten its
ability to insure a clean bloodstream; for the same blood which now passes
through our cerebrum and our heart, moments later passes through our
intestinal villi and kidney tubules.

As noted eslewhere, in thousands of patients, Dr. Richard Schulze has
routinely observed that more than 85% of disease conditions resolve
spontaneously after a thorough bowel-cleansing program is completed.

It would be beneficial for virtually everyone in a human body living in
the late twentieth century to have the benefit of a periodic colon cleansing,
either in a facility equipped for such procedures or with one of the very
reasonably priced home-units. A minimum of five gallons of tepid water -
sometimes with various cleansing aids added - is gently circulated through
the colon, and periodically eliminated by natural reflexes, unburdening the
lower intestinal tract of age-old wastes and accumulations, freeing the
body of the necessity of absorbing or eliminating these poisons.

While an enema provides some cleansing as well, it is, by comparison,
shallower in penetration and weaker in flow capacity; one should estimate
six enemas roughly equaling a single colonic irrigation.

Colonic irrigation has an immediate purifying effect on the bloodstream, freeing it of systemic breakdown products and ridding it of a great
number of pathogens. While not to be overdone, it is an invaluable aid to
healing and energy-optimization, best undertaken along with a comprehensive modality of diet, exercise, massage and supplementation.

Further reading:
Jensen, Bernard, D.C., *Tissue Cleansing Through Bowel Management*,
    Escondido, CA, 1961.
Reid, Daniel P., *The Tao of Health, Sex & Longevity*, Simon & Schuster,
    NY, 1989.
Walker, Norman, *Become Younger*, Norwalk Press, Prescott, AZ, 1987.

Oral Detoxification

There are certain substances which, due to their highly charged negative polarity, have an affinity for the toxic molecular matter within the body, which is often found to carry a positive charge. Two of the finest of these are clay and charcoal.

Clay

A superb detoxifier, montmorillonite clay will, within a matter of hours, render sterile even highly contagious bacteria and inactivate cultures containing such pathogens as diphtheria, typhoid, cholera and pneumonia. A single quart of liquid bentonite carries the ability to cover and detoxify a surface area of ten football fields.

Regular oral consumption of clay has long been a practice of native cultures, some of whom were found by medical anthropologist Weston Price to always carry portable bags of it on their person, considering it invaluable to their well-being. When Price investigated further, he found that it was blended with water into a thick fluid, then used for dipping foods into immediately prior to consumption, rather like a sauce.

A potent biological catalyst, even a little clay may facilitate major metabolic transmutations within the body, permitting and encouraging nutrient-exchanges on a subtle but broad order of magnitude, and resulting in homeostatic enhancements too numerous to mention. Among them: internal cleansing, better elimination, the resolution of ulcerations of the gastrointestinal tract, improved digestion and assimilation, immune system stimulation, higher resistance to infection, clearer complexion, a marked decrease in pathogenic bacteria in the bowel, decreased body odor, elimination of parasites, and increased energy. In short, clay triggers a full-spectrum physical renewal proceeding from the cellular, to the organic to the systemic level.

Possessing over 70 trace minerals without which the body cannot properly metabolize and utilize nutrients, clay is a micro-crystalline structure which, chemically speaking, is alive; its constituent particles carry a negative electrical charge which bears a natural affinity for the positively charged particles of toxic substances, attracting and binding them to itself first by adsorption (external magnetic bonding), and then by absorption (internal magnetic bonding). A graphic illustration of this effect is that of the typical kitty-litter box, which is sprinkled with a layer of what, upon close inspection, turns out to be largely a derivative of various kinds of clay. This is no accident, but due to clay's inherent ability to act as a living sponge for impurities, adsorbing and absorbing the noxious odor molecules before they escape the immediate area.

Externally applied, clay is no less beneficial in its health-enhancing properties, often working in a manner which so defies explanation as to be called miraculous. Upon wounds, ulcerations, external growths and tumors, skin diseases, rashes and bruised, fractured and broken bones, clay's action is both gentle and powerful, dramatically drawing an increased blood flow into the tissues upon which the clay poultice is applied. Its seemingly 'miraculous' benefits stem largely from this flood of fresh blood, with the enhanced processes of dead-cell removal and tissue regeneration occurring as a result of the increased flow of rapidly arriving oxygen and nutrients.

In a similar manner, clay facial masks effect their cleansing properties, literally drawing toxins out from the pores while pulling the circulation powerfully toward the surface of the body.

Native Americans made extensive use of clay deposits in their healing practices, having observed the instinctual behaviors of wounded and sick animals seeking out clay deposits immersing their wounded bodies in them, as well as consuming it internally.

Further reading:
Abehsera, Michel, *The Healing Clay*, Swan House, Brooklyn, NY, (date unknown).
Dextrait, Raymond, trans. by Michel Abehsera, *Our Earth, Our Cure*, Citadel Press, 1979.
Knishinsky, Ran, *The Clay Cure*, Healing Arts Press, Rochester, VT, 1998.
Pendergraft, Ray, *More Precious Than Gold*, Borderland Sciences, Bayside, CA, 1994.

Activated Charcoal

Activated charcoal is a highly absorbent, gritty black material with a host of highly beneficial uses: 1) as a universal antidote for drugs, chemicals and poisons, 2) as the finest substance for the systemic clearance of drugs and intoxicants, 3) as a general detoxifier, 4) for purposes of anti-aging and life extension 5) for reducing cholesterol, coronary disease and arteriosclerosis, 6) for counteracting pathogens, 7) for counteracting intestinal complaints. It is created by carbonizing organic matter in a kiln under anaerobic conditions.

Charcoal should immediately be taken in a 10:1 ratio with any poison ingested. For systemic clearance of drugs and intoxicants, activated charcoal purifies the 6-8 liters of digestive fluids secreted daily, removing foreign substances from the blood. It absorbs intoxicant substances and their metabolites, excreting them into the small intestine, preventing their reabsorption. Likewise it adsorbs drugs that diffuse back into the stomach and intestines, and it decreases the detoxification work load of the liver. It is the best single substance for systemic detoxification.

Activated charcoal was found by Dr. V. V. Frolkis, a Soviet gerontologist, to extend the mean life span of older test animals by approximately 50%, and their maximum lifespan by approximately 34%. Activated charcoal decreases age-related increase in the brain's sensitivity to drugs and toxins, and has been reported in *Lancet*, the British medical journal, to lower high cholesterol and triglycerides in the bloodstream.

An effective treatment for dysentery, cholera and many infectious conditions of the digestive tract, activated charcoal is nonetheless safe and biologically harmless. It is available in capsules and bulk powder for purposes of daily supplementation.

Further reading:
Cooney, David D., *Activated Charcoal in Medical Applications*, Marcel Dekker, 1995.
Cooney, David D., *Activated Charcoal: Antidotal and Other Medical Uses*, Dekker, 1980.
Cooney, David D., *Activated Charcoal: Antidote, Remedy, and Health Aid*, (out of print).

Psyllium (seed or husk)

Psyllium is a tasteless fiber-like substance which can be added to water or juice, acting very much like an internal broom through its immediate bulking and bonding action with uneliminated intestinal elements, carrying them through and out of the system in an extremely thorough-going fashion. Through its adhering properties it attaches itself quite forcibly to the coatings of mucoid plaque overlaying the internal walls of the intestines, dislodging and eliminating them. For best effect, this should ideally be done in conjunction with various bowel-cleansing herbs and botanicals several times a year. Many uneliminated metabolic byproducts will be removed from the system, and the body will be freed from long-standing toxic burdens (or stagnant chi) with a lightness and clarity indicative of clean, fresh chi.

CLEANSING THE LYMPHATIC STREAM

The lymphatic system is the great unheralded network of channels, ducts and glands responsible for unburdening the bloodstream of its wastes, replenishing the cells with fresh nutrients and transporting metabolic catalysts through the body.

> The lymphatic system represents an accessory route by which fluids can flow from the interstitial spaces into the blood. And, most important of all, the lymphatics can carry proteins and large particulate matter away from the tissue spaces, neither of which can be removed by absorption directly into the blood capillary. *We shall see that the removal of proteins from the interstitial spaces is an absolutely essential function, without which we would die within 24 hours.*
> (*Textbook of Medical Physiology*, Dr. Arthur C. Guyton, p. 351, W.B. Saunders Co., 1986.) (Author's italics, J.M.)

While just 12% of one's body fluid is blood, another 62% of all body fluid exists within the cells of the body itself; lymph constitutes 36% of that fluid, and forms the cell environment. All cells thus depend on the lymph fluid and its circulation, including even such cells as bone cells. Lymph is filled with nutrients en route to cells as well as enzymes and hormones generated by the cells, and waste products excreted by the cells. Thus, constant motion of the lymph-stream is essential. However, there is no lymphatic corollary for the heart in the circulatory system by which to propel this massive quantity of lymphatic fluid through the many ducts.

> While intrinsic contraction in the lymph ducts occurs with their filling with fluid, the major stimulation and pumping action is derived from exogenous (external) factors:
> Almost anything that compresses the lymph vessel can also cause pumping, such as the contraction of a muscle, movements of body parts, arterial pulsations, and even a body massage. Obviously, the lymphatic pump becomes very active during exercise, often increasing lymph flow as much as ten to

thirty-fold. On the other hand, during periods of rest, lymph flow is very sluggish. (*Textbook of Medical Physiology*, by Dr. Arthur C. Guyton, p. 351, W.B. Saunders Co. 1986.)

From the above, it should be clear how crucial the lymphatic system is in the elimination of metabolic wastes, the purification of the bloodstream and the inter- and intra-cellular environments, and further, how dependent these processes are upon mobility, activity and stimulation of the physical body and its processes. Following are discussed three of the most potent modalities for galvanizing enhanced lymphatic metabolism.

Skin Brushing

An excellent, quick and pleasurable way to externally stimulate the lymph flow within the body, a mere 5 minutes of skin brushing with a natural bristle body brush will remove dead epithelial cells while delivering a galvanizing current to the intracellular lymphatic fluid. Performed just after rising, it will create an enlivening tingle throughout the body. Brushing is best done from the extremities toward the main nexus of lymphatic ducts in the thoracic cavity. The great value and effectiveness of this simple tool should not be underestimated.

Rebounding (Trampolining)

The National Aeronautic Space Administration has confirmed rebounding to be the most efficient cardiovascular activity known to man. 67% more efficient in its circulatory and respiratory effect on the body than jogging, rebounding occasions no resultant stress in the joints, tissues or organs, despite the fact that it delivers the maximum biological stimulation of any human activity. Causing the body - and every cell within it - to pass many times each minute through extremes in the gravitational spectrum spanning from zero G's to 3 or 4 G's, rebounding forces a highly accelerated process of cellular respiration, assimilation and elimination, which routinely reaches 400% over normal capacity. In other words, the cells are exchanging fluids, gases and particulate matter (protein waste products) at a vastly increased tempo, optimizing the transport of nutrients and nuclear material for tissue repair and blood cleansing.

Numerous parameters of function are highly beneficially influenced by regular rebounding, including cardiovascular function, respiratory capacity, neurological response, balance, endurance, muscle tone, sleep quality, vision, mood and immunity. It presents a simple, inexpensive profoundly effective exercise activity which is available to all people - young and old, energetic and delicate, healthy or seeking health - year-round, weather notwithstanding.

Further reading:

Carter, Albert E., *The Miracles of Rebound Exercise*, A.L.M. Publishers, Scottsdale, AZ, 1988.

Walker, Morton M.D., *Jumping for Health, A Guide To Rebounding Aerobics*, Avery Pub., Garden City Park, NY, 1995.

Brooks, Linda, *Rebounding for Better Health*, KE Publishing, 1995.

Self-Massage - Sculpting One's Health with One's Own Hands

One of the most ancient and powerful of healing techniques, practiced by many cultures and evolving into numerous diverse systems, massage - in this case, self-massage - can produce truly miraculous benefits in relieving the organism of stress and ridding it of toxins; due to the enhancement of lymph drainage and blood flow, conditions which might have required days or weeks to remedy, have been reversed in a matter of hours or days. The spectrum of effects generated by massage is vast and profound, embracing virtually every system of the body: nervous, circulatory, lymphatic, musculo-skeletal, respiratory as well as chakral and chi-carrying.

Facilitating immediate metabolization of fatigue acids and crystallized toxins, massage aids the bloodstream in its work of penetrating tissues and ferreting out offending substances, not least of which are unassimilated protein by-products; additionally, it enhances the flow of clean blood into these same areas. Lacking its own pump, the lymph system depends on external stimulation to insure its continual drainage of body wastes, achieving these mainly through motion, exercise and deep breathing. Massage lends a mighty hand in stimulating and conducting the flow of lymph into, through and out of its repositories in the numerous lymphatic ducts and channels. One of the most effective physiological cleansing modalities is a 30 to 45 minute massage with an equal blend of unrefined olive oil and peanut oil, commencing at the crown, down the spine, over the head, face and shoulders, into the soft tissues of the abdomen and pelvic girdle, proceeding to the limbs, palms and soles of the feet. It is advisable to first stimulate the hands, taking care to enliven the energy centers in the palms and fingers before proceeding to other areas.

Following such a massage (and requisite shower), there is a notable, sometimes copious drainage through the various mucous membranes - occasionally for hours - and a glow of energetic warmth throughout the system, as well as a great exhilaration and serenity of mind and body, denoting that neurological as well as musculo-skeletal systems have been stimulated, de-stressed and harmonized.

While many esoteric and involved approaches exist in the realm of self-massage, such as shiatsu and Chi Nei Tsang (which targets the Vital Center as its focal point of systemic clearing), the essential thing is to develop a simple, practical wisdom which will enable one to intuitively identify, locate and address physiological stresses, tensions, tenderness and blockages, to a great extent freeing them manually, and enhancing the body's efforts to clear itself and remain energetically open to the universal forces.

After a time, a spontaneous rhythm and sequence begin to evolve, and one's hands almost take on a life and intelligence of their own, moving swiftly and surely from place to place – not always sequentially or logically – but with great assurance and skill. Sometimes the session may be brief and light – requiring a mere ten or fifteen minutes, while at other times the body may not be content with anything less than thirty or forty minutes of penetrating massage, or even longer. One will instinctively know the moment to end the process, by the balance and peace one experiences.

This may very profitably be followed in the morning by an alternating hot and cold shower, shifting the temperature every 30 seconds for several minutes; this provides a potent shifting polarity of stimulation to the blood and lymph, forcing them first to the surface and then deep within the body, with profound cleansing effect. In the evening the massage may be followed by a hot bath into which a cup of unrefined sea salt has been added. Remain until the water cools, resting or retiring for the night afterward. These practices will further purify the energy field of any residual stress.

Further reading:
Chia, Mantak, Healing Tao Books, *Chi Nei Tsang*, 1990.
Chia, Mantak, Juan Li (Illustrator), *Chi Self-Massage: The Taoist Way of Rejuvenation*, Healing Tao, 1991.
DeLangre, Jacques, Ph.D., *Do-In 2: A Most Complete Work on the Ancient Art of Self-Massage*, Happiness Press, 1989.
Reilly, Harold J., Ph.D., D.S. and Ruth Hagy, *The Handbook for Health Through Drugless Therapy*, MacMillan Pub. Co., Inc., NY, 1975.
Tulku, Tarthang, *Kum Nye Relaxation*, Dharma Pub., Emeryville, CA., 1978.

Palma Christi: Castor Oil Packs

Dr. William McGarey, holistic physician and founder of the Association for Research & Enlightenment Clinic in Phoenix, Arizona has this to say of his nearly fifty years of healing experience:

> Of all the many therapies I have used in my practice, none can compare with castor oil in its healing qualities and its variety of therapeutic applications. Sometimes it seems as though castor oil is good for everything that ails us. At the clinic we use it externally and internally, often experimentally, and we almost never fail to get good results.

Its Latin nomenclature translates as 'The Palm of Christ' and derives from its long standing as a traditional healing modality of many ancient cultures.

McGarey goes on to explain that ' . . .the elimination internally and regeneration of the tissue are primary effects when castor oil is applied to the body. If this principle is exercised in therapy, much can be accomplished in the body's healing process.'

Applied externally, as poultice, three to four layers of wool or cotton flannel soaked in warm castor oil are applied under a heating pad directly to virtually any part of the body requiring help or healing. Castor oil packs catalyze a dramatic reversal of many injuries and disease conditions, among them: abrasions, adhesions, appendicitis, arthritis, cancer, cholecystitis, cirrhosis of the liver, colitis, constipation, contusions, cysts, epilepsy, fractures, gallstones, gastritis, hepatitis, hernia, Hodgkin's disease, hookworm, incoordination, intestinal impaction, lesions, lumbago lymphitis, migraine, multiple sclerosis, neuritis, Parkinson's disease, pelvic cellulitis, poor elimination, scleroderma, sluggish liver, sterility, strangulation of the kidneys, stricture of the duodenum, toxemia, tumors, ulcers, and uremia.

Castor oil packs are a particularly excellent systemic lymphatic stimulator, especially when placed upon the lower abdominal area.

Further reading:
McGarey, William A., M.D., *Healing Miracles*, Harper & Row, 1993.
McGarey, William A., M.D., *The Oil That Heals, A Physician's Successes With Castor Oil Treatments*, A.R.E. Press, 1993.

Contemporary Blood-Lymph Purification Technologies

Colloidal Silver

The most effective germicide known, colloidal silver will kill over 650 pathogens and viruses on contact - a stunning statement in light of the ability of most common antibiotics to deal with only six or seven infectious conditions. Considered the most universal antibiotic substance, it is non-toxic in micro-concentrations of 3-5 p.p.m..

Many forms of bacteria, fungus and virus utilize a specific enzyme for their metabolism. Silver acts as a catalyst, effectively disabling this enzyme. Toxic to all species tested of fungi, bacteria, protozoa, parasites, and many viruses, to primitive life forms silver is as deadly as the most powerful disinfectants.

There is no known disease-causing organism that can live in the presence of even minute traces of the chemical element of simple metallic silver. Based on laboratory tests, destructive bacteria, virus and fungus organisms are killed within minutes of contact.

E.M. Crooks has stated ". . . colloidal silver kills pathogenic organisms in three or four minutes upon contact. In fact, there is no microbe known that is not killed by colloidal silver in six minutes or less . . . and there are no side effects whatever from the highest concentration." (Crooks, E.M. *Metals and Enzyme Activity*, The University Press, Cambridge, 1958.)

Among the conditions it has been used successfully on: acne, athlete's foot, arthritis, bladder inflammation, B. Tuberculosis, burns, colitis, cystitis, dermatitis, diabetes, diphtheria, dysentery, ear infections, eczema, fibrositis, gonorrhea, gonorrheal herpes, impetigo, influenza, intestinal trouble, keratitis, leprosy, lupus, malaria, Menier's Syndrome, meningitis, pleurisy, pneumonia, pruritis ani, prostate problems, rheumatism, rhinitis, ringworm, sepsis, septic ulcers, septicemia, shingles, skin cancer, staph infections, strep infections, tonsillitis, toxemia, trench foot, tuberculosis, typhoid, ulcers, warts, whooping cough and yeast infections. (*H.E.L.P. ful News*, Vol 9, No. 12, pp. 1-3)

While the cost of commercial colloidal silver is prohibitive, affordable home units exist capable of producing colloid of comparable or better quality than store-bought products for pennies per quart.

Further reading:
Baranowski, Zane, Colloidal Silver, *The Natural Antibiotic Alternative*, Healing Wisdom Pub., 1995.

Coburn, Dhyana L. and Patrick D. Dignan, *The Wonders of Colloidal Silver*, Plastic Comb, 1995.
Sota Instruments, P.O. Box 1269, Revelstoke, BC, VOE 2SO Canada, 1-800-224-0242 (for home production units).

Blood & Lymph Electrification

A recently implemented modality, the application of cyclic, low voltage electrical currents along relevant pulse-points for several hours each day has produced remarkable reversals in viral, pathogenic and parasitic infections ranging from AIDS and cancer to the common cold. Too remarkable to be readily credible, this healing protocol is the implementation *in vivo* (inside the body) of a technology first devised *in vitro* (outside the body) following a discovery by William Lyman and Steve Kaal, two physicians in 1988 at Albert Einstein School of Medicine, in which the blood of an AIDS-infected patient was drawn, exposed to such electrification, reintroduced into the patient's body, and found to have inactivated the virus' ability to bond to certain life-sustaining enzymes necessary for its existence.

The physicians were quick to qualify the implications of this potentially sensational discovery by describing it as experimental, and predicting an approximate price tag of forty to sixty thousand dollars for the medical cost of implementing a series of treatments in which the blood would be routinely extracted, electrified and reintroduced into the patient. However, physicist Dr. Robert Beck ingeniously devised a non-invasive variation on this modality which uses two relatively simple and inexpensive devices and achieves identical results without complex biomedical procedures or surgery.

Dr. Beck, a victim of lifelong obesity and extremely high blood pressure, points to his own reversal of ill-health through these same modalities, cleansing his bloodstream of parasites, shedding 125 pounds and normalizing his blood pressure in the process. The experimental results obtained to the present warrant a thorough exploration of this information.

Further reading:
Beck, Robert C., *Take Back Your Power*, Sota Instruments, P.O. Box 1269, Revelstoke, BC, VOE 2SO Canada, 1997, 1-800-224-0242 (for Beck materials and home production units).

Bio-Magnetic and Far Infrared WellnessTechnology

While only recently recognized by Western medicine – and now heavily utilized by professional sports physicians - the use of magnets for healing dates back many centuries. Such companies as Nikken of Japan have enhanced magnetics to the point of cutting edge biological effectiveness, with many reports of the eradication of, amongst others, longstanding chronic auto-immune, neurological and circulatory conditions. The key dynamic at work appears to be the restoration of the intra- and extracellular postive-negative polarity, with the resultant facilitation of blood, lymph and chi flow through enhanced bio-conductivity; this assists the body in more rapidly accomplishing its metabolic agenda through deepended physiological rest and heightened tissue repair, through the efficiency afforded by lowered endogenous energy expenditure on the part of the organism while in the presence of benign force fields.

Further reading:
Payne, Buryl*Magnetic Healing; Advanced Techniques for the Application of Magnetic Forces*, Lotus Light, 1999
Nikken Bio-Magnetic Products Information: (Phone) (413) 498 5716

OTHER LIFE SUPPORTIVE PRACTICES

Toning, Chanting and Singing
The Power of Vibrational Vocalizing

Quite apart from any religious or conceptual frameworks, the use of vocalized sound can have a profoundly centering and balancing effect on the human energy field. The human body is sound-sensitive in the extreme, its whole skeletal framework being one huge highly conductive sounding board, while its tissues are composed of crystalline micro-structures whose fundamental purpose is the transmission of impulses and vibrations throughout the entire system. The human body may also be seen as a series of interconnected resonating chambers - the skull, thoracic cavity and pelvic diaphragm - which harbor and amplify the frequencies generated to and by them.

Chanting, sounding and intuitive, creative toning are all effective means of stimulating the neurological and energetic centers and pathways, dissolving subtle blockages, both physiological and psychological, mobilizing dormant energies, and accumulating and directing internal forces for purposes of self-healing, vibrational enhancement, cleansing of psychic environments, and devotional empowerment.

The area of sound embraces dimensions seldom accessed by means of any other modality, and constitutes one of the deepest dynamics of our being. It's sincere exploration will not fail to yield inner rewards.

Further reading:
Campbell, Don, *Music, Physician for Times To Come*, Quest Books, 1991.
Campbell, Don, *The Roar of Silence*, Quest Books, 1989.
Gardner, Kay, *Sounding the Inner Landscape*, Caduceus Pub. 1990.
Gaynor, Mitchell L., M.D. *Sounds of Healing*, Broadway Books, 1999.
Keyes, L., *Toning, The Creative Power of the Voice*, DeVorss & Co., 1973.
La Voie, Nicole, *Return to Harmony*, Sound Wave Energy Press, 1998.

Music - Spirit in Sound

The use of music for the purposes of raising the vibrational levels of oneself, others or environments is of great value; it is also a powerful psychological and emotional catalyst, causing dissociated areas of the psyche to be spontaneously processed, integrated and liberated with the entirety of a person's psychophysical being. An entire modality exists within this realm, known as Guided Imagery in Music, which explores such processes with the aid of a facilitator trained in the relevant techniques.

Further reading:
Campbell, Don, *Music and Miracles*, Quest Books, 1992.
Campbell, Don, *The Mozart Effect™*, Avon Books, NY, 1997.
Lingerman, Hal A., *The Healing Energies of Music*, Quest Books,
    Wheaton, IL, 1995.

Tapping the Energies of the Earth

The density of chi is dramtically higher in the world of nature than the world created by man; thus we can understand the statement regarding the much greater ease of performing wall squats beside a mature tree rather than indoors, due to the ambient chi field emanating from the tree and augmenting our own field. This is a distinct and pronounced phenomenon which can easily be experienced by any sensitive practitioner with relatively little effort. Chi emanates omnidirectionally from the greater universe, but it is most palpably experienced as it issues upward from the earth, downward from heaven, and outward from manifest forms and beings. There are many Taoist practices designed which effectively enhance and augment this man-nature synergy.

A simple, yet potent practice for the restoration of depleted energies or simply the healthful augmentation of one's normal field is to lie upon the ground, preferably over grass, moss or other low vegetation, relaxing one's tensions, and to quietly rest, breathing softly, while gently maintaining the intention of opening and expanding one's field into the greater field of the earth. An immediate process of subtle recharging begins to occur, with energetic and neurological imbalances and excesses coming into equalization, overstimulated areas becoming pacified, and overly intense psychospiritual states dissolving into peaceful awareness.

Should the student find herself in an especially disturbed state, and unable to easily release compulsive thinking or powerful emotions, and to simply yield herself to the earth-field, she should lie face down, pouring her every breath and her consciousness itself into the depths of the ground, with the intention of deeply emptying herself of the conflicted inner energies or stresses; this position encourages and allows for very rapid unburdening of psychic and emotional excesses, as well as the implementation of total trust and surrender, followed by the release of overcharged, uneliminated forces within the system.

Eventually, if done in earnest, this emptying process will come to a natural closure, with a simultaneous sense of relief on all levels, and one will no longer feel inclined to remain in the prone position. It is then time to turn onto one's back and to allow the refilling or recharging process to naturally occur. After a time, the body will instinctually feel like moving, stretching and eventually rising as its reserves and inner balance are replenished.

Further reading:
Chia, Mantak, *Chi Nei Tsang Healing*, Tao Books, Huntington, NY, 1990.
Chia, Mantak, *Awaken Healing Light*, Tao Books, Huntington, NY, 1993.
Kok Sui, Choa, *Pranic Healing*, Samuel Weiser, NY, 1990.

Sexual Energies and Self-Development

While touched upon only briefly in the present text, Professor Pang has expounded elsewhere in much greater depth upon the importance of nurturing and directing one's sexual energies in the course of undertaking the practice of Zhineng Qigong.

The importance of vigilance and care in directing the course of one's sexual energies is paramount. Whereas the common world view of this domain emerges from a concept of fragmentation - as it does with regard to all areas of life - and conceives of reproductive energies as separate and self-contained, with only negligible or peripheral impact on the body-forces proper, the view presented by an entirety-perspective yields a radically different picture.

The sexual and reproductive forces are, in fact, intimately connected with and primary to the integrity of the total energy field of a person, as directly as is a well to a pump. This system provides the root forces which, through a sequence of deeply subtle transmutations and transformations, eventually become our generic life-energy or chi. While there are various complex and ingenious traditional solutions to the challenge of conserving these core energies while still maintaining a life of natural sexual relations - and while the very word 'natural' has itself come to represent many things alien to its essential meaning, due to the severely eroded connection of modern man with primal nature, the safest initial course in these areas is simply a sustained conservation and sublimation of these forces for the purpose of enhancing the body's reservoirs of root energy, or vital essence.

A wisdom not easily accepted or assimilated by those for whom instinctual sexual satisfaction, sensory pleasures, and shared physical intimacy have provided the major gratification, incentive and meaning in life, the idea of harboring the sexual essence may bring forth a distinct rebellion from one's inner being. Even so, such a periodic redirection of these energies may lend a man or woman unexpected internal prowess in a number of unsuspected areas, but this is a matter more for personal exploration and less for specific promises of one kind or another.

This need not be misconstrued as a life-sentence of monasticism or self-denial, but rather an invitation to come into conformity with obscured natural laws by which mankind may harmonize itself with the cyclic progression of nature and the cosmos - not by enforced celibacy and private frustration, but by the participation in seasonally and energetically sensitive relations which respect both human need and human capacity. A deeper study will yield the realization that sexual and reproductive forces and relations ebb and flow in sympathetic resonance to larger natural and cosmological cycles which deeply impact human bio-rhythms and vitality.

Also, it is important to bear in mind that, for those in contemporary Western culture whose entire lives have been openly or subliminally subject to the unceasing persuasions and pressures of mass media and marketing strategies which repeatedly and relentlessly target these vulnerable dynamics in human nature for one's own exploitation, there is a distinct disadvantage already built into their psychic conditioning with regard to sex. In such people, amongst whom may be counted the great majority of Westerners, the pristineness of original sexuality has long been eradicated and replaced by the strategized cosmetic sexualism so rampant in our era. The truly and gently erotic has largely been infected by the manifestly and violently neurotic, and what was once the most natural and chaste of human expressions is in danger of becoming the most unnatural and corrupt.

Further, aside from the immediate enhancements to one's own life and practice, the adoption of a certain respectful distance from the immediacy of sexuality - either one's own or that of others - is the freeing of one's psychic and spiritual energies from compulsive reliance upon the energies of others - either in order to fulfill one's own needs, or the expressed needs of others. In this way, if one does come to choose a life of sexual activity, it may be done in a more conscious and discerning manner, and without the burden of a routine obligation or the drain of unceasing imperative.

Lastly, with the sensitive pruning and watering of this tree of sexuality, it is possible for new outbranchings of heightened aliveness, feeling, perception, insight, empathy and creativity which one might never have imagined, to emerge and blossom.

Further reading:
Chang, Jolan, *The Tao of Love and Sex*, E.P. Dutton, NY, 1977.
Chang, Jolan, *The Tao of Loving Couple*, E.P. Dutton, NY, 1983.
Chia, M. & Winn, Michael, *Taoist Secrets of Love*, Aurora Press, NY, 1984.
Chia, Mantak & Chia, Maneewan, *Cultivating Female Sexuality*,
    Healing Tao Books, Huntington, NY, 1986.
Reid, Daniel P., *The Tao of Health, Sex & Longevity*, Simon & Schuster,

Communion with Oneself -The Inner Smile

Whatever seeming causative factors there may be originating outside of ourselves which affect our lives to different degrees achieve their effect upon us by first finding resonance with conscious or unconscious aspects of our own being, which then proceed to act as catalysts, transmitters or transformers, relaying the initial impetus from the outer to the inner world. To the extent that our systems succeed or fail to yield resonance or conductivity to these initial stimuli is precisely the degree to which we shall or shall not find ourselves impacted by them.

Although it is tempting to attribute praise or blame for our inner condition to the phenomena of the objective world, such a belief encompasses only a very narrow view of the truth.

While the number of levels upon which this phenomenon occurs is far greater than many are presently capable of believing, and is a subject with profound implications in every dimension of life, it may be helpful to approach such an exploration on the simplest level, where one can more easily work with it and perceive its deeper and extended implications.

Many studies have demonstrated the beneficial effects of positive relationships, peer-support, social bonding, friendship, and the presence of pets and many other factors in reinforcing the emotional, psychological, physical and spiritual health of human beings. No one can truly dispute that these represent natural fulfillments for the great majority people, yet few realize the mechanism by which they achieve their healing effects.

In each case, the value or virtue of the contact or relationship emerges from its ability to enable us to feel, to think or to be in a more desirable way. Through such contact, aspects of ourselves are called forth which we ordinarily feel incapable of accessing on our own; in fact, we may well be convinced we do not even possess them. The warmth, the safety, the love or the trust all clearly seem to be entering into our being from without, as gifts of the various people, places or events we are privileged to be experiencing. We have never known it to be any other way, nor has anyone ever intimated that it might be seen any other way.

Yet, there is another perspective, easily missed because it lies so close to us. Modern kinesiology has, through very visible techniques, demonstrated that everything in our immediate environment has a measurable effect upon the energy flowing through our meridians - from the food we eat to the way a certain musical conductor performs a symphony. One very important such test involves monitoring the thymus gland's energy output in response to various stimuli presented, as this gland is the master-controller of life energy and of the body's immune response, as well as the seat of one's personal experience of love. By either enhancing or distorting the natural flow of energy therein, the various stimuli in our lives impinge upon us and cause a similar enhancement or distortion. Likewise, the facial expressions of those about us subconsciously impact our vitality and mood, though we may be entirely unconscious of the process. A frowning face can severely curtail the amount of chi coursing through the meridians, weakening our field and our vitality, while a smiling face can greatly enhance the chi and vitality.

Though we would prefer to think of ourselves as immune from such seemingly innocuous influences, the fact remains that, being interconnected with all things, we are knowingly or unknowingly affected by them. However, the most important factor in this chain of events is the final link - the one closest to us - ourselves. Whatever may or may not be going on in the outer sphere, we have the choice of creating the ideal inner environment for ourselves. This may most easily be done initially through the awareness of one's visage. While wearing a defensive face may succeed in warding off potential predators and threats, it does little to nourish our sense of inner happiness; for we have sacrificed that too for our perceived need for self-preservation. But it may be that a different visage will both deter unwanted interference from outside and yet nourish the internal need for positive energy.

The Taoist sages have long taught the value of what they have termed 'the inner smile'. They teach that when we smile, our organs secrete a sweet essence which nourishes the entire body, and that when we are stressed, or in states of fear and anger, the organs secrete toxic substances which obstruct the energy channels, decreasing the flow of chi, and causing tension, indigestion, insomnia and other problems.

As the eyes are the primary locus of one's psychological and autonomic functioning, they are pivotal in initiating and sustaining the tone of all one's inner states; thus the Taoists advise that the practice of the inner smile begin here. As the eyes are the first to perceive and respond to signals and stimuli, they function as triggers in galvanizing or tranquilizing the processes of the entire human system - psychological, neurological, glandular, cardiovascular and respiratory - in response to life situations.

Allowing the eyes to relax begins a chain reaction throughout the body. The eyes convey the assurance of ease to the face, which relaxes in turn and assumes a softly smiling countenance only faintly detectable from without. This 'inner' smile proceeds to impart a fuller sense of self-fulfillment to the inner person and establishes a living communion with one's own being, bestowing a sense of gentility, love and care, no matter what may be occurring outside ourselves. As this natural sequence of benign gestures is implemented, one's physiology will be restored to balance and free-flow, relieving itself of the crystallized stresses and rigidities.

Whatever one's activity or endeavor, light or heavy, casual or intensive, one may profitably practice the transformation of one's visage into a softly smiling one. If undertaken in a natural way, without force or artificiality, it can relieve both one's persona and one's spirit of accumulated defenses and inhibitions, restoring a sense of self-esteem, trust and joy in living.

When adopted prior and during the practice of Zhineng Qigong, it insures that the exercise is done in a spirit of warmth, enjoyment and serenity and prevents it from becoming harsh or mechanical.

Lastly, and perhaps most important, the practice of the inner smile frees us from the reliance upon outer circumstances and other people in order to access our own joy in living.

Further reading:
Chia, Mantak, *Transform Stress Into Vitality*, Healing Arts Press, Huntington, NY, 1985.

Meditation - Allowing the Primordial Silence to Emerge

The practical benefits of meditation are many, quite apart from its spiritual value. A study of two thousand meditators demonstrated an across-the-board superiority to non-meditators in over thirteen major health categories and disease conditions; among these categories, meditators had 80 percent less heart disease and 50 percent less cancer. Levels of DHEA, (a hormone considered a marker of aging, which, by the end of one's life, normally dwindles to only 5 or 10 percent of its levels during one's twenties), is 23 percent higher in men over age forty-five who meditate than in non-meditators, and 47 percent higher in women who meditate. A great wealth of further clinical studies concerning other extended benefits is available, insuring that the adoption of meditation into one's daily life constitutes a primary means of health-enhancement.

Meditation is our natural state, but our use - and overuse - of the faculties of cognitive consciousness has made it seem rare and elusive. Just as roiled waters spontaneously calm when the wind ceases, so too does the surface of the mind become still when not compulsively driven by thinking.

A lifetime of over-addiction to thought - and a repression of the intuitive realms of our being - has caused the mind to take an almost obsessive role in directing and driving human life.

Meditation, then, is not so much the laboring to build a new 'castle in the sky', or the concentrated effort to implement or construct a 'higher reality' based upon one's private psychospiritual concepts, be they humble or lofty, but rather the plunging of the torch of consciousness into the sea of quietude.

325

Felt at first as a sacrifice, an unfortunate self-loss, this plunge is an act of initial surrender and trust, a release of one's grip upon the lesser life and an invitation to the Greater Life to infuse one's being.

In this dimension, silence reigns. Consciousness ceases to speak to itself, and in the clearing of that airspace one's awareness begins to perceive much to which its compulsive self-dialogue had deafened and blinded it.

The mind moves into relaxation, the nervous and glandular systems shift into balance, the cardiovascular and respiratory systems become quiescent, and an inner poise possesses the whole person.

Once the initial layers of mind and body are becalmed, the indwelling awareness is freed to move further into the regions of silence. On these levels, spontaneous insights are forthcoming, a result of both the emergence of deeper and far more intuitive levels of the psyche as well as the interfacing of one's extended consciousness with transpersonal, universal and transcendent fields of existence and information. This is not, however, a process to be forced or aggressively pursued, for such an effort will only insure the mind's restriction within the very functional levels from which it is seeking to become free - the prison of personal will.

In this sense, if one truly wishes to venture forth into freedom, there is nothing at all that one can do but yield. The pilgrim must travel lightly, with no backpack, wilderness manual or road map, lest she be tempted to prematurely interpret the experiences and insights of the meditative journey by means of her cultural or psychospiritual binoculars; these will only frame and filter the borderless reality which engulfs her until she mistakes it to be encompassed by the aperture through which she views it.

Like the blind men feeling the measure of the elephant - each one adamant as to the contour of its totality – the overly 'well-equipped' seeker will come away from her experience with the numinous with only as much of it as will fit into her spiritual measuring spoon. Touched by the hem of its mystery, she will know that something rare, something special is held within it, yet, incapable of allowing that mystery to live unviolated within her, she may yield to the temptation to define and privatize it: Christian, Buddhist, Judaic, Islamic, yogic, Holy Mother, Divine Feminine, Father God, Great Spirit, and a thousand other human archetypes - heavily colored stained-glass windows - through which mankind has filtered the Light Too Brilliant to Behold.

Yet the Light knows nothing of this human twilight, for the dimness and gloom cast by the many-colored lenses are not so much the presence of darkness as the absence of illumination. With impaired transparency there comes lower conductivity of That which is the essence of life itself, and with the endurance of that obscurity over time the consciousness of mankind becomes convinced that the darkness itself - inner or outer - has the quality of real and essential existence.

In fact, while it is certainly everywhere apparent, paradoxically - darkness does not exist. It is only a transient interface embodying the unmanifest potential of the Source-Light as it, in its expansion, encounters the cognitive differential of lower forms and frequencies of manifestation as yet incapable of rendering It partial or complete penetration.

These ever-resolving layers of transmutational differential comprise the endless process of physical and spiritual evolution of mankind and the cosmos upon all levels.

To attempt to embrace God or to be embraced by God? These are two radically different processes, and our destiny pivots upon which we allow to occur within our lives. The first will return us to ourselves with the deepest convictions of Who and What we know God to be - only to discover that, somehow, as in a bad dream, we are in endless open or covert conflict with a world of others who, deeming that they too have tasted the Divine wine, are equally adamant or even arrogant about their own hard experiential data.

The second will not return us to ourselves at all - something will be missing - or even someone. The highly prized lens will somehow have been stolen, the stained-glass window discovered to be strangely absent, and the aperture to heaven slid startlingly wide open, with ourselves left wordless and undone in the wake of its shed light. Mute, and at a sacred loss to summon the psychological tools created by mankind to even begin to approach or describe this Mystery, we nevertheless sense a thrilling undercurrent running beneath the apparent surface divisions of our world. Our long-grieved isolation from each other is underlit by an inescapable sense of connection and unity - even when our world insists upon and enforces separation upon us.

The sincere practice of meditation, beginning as simply as the cultivation of interior silence and physical stillness, day-by-day, can offer us an unexpected opportunity to step off of the wheel of necessity and into the realm of Grace.

Further reading:
Thakar, Vimala, *Silence In Action*, E.A.M. Frankena-Geraets 1968.
Thakar, Vimala, *Mutation of Mind*, E.A.M. Frankena-Geraets 1966.
Harding, Douglas E., *On Having No Head, Zen and the Rediscovery of the Obvious*, Viking Penguin, NY, 1986.

Khalsa, Dharma Singh, M.D. & Streuth, Cameron, *Brain Longevity*,
    Warner Books, NY, 1997.

As stated earlier, everything we do - every act we perform - whether in the domain of Zhineng Qigong or beyond it, either enhances or depletes the energy with which we live our lives. If the quality of our daily lives – physical or spiritual - can enhance or deprive us of life-force, and thereby yield health and life or disease and death, then it must come to assume major importance in enhancing our practice and our life overall. To that end, this section has offered the serious student an overview of a high chi diet and lifestyle designed to maximize the energy and conductivity in the human life-field. It represents a broad cross-section of the profoundest explorations, both East and West, into human health, well-being and vitality.

While this has been a relatively brief cross-section of a number of such valuable practices and substances, it is in no way intended to be a comprehensive overview of this rapidly expanding field. For that endeavor, further reading is suggested.

Alternative Medicine Digest, Bi-monthly holistic periodical, P.O. Box 1056,
Escondido, CA 92033-9871,   1-800-333-HEAL.
Brennan, Barbara Ann, *Light Emerging*, Bantam Books, NY, 1993.
Goldberg, Burton, M.D., et. al., *Alternative Medicine, The Definitive
    Guide*, Future Medicine Pub., Inc., Tiburon, CA, 1999.
Myss, Caroline, Ph.D., *Why People Don't Heal, and How They Can*,
    Harmony Books, NY, 1997.

Life More Abundant

It is not enough to want life, health and happiness alone - for these may be only empty abstractions which fail to impart power to our spirits, or to galvanize our actions with the passion and purpose of one who truly loves life. Even great force of will and relentless discipline are not sufficient, for these alone may become subtle forms of self-abuse which paralyze the spirit and weary the soul.

It is deeply, crucially necessary to have something to be alive, healthy and happy *for*. The goal of our endeavors needs to encompass a horizon loftier and further than the immediate letter of the laws of practice, however esoteric, dramatic and impressive those principles may be. The human spirit is simply not capable of surviving on a diet of pure functional rationalism - even one of the profoundest kind - and to the extent that it does, what survives is not the essence - but rather a severe compromise - of that which is most truly human in us.

In the end, despite the crush and press of outer fact, man is nothing if not a dreamer. There is no dimension of his being which is not born of dreaming on some level, and his life knowingly or unknowingly becomes the crystallized essence of dream – sustained creative imagination – by which, as in a waking trance, he lives out the role he has fated himself and his world to enact. The abiding irony – if not outright tragedy – of this truth is that we have never been told that we are dreaming, and that our life-experiences - whether tragic or triumphant - are the fruit of our awesome powers of spiritual creativity. And so may pass a lifetime.

No matter how stringent and repressive the personal, social or spiritual structures we find ourselves living within, or how dutifully, fearfully or fanatically we attempt to conform to their demands, protocols and patterns, we are but holding failing fingers in a dike soon doomed to collapse under the immense torrent of creative force dammed within the spirit of mankind. There is nothing and no one that can withstand the unleashing of the evolutionary power of creation. It is the very means by which the universal communes with and conveys its power to the individual.

In the end, one's spiritual life needs to become as spontaneous and instinctual as one's breathing, if it is ever to arrive at true freedom.

Then let us dream noble dreams, dreams of the heart, of the soul, and of the endlessly expanding spirit, and let us have the courage to hold these dreams in an abiding embrace, lest, through weakness of faith, we too soon betray them. And let us allow our dreams to inspire and support our moment-to-moment actions, words and attitudes, lest they remain only dreams. Then will the true meaning of the word 'discipline' come clear - for a disciple is one who learns - not because one must, but because one thirsts for the Greater Life. Such a discipline - a learning - will neither be dead nor empty, but dynamic and full, because it will be ceaselessly expanding throughout all the levels of one's being and of the greater universe. And then our labors truly *will* be light, because they will be those of love.

'I have come that ye might have life, and have it more abundantly.'

- Jesus

Afterword

THE SPIRIT OF WHOLENESS

THE SPIRITUAL DESTINY OF MANKIND:

From Self-Consciousness to Cosmic Consciousness

It may be wondered that, in a book exploring an esoteric Eastern energy art, the subject of spiritual awakening should arise, especially in view of the omission of any such discussion by its founder in the main body of the teachings. Is Zhineng Qigong an esoteric practice without a spiritual dimension? It might at first glance seem so. This may, however, be only a matter of form and not of substance.

Just as the reality of a thing resides in its essence and not its appearance, and the truth of a word or a gesture lies in its tone rather than its form, so too can the spirit of a practice, a way, a discipline or a path dwell as much - and often more - in those things which are not spoken than those which are uttered.

Perhaps the simplest means of determining the genuine quality of a thing or person is by the awareness of their cumulative effects on ourselves or others. "By their fruits ye shall know them" is no philosophical cliche, but an acid test of the most probing kind.

If, while espousing love, an individual or an organization succeeds in injuring, abusing and violating the humanity of another, or the sanctity of life at any level, we may be certain the deeper layers or structure of such an individual or organization is not truly aligned with the ideals expressed, for ends always run true to means.

If, however, without pronounced emphasis on any particular virtues or ideals, we find an individual or organization leaving a path of restoration, healing and deep gratitude in its wake, we can only conclude that, in spite of the notable absence of patent ideologies concerning love and compassion, these have indeed been the fruits bequeathed, again, because ends must run true to means.

If one inclines to objectively examine the fruits of Zhineng Qigong amidst its many beneficiaries and adherents, and also in its institutional, social and financial - as well as its human - domains, it might well present a picture of having given the greatest benefit and the least injury - on many different levels - to the greatest number of people. Can we say that these benefits have not extended into the spiritual realms of those involved? Is not being lifted from death into life necessarily an experience of the deepest spiritual nature? Is not moving from hopelessness into hope a resurrection of the soul? Is not feeling the genuine and abiding care of one's fellow seekers - strengthening what was weak and mending what was broken - the profoundest embrace of one's being?

The Entirety Theory so deeply plumbed by Professor Pang does not cease at the borders of science, because, as that very principle affirms, in reality there are no borders. What borders there may seem to be are only the dotted lines placed upon the unfathomable totality by the minds of explorers who did not know how else to begin to take the measure of Infinity. But entirety is nothing if not whole, and wholeness is not merely an aggregate of parts synthetically juxtaposed into a nightmare of artificial togetherness - it is an intrinsic indivisibility, a presence whose center is everywhere and whose circumference is nowhere. In that everywhereness is everything - every *thing* - that is, or was or will be, on every level and in every dimension, from alpha to omega, in substance and spirit, now and forever. This is none other than the 'world without end' whose mystery has defied every mortal attempt to unveil it.

When humanity comes into a sustained dynamic awareness of this entirety, and of its participation and the participation of all other beings in this entirety, its daily existence will, without design or premeditation, come very close to being a sacrament of living reverence.

But this is not yet, at least not for most, for there are shadows to be dispelled. The greatest tool and the most brilliant faculty of humankind, by which it insures its survival, its adaptation to life, and its future growth, has threatened to become its greatest liability - the intellect.

The gift of the ages, the image-making facility so unique to human consciousness, has become the most brilliant and the most dangerous of double-edged swords. By it, man can remake his world in accordance with his self-created thought-forms, and by it also he can blind himself to the unity of Being and 'put asunder what God has joined', misconstruing the idea for the very thing it represents.

Since the dawn of the mind, humanity has mistaken its belief systems for reality, and has confused its cultural icons for the truth. So precious have been the archetypes by which humanity has steered its perilous course through the unknowns of the universe - its racial, cultural and creedal identifications - that it has been willing to sacrifice its very existence rather than relinquish and go beyond them.

The transcendence of all fragmentary identifications - racial, societal and personal - is the ultimate mandate and destiny for humankind, carrying with it the promise of a life unimagined; then and then only will the human race begin to tread the path of true freedom, and to move into the dimension of its highest potential.

This transcendence of limited identification is not a matter of cold detachment from - or monolithic impersonality to - the world, but rather the liberating of thought and feeling from their entrenchment in self-invested fragments of life - whether family, church or political ideology - and a choiceless extension of our humanity throughout the totality of existence. In this opening, one's family remains as dear as it ever was, but one finds oneself possessed of a spontaneous affection and concern for others and one's world which consistently call forth the deepest levels of care and compassion commonly reserved solely for intimates.

In its profoundest aspect, love is neither a deep feeling nor a fond sentiment, neither an ardent passion nor an overpowering attachment - for in the name of all of these humanity has justified division, conflict, alienation, and even genocide. The Creator's lament, 'The voice of thy brother's blood crieth to me from the ground' is as true today as it was when it was first uttered (Genesis 4:10).

In its essence, love is rather the silent, overwhelming awakening to the absolute and indivisible oneness of all creation - cosmic, terrestrial, human and non-human. Without this perception, humankind will continue to mistake the reflection for the reality.

Humanity is now poised - as it has ever been - on the razor's edge of extinction and survival, torn by the dual forces of human bonding and mortal strife, affinity and alienation, and what it is pleased to call love and hate.

A multi-dimensional being of spirit and light beguiled by evolution and the limitations of embodiment into the illusion of being merely a tiny, circumscribed and localized entity totally identified with and conditioned by the cultural matrix in which he dwells, man has become the prodigal son, abandoning his infinite inheritance for a pauper's estate.

Fearful that true awakening from the dream of selfhood will spell the end of its private reality and personal existence, humankind has both consciously and subconsciously avoided its inevitable confrontation with truth, attempting to move against the momentum of evolution, in order to cling to a few brief moments of illusory safety. Unable to see further than the walls it has built, humanity doesn't realize that just beyond its self-made interior world lies a realm undreamed of - and only obliquely hinted at in the teachings of the awakened. Man - as do all fearing beings - is only able to see the contents of his own consciousness; and if perchance he does dare to look beyond them, glimpses only an abyss - a fathomless void whose terror drives him back upon himself, to re-occupy the safety of his prison.

The knowledgeable and the clever are not spared the awesome threat of this vision; they merely possess a great many more psychological tools and toys with which to preoccupy themselves, lest they inadvertently see what they would rather not have seen. Foremost among these are those who purport to be explorers of truth themselves, the 'wise' and the 'spiritual', the 'intellectual' and the 'philosopher', and those of the church, the mosque and the temple, as well as the temples of the secular world - the university and the 'halls of higher learning'.

After fear, knowledge reigns as the most powerful deterrent to a direct encounter with reality. The psychic evolution of humanity has reached a fateful point, a place in which the abiding intensity and compulsiveness of his conceptual life has superseded the perceptual openness and clarity which is the indispensable prerequisite to an experience of Primal Being. Deep within humanity, at the level of the racial unconscious, there dwells an abiding fear of self-loss. At this level, man instinctively knows that to become the whole is to relinquish the part, and that to be all is to lose oneself. Like a swimmer suddenly lifted by a wave into an overpowering inter-continental current, he senses the immanent danger of being deprived of the safety of the shallows and thrust irrevocably into the fathomless depths to be carried he knows not where.

Religion is helpless to rescue here, for it belongs to the realm of thought, belief and memory, the relative surface layers of humanity's being, and is of little use to one who has been carried out into deeper waters. To know the truth - yes, means to be free - but to be free through being completely denuded and divested of all unreality, all falseness and all illusion, whether inborn or acquired, culturally-sanctioned or personally compelled. Going further, it implies the dissolution of the myth by which - as a parasite - illusion thrives: the autonomous, separate self.

If cultures - seeking safety - will not do it, if nations - seeking supremacy - will not do it, and if individuals - seeking security - will not do it, who in our world will do it? Who will trade the claustrophobic chamber of self-hood for the infinite horizon of freedom? To dare to strip away not only one's social conditioning, but also one's pedigree of race, cultural loyalties, gender pride, and even one's personal ego, and to immerse oneself in the depths of pure Being or Original Consciousness - in which no self-reflectivity survives - is this not asking too much of ordinary mortals?

No one will do it - until the ache and the torment of the self-conscious life reaches its terminal phase, until the separation and alienation from the greater life becomes impossible to bear, and until our very being spontaneously convulses and shatters the side show mirrors of the illusion of self.

The truth is - without access to our source and origin - or in more traditional language, without God - we are not merely discontent and destitute - we are in a state of spiritual suffocation - of living death. In this light, God becomes not merely a sacred idea, a secret refuge or even a divine touchstone - but a desperate and blinding necessity.

Religions, despite the loftiness of their principles and agendas, and the moral virtues of their adherents, have to a regrettably great degree failed to embrace and embody the very lights by which they have come to exist, shattering into a maelstrom of warring belief-systems and factions, in which their most sacred ideals are severely compromised.

Sensitive and caring people existing within these structures intuitively sense and suffer from an unspoken isolation from the living numinous presence, despite their depth of faith, denominational loyalty and purity of intention. Humanity's deeper being instinctually apprehends the provisional and restrictive nature of the institutional structures and concepts by which his surface self attempts to frame the Infinite, and according to the capacity of his self-honesty, he either constricts further within these pillars of security which reinforce his inherited beliefs, or he expands outward, together with all the rest of creation, into the unknown.

While these two options are always available to all who tread the path of life, there comes a moment in the journey of the true seeker when she can no longer be satisfied or enticed by safety and sameness, or for that matter, by restriction to or within any form of structure at all. At this point there is no longer any choice, and the cocoon opens, never to close again.

At present, the evolution of the overwhelming body of humankind is still snared in self-protective structures which, like nested concentric circles, encompass its potential universality: the self, the other, the family, the institution, the social framework, the national identity, the racial portrait and the species pattern, with the immediacy of true human care and compassion falling away in parallel perspective with these receding rings of identification.

Yet, dimly or brightly, the flame of infinity is at work in all its creatures, kindling an unrest which can never quite be extinguished, even as we find ourselves entangled in self-illusions and denials. Every moment of open wonder, every glance that dares to look beyond its own portal, every flash of listening that awakens to a song beyond its own imagining, every instant in which the mind risks emptying itself of its ancient, jealously kept heirlooms of memory and knowledge - are the breaking forth of eternity within us, and the invitation to release ourselves from out of the shoals and into the deep.

It is here that the concealed spirituality of Zhineng Qigong may providentially reveal itself, in offering self-enclosed humanity the simplest of tools for unlocking the shackles of separatism and enforced confinement in the world of duality. Through its humble exercises and visualizations, it may kindle the long-forgotten memory of freedom, of greater being, and foster an awareness of life which transcends the narrow corridors of self-interest and self-preservation which have become the hallmarks of humankind, launching it into an awakening which takes in the shimmering totality of existence - cosmic consciousness.

And so it is for freedom, awakening and enlightenment. Ours it must be - whether now or at the end of all time. The 'when' is for us and us alone to decide. But one thing is certain, whenever that may be, we shall see the world and all its inhabitants magically metamorphose before our eyes from separate and alien creatures into living extensions of our very own being.

And then there will be compassion without effort, love without boundaries, and life without end.

> . . . *Lead me from the unreal to the real,*
> . . . *Lead me from darkness to light,*
> . . . *Lead me from death to immortality* . . .

- Brihad Anranyaka Upanishad (c. 1200 B.C.)

Joseph Marcello
May 10, 1999

Appendix A

THE VITAL CENTER OF MAN

Kaneko Shoseki: Nature and Origin of Man

Turning to the writing of Kaneko Shoseki, who became a powerful healer after a partial enlightenment experience in 1910 after many years of practice of Zen Buddhism, we find further cross-cultural corroboration of the primal role of the Vital Center of Man, and the revelation of a further level of meaning approaching its transcendent aspects:

If one concentrates all of the activities of the mind which are normally directed outward, that is, ideas, judgments, feelings, volitions and even the function of breathing, in fact if all the life energy is concentrated in the center of the body, in the tanden (*dantian*), a new sphere of consciousness arises within us which completely transcends the opposition of objective and subjective, of outward and inward and even our usual, vague sleep-clouded consciousness. This leads to the absolute and final stage of spiritual experience in which one realizes that God himself lives and works as the highest principle and the Primordial Source of life in every single being, as well as in Nature as a whole. That which reigns in the individual as the unmediated administrator of the Divine Law within every human being is what I call the 'primordial I' or the original One. For it is not only that from which all man's activity, whether conscious or unconscious, proceeds, but also it is the one thing in man which belongs completely and directly to the highest Being. Realization of this is the deepest experience which the human mind can reach.

To every activity of body as well as of mind the function of breathing stands in the closest relationship, a relationship which is not only a physiological one but an immediate essential one. For between the original One and the external ego there are two connecting links, namely breathing and the system of the 14 keiraku (energy channels).

By keiraku I mean those imperceptible fine passages in the body which connect bones, muscles, brain, intestines, the senses, etc. with each other and eventually reconnect them all with the primal Life Force. Like the blood vessels and nerve fibers connecting all the inner organs, they run through the whole body, mostly alongside the blood vessels. But in relation to their function the keiraku are quite different - their function is in the nature of supervising the circulation of blood and the movement of thought and allowing each individual organ to work harmoniously with all the others. They neither nourish the organs nor are they controlled by the brain. They are, so to speak, a network of passages which transmits to all parts of the body the spiritual-physical rhythm of the Life Force. Thus the keiraku working together with the Life Force, which unites them in itself, are the only parts of man which belong unqualifiedly to the universal Life. Furthermore we can apprehend them by this - that in death they disappear completely, that no trace of their existence can be found in a corpse. . .

Apart from the normal communication between men through language and action there is another quite different sort of mutual influence. It is that of the rhythm of the Original strength which permeates all human beings and all Nature. Through it every individual thing in essence and, as it were, underground, is connected with every other. If then one who is further removed from the working of the Primordial Force is close to one who lives more in accord with it, the rhythm of the Primordial Force will certainly be transmitted from the one to the other. The latter, without knowing it, exerts a good influence on the former. . .

The relation between artistic creation and the tanden, the seat of the Primordial, is immediate and essential. Neither the hand nor the head should paint the picture. It is a necessary condition for the expression of the essential in all art that the artist should empty and free his head, and then concentrate his whole energy in the tanden. His brush will then move of itself in accord with the rhythm of the Primordial Force.

When the Primal Force, ever working gradually within us, finally reaches the highest peak of its activity, then out of the thick heavy fog of ordinary consciousness there bursts forth from the eternal Being the clearest possible state of consciousness . . . Here no fixed form is perceptible, neither an object nor an I, neither an inner nor an outer, breathing is suspended, the bodily shell completely vanished. Here no body exists, no mind, neither man nor world. The ego is completely at one with the world. What alone reigns in this experience is Universal.

The primal Force of Life, exactly like water rushing swiftly through a tube, streams from eternity to eternity whirling around in the lower part of one's body. . . .

Reference:
Von Durckheim, Karlfried Graf, *Hara, The Vital Centre of Man*, Allen & Unwin, 1962.

Appendix B

THE VITAL CENTER OF MAN

Hakuin Zenji: Yasen Kanna

Perhaps Hakuin Zenji (1685-1768) is most eloquent on the primacy of the Vital Earth-Center in restoring the balance of the life-force, in his justly admired treatise, *Yasen Kanna (Tales Told In a Barque of an Evening)* This document details his near-death prostration from severe psychophysical exhaustion as a young man, in the wake of years of extreme spiritual efforts, and his apocryphal pilgrimage to one Hakuyshi, a Taoist master of great wisdom and accomplishment, from whom he receives the secrets of life. An uncanny embodiment of the profoundest essences of Taoism, Chinese medicine, and ultimately, of natural Zen or spontaneous awakening, this rare treasure has come to assume the stature of a spiritual classic.

Yasen Kanna
Various Tales Told on a Barque of an Evening
by Hakuin Zenji

Foreword by Kito (the Starving and Freezing One),
of the Hermitage of Poverty, a pupil of Master Hakuin.

In the spring of the seventh year of the Horeki era (1757), at the Zodiacal sign of the Ox in the fourth duodenary of the Calendar, the proprietor of the book store in the capital, called Shogetsu Do, sent a letter written to the close disciples of our Kokurin (Hakuin), written in the present handwriting, begging us in the following words:

"With humble respect I have heard of the existence of some old manuscripts by the Master - and among these papers, also a draft by the name of *Yasen Kanna* (Various Tales Told on a Barque of an Evening). In this work, so it has been said, he has very carefully written down precious mysteries - the secrets of how to nourish the soul, and to exercise and provide power for the spirit, to further the circulation and to keep one's elasticity, thus enabling one to live to a very old age. Indeed, this work possesses the secret of the saints, the essence of 'Rentan' - or what is termed the divine elixir of life. There are those who are greatly curious and desire so much to look into this book - the wise men of the world who know the good things of life. Their desire is as strong as the desire for rain in the driest of times, who think of this document as of a rainbow glowing in the firmament after a long draught. Several itinerant monks have betaken it upon themselves to transcribe this work furtively, keeping it as a great secret, but would never have shown it to others. It is as if mighty treasures of heaven were being uselessly preserved in a great chest. Therefore, this editor humbly requests that this precious draft be published and given as long a life as the catalpa tree, in order that the thirst of the people be quenched.

I understand that your revered master, even in his elder years, is ever willing to be of help to the world. Thus, if you feel there is something in this draft which may be of aid to us ordinary mortals, assuredly, he will not deny it to us."

This letter was then dispatched in duplicate, and the pupils went to their master to give him the letter. The old man only smiled. Then his pupils rummaged inside a chest full of old manuscripts, most of which were almost completely worm-eaten. From them the pupils took the manuscript of 'Yasen Kanna' and copied it out, until it had reached 50 pages. They are being bound in paper covers and sent to the teacher in the capital. But before we send it to Kyoto, I, as the oldest among them, am obliged to write a foreword.

The teacher said:

"Already this teacher (myself) has been living in this temple of Shoinji for about forty years. Since I first took up my alms-bowl three generations of hemp-robed monks have crossed this threshold. They have endured my poisonous spittle and the painful strokes of my rod, but they have neglected to go away, some staying on as long as twenty years now. Some seem undaunted by the prospect that they may become part of the dust beneath the Swan-Grove of this temple. They are the 'Fairest Flowers' of many regions, eminently good Buddhist monks of the first class. They live in old houses, dilapidated huts, and broken down shrines around our temple, and live miserably, going hungry by day and freezing by night, eating nothing more than leaves of vegetables and oats, winning from the Master Hakuin only admonishments and reprimands, feeling only the blows of his hand and his stick, that which they see causes them to furrow their brows, and that which they hear causes them to perspire. The very gods must surely weep for them, and the demons can only put their hands together and pray for them.

"When these beautiful young men first came here, they looked like Sogyoku and Ka-an, so attractive were their appearances, and so like fine oil did their skin shone. But even they soon became meager and pale, like To-ho and Ka-to, their bodies drying up and their faces becoming haggard. If one were to meet them on the shores of the lagoon they would appear to be bent and wizened old things. If they were other than in essence the very Bodhisattvas of beings, bold and strong of spirit, disregarding the comfort of their bodies, what reward could there ever have been for them in huddling together here for such a long time? But because these men have been too harsh in their disciplines they have suffered excessively, their lungs shrinking and their bodies becoming weakened. They suffer with indigestion, pains in their loins, and other illnesses difficult to cure. Even I, who had never been too well, and pale, can no longer restrain myself, but must rouse my hoary old head and attempt to give them nourishment from my ancient breasts by sharing with them the secret of what I have come to call inner-reflection.

"Allow me to here say also that if there is anyone who has practiced meditation and knowledge of the Way, and who is an advanced disciple, who yet experiences bouts of dizziness and great weariness - as if the five internal organs are out of harmony with each other - that if he attempts to cure his sufferings by the use of the three arts of acupuncture, moxibustion and drugs, it would be most arduous for him to heal the worst illnesses, even were he Ka-da or Henso. However, I possess the secret of the hermit's elixir of life. My friends, I do hope you will give it a fair trial, for early will you see wonderful benefits. It would be for you as if the sun, emerging through the obscuring cloud-mists at night, were breaking over the earth in its full glory.

"Who wishes to try it should cease all thinking and all koans. First, learn to sleep your fill. But before you sleep, before you close your eyes, stretch out both legs straight and equally, pressing them together tightly and concentrating the spirit force of the whole body under the navel (Kikai-Tanden), in the loins and the legs, and also in the middle of the soles of the feet, allowing these all to become full, while at the same time reflecting upon the following ideas:

"This, my body, - my Kikai-Tanden - and all areas below my navel - my loins, legs and foot-soles - these are the true face of my primal and essential Being; what need have I then of nostrils here?

"This, my body - my Kikai-Tanden - my loins, legs and foot soles - these are the clear country of my origin - my true home - and what need is there of knowledge of any other home?

"This, my body, - my Kikai-Tanden - and all areas below my navel - my loins, legs and foot-soles - these are in very truth the pure landscape of my soul - and what need is there of any other splendor?

"This, my body, - my Kikai-Tanden - and all areas below my navel - my loins, legs and foot-soles - these are truly my very own Amida Buddha, and what principle of wisdom does he teach me?

"If one continues to ask these questions, bringing their ideas again and again into one's mind, looking for these and asking these of oneself, one will then find that, when the success of this continuous looking within accumulates, as if unconsciously, it happens that all of the spirit forces come to fill the Kikai-Tanden, the loins, the legs, and the soles of the feet, until the area below the navel will become firm, like a ball of leather which has not yet been pounded to softness. And if you use inward-looking in this manner and continue for five or seven days, or perhaps even unto twenty or thirty seven days, then all the hitherto existing griefs, weariness, and illnesses (the five aggregations and the six accumulations of sickness) will be healed, until nothing remains of them. And if not, cut off the head of this old priest and carry it away with you.

"When my pupils heard this, they were overjoyed and filled with gratitude, bowed and began to practice as the master admonished. And each of the pupils personally undertook this teaching and saw great success. Whether they succeeded quickly or slowly depended upon the degree of correct practice, but almost all were healed. And each monk praised the success of this exercise of looking-within. Then the Master added: Don't be satisfied with the healing of illnesses, but go further. If the illness heals, exercise further! And if you get satori, exercise yet again! As an old priest I say to you: when I was on the beginning of my path as a Zen pupil I myself developed a serious illness and suffered pains and griefs ten times worse than you. I became unable to move. In this way I came to the verge of despair. And I thought to myself: I would like to come to death. It should be better to put away this old leather-bag of bones as soon as possible, rather than to carry on, living with all these pains and griefs. But, oh what joy, then, when I was taught this secret method and I completely healed myself, as it should be with you. My joy was like yours.

"The master of all masters, Hakuyushi, teacher of this Hakuin, once said: 'This will be the technique of the saints to gain eternal youth and to attain a great age. Already men of middle and lower classes could live a span of 300 years if they would master it, and men of the first class could live without seeing the end.' I myself was glad to hear about this technique and I practiced it during some three years; as a result both spirit and body, my health and my vital forces had gained extraordinary power.

"But I began to wonder within my mind that although I might succeed in this exercise and could now live 800 years like Hoso, would I be more than a cadaver without a soul? More than an old badger sleeping in his nest, leaving behind only the dust of dissolution? Also, I would come into ruin and to death sooner or later. Why have I never had companions such as Kak-ko, Tek-kai, Cho-kwa, and Hi-cho (the immortal ones!)? Therefore it would be better for me to enact the four great vows, to acquire the dignity of a Bodhisattva, fulfilling the works of the law, and to perfect for myself a great body of Truth made of diamond-substance, one which never dies because it is without birth.

"Thus I found several like-minded persons - Bodhisattvas -who came to probe these mysteries with me. With them I practiced the method of looking within, and also meditation. With them I cultivated the hermetic virtues, and with them I strove for more than thirty years. Every year several more have increased our number, until now there are more than two hundred who have gathered here. There are, in our community, monks who have hailed from all parts of the land, those who have undergone work, weariness, sorrow, those of pity, whose souls cause them dizziness and near madness. I taught these monks, who, because they have become ill by too much wrong spiritual exercise, the practice of looking within and quickly healed them. The more they understood, the more they practiced, in order to further experience satori.

"This year I am seventy years old, but I don't see the shadow of an illness; the teeth are strong and good, the eyes and ears become better and better. Mist in my mind is forgotten now. Twice a month I hold sermons and never become tired. Also, I have preached to three hundred or five hundred men and sometimes have spoken to assemblies of monks about the sutras and the words of the patriarchs during the course of fifty to seventy days. And I did this from fifty to sixty times without ever missing a day, never once having been obliged to foreclose any meeting before concluding it in proper fashion; but yet the spirit and bodily forces are now more eminent than when I was twenty or thirty years old. And I believe it all comes from the experience gained by looking within. The pupils living in the temple pleaded, 'Please write down the plan of the precept of looking within. Teacher, please, please, out of your deep compassion and by this treasure save our newly arriving brother students of Zen, who may in future suffer from the self-exhaustion that comes with hard za-zen.' The master acceded to this request and the draft was soon ready.

"What is the essence of that which is embodied in this document? To nourish life and to live long, one must exercise the right form. To exercise that, one must concentrate the spirit in the Tanden, pressing it down deeply under the navel. Only if the spirit is sitting (situated) there, is the mind's force thus concentrated. And if it is concentrated there, then the elixir of life can be produced. And if the life-elixir is thus produced, the outer form becomes strong and firm. And if the form becomes strong, then the spirit becomes perfect, and life becomes long. And this is the secret of the saints to gain the True Tan (Tanden), as well as of the nine revolutions of the elixir of the hermits in its most perfect form.

"And you should know that the True Tan is nothing emanating from outside, that is, not from finite things. By it, it is intended that you should descend your heart's fire (spirit-breath) a thousand times into the Tanden, the space below the navel, filling it with force. If those of you here and all of my disciples in this Temple are diligent in undertaking this and practice this exercise with care, further in this wise, not only will the over-meditation illness be healed and the weariness of body be eliminated; and not alone this, but the awakening process of Zen itself will be greatly enhanced with it, and in times to come those who had despaired for so many years will clap their hands, because they will see great things and great joy. And why? Look!

If the moon is high,
The shadows of the castle disappear.

'On the twenty-fifth day, fourth calendar insignia, in the seventh year
of the Horeki Era (1757)
By the Master of the Refuge of the Starving,
Penniless and Freezing,
Sitting in Incense, bowing his head.'

"On the beginning of my Buddhist journey - the very first day I went into the mountains to study and meditate, I swore to exert my full powers and to be bold in faith, working hard in my pursuit of the discipline of the Way of Truth. But after two or three wintry seasons had come and gone, during which I undertook the most arduous exercise, suddenly, one night, the breakthrough came. Doubts that had hitherto existed melted completely away, like ice in warm water, and the root of karma, of the cycle of life and death, disappeared without a trace, like froth on the face of the sea. I thought to myself: So the Way is not so far off from man! But my

343

predecessors have toiled for twenty and thirty years; what a swindle this story is! I danced in happiness for a few weeks.

"But as I looked upon my daily life, seeking clarity, I saw that my movement and my stillness were not in harmony. Both in action and in inaction I wasn't free. I thought to myself: 'Begin once again; take courage once more and practice in the name of Life, with all that you have.' I clenched my teeth, opened wide my eyes, and determined to avoid sleep and to fast. Before a month was gone the blood climbed from heart to head, the lungs became weak, and the legs like ice. In both ears was a rushing sound, like a stream in a valley. Liver and bile did not function. During the day I was afraid. Heart and soul were so weary. In sleep and waking, illusory worlds arose; sweat broke out from my armpits and both eyes filled with tears. In this condition I applied to a few of the Zen masters and asked the help of various doctors. No medicine helped.

"Somebody had said: 'Beyond the mount of Shiowhawa (White River), beyond the capital, dwells a hermit high up in a cave of rocks. People call him Hakuyushi. He is very old, people believe from 180 to 260 years old. He lives some miles from human habitation, for he does not like to see people, and if they go he will run away and conceal himself. People do not know if he is a sage or a madman, but the villagers say that he is a Sennin - a mountain immortal. They say he was once the teacher of Ishikawa Jozan, and that he is deeply versed in the science of the stars and the lore of medicine. And if somebody asks him very respectfully their questions, he will answer, but only very seldom, and in few words. But if you reflect upon what he has said during the homeward journey, you will derive a deeper wisdom from it, which will enrich your life with great benefit.'

"In the middle of January 1710 I quietly put together some traveling things and undertook the journey. Carrying my baggage on my shoulders I went from the province of Mino through The Black Valley finally coming to the village of White River. There I left my baggage in the tea room and asked for whereabouts of the hermitage of Hakuyushi. A villager pointed at a mountain brook which looked, from afar, like a branch of wood. I followed the rushing of this brook further into a remote mountain valley. Following it straight up for a couple of miles, I found that it suddenly disappeared. There was no path and I was at a loss; unable to go on, I stood in dismay. Helplessly I sat down on a stone to one side, and with closed eyes and palms joined repeated a Sutra. Like a miracle there fell upon my ears the far-off sound of ax-blows in the distance; following the sound through the woods, I came upon a wood-cutter. The old man gestured toward the mountain mists looming from afar, and I could distinguish a tiny patch of white-yellow color, which appeared and disappeared at the whim of the mountain wind. 'That,' the old man told me 'is a reed shade which Hakuyushi himself made to cover the entrance of the cave.'

"Then I tidied up my clothes and climbed up the rocks. Water, cold like ice and snow, soaked into my sandals! In the mist and cloud my clothes became wet through and through. Soon I was covered with sweat as a result of my pains and efforts. Then I came into the shade.

"Up there the landscape was of unearthly clarity and beauty so that I felt as if I had left the world of men. A dread gripped my heart and spirit, and I was shivering as one who was stripped naked.

"I leaned on a rock and collected my breath for several hundred respirations. Then, after a time I ordered my clothes, arranged my collar, and went ahead with reverent awe. Taking the reed shade aside, I bowed respectfully in the semi-darkness. I saw the master sitting in meditation with half-closed eyes. His hair hung, black, to his knees; his cheeks were red, full of life, like rose buds. From his shoulders draped a cloth, and he was sitting on a soft pillow of grass.

"In the cave, about three yards square, there was nothing of household items or foods; on a low table were three books: Lao Tzu's *Tao Te Ching*, the *Doctrine of the Mean of Confucius*, and a Buddhist book, the *Diamond Sutra*. I began to speak very politely to tell him about my illness and to beg him for salvation.

After some time he opened his eyes, looked at me, and slowly began to speak.

'I am only a man driven into these mountains, half-dead, old, and useless. I eat only chestnuts, wood apples, sleep with stags and does, knowing nothing for the rest. I am in shame for such a great priest having taken pains in coming to me, with no answer for him.'

"So nothing remained for me but to again bow to him and more urgently repeat the entreaty. Finally he looked at my hands and examined my whole body - the various openings therein and the five internal organs, and continued on, examining the nine markings on my fingernails; these were only half an inch in length (or half of what they should have been). And then, as if in pain, his face was furrowed with critical wrinkles. His long-nailed fingers passed over his forehead, as if in empathy. He said,

'It is a pity the illness went so far. There was too much overly strenuous concentration and strict ascetic practice, and you have lost the natural rhythm of spiritual growth; therefore you have got this serious illness, which appears too difficult to heal. The chance of recovery may be lost. Really, this meditation sickness is something difficult to help, even by using the three methods, acupuncture, moxibustion and medicine - and by taking pains under the care of the best doctors, like H and K, nothing would succeed. You must cure it by looking within yourself (Nai-kan), because you have come to this illness by too much thinking on truth (Ri-kan); in any other way you will never recover. It is said, "If you fall down to the ground, you must begin to rise once again from the very ground from which you fell," and the method of Naikan - inward looking - is a demonstration of this principle. Unless you now gather up the goodness of this method of introspection, you will see that finally you will not be able even to stand.' - And this he meant literally.

"I replied, 'How I would like to learn the secret of looking inward from you, and once having learned it, to carefully practice it in the temple also.'

"Hakuyushi sat solemnly and answered with great quietness: 'Ah, such a man are you - a true seeker - who really wishes to hear these things? Then I may pass on to you a little which I myself have heard in earlier times. The secret of replenishing the life is something known only to a few men; if you are not too remiss in carrying it out, you will receive not only a wonderful effect, but also you may hope for a long life.

" 'The Great Way (Tao) divides itself, manifesting in two forces: Yin and Yang, from whose harmonized interaction emerge all living things, human beings and all else. Due to the harmonious interplay of their innate forces, all the inner organs are ordered and connected together by the innate vitality (ki-energy) moving silently in the Vital Center, through which the natural rhythmical movements of the pulses are carried on; in this way do the internal channels function well. The inner vitality, the breath - which protects the body, and the blood, which provides it activity, rise and fall cyclically about fifty times in the course of a day. With each complete exhalation there is a rhythmic movement of flow of this energy of approximately three inches, and so also for each inhalation. There are some thirteen thousand five hundred full breathings in and out during the course a one full day and night. In this way, the heart does its work rhythmically and easily. The lungs do not become overheated or weary by ceaseless efforts to keep apace with an overexcited heart. None of the forces which govern the body are worked to exhaustion. And all the processes of life - attaining nourishment, movement, perception, study and enlightenment - are carried on effortlessly. Nor do the six sense organs which depend upon the inner organs become victim to stagnation. The lungs, under the sign of metal, are feminine and are situated above the diaphragm, the liver, under the sign of wood, is masculine and is found below the diaphragm; the heart - fire - and the breath are the sun - the great yang, while below are found the kidneys - rainwater - which is yin. Inside the five organs seven ruling deities are sitting; in both the spleen and the kidneys two gods each reside. Breathing out comes from the heart and lungs, while breathing in comes into the kidneys and liver. The fire is light, and likes to go upwards; the water is heavy and seeks to flow downward. And if you look after them too much, the heart will be too active and the lungs become weak. If the lungs suffer, then the kidneys weaken. If the mother (lungs) and children (kidneys) together are damaged, then all relations of the vital organs experience difficulties and they lose their force; the four elements augment or diminish and a hundred and one illnesses appear. No medicine will succeed, and no salvation is possible, though all the physicians in the world come together on your behalf.

" 'Caring for life is like protecting a nation. Wise kings and holy rulers will, under these conditions, concentrate their concerns on all those beneath them; meanwhile, the unwise kings recklessly give play to their thoughts in the upper regions; but if you only function in the upper regions, then the many noblemen or 'Nine Lords' become too proud and assert their power, the lesser officials draw special attention to themselves and feel dependent only on the force of the King, without looking after the troubles of the people; thus, though the land may look verdant, the people become poor and thin, because hunger and starvation follow. At that time the men of virtue conceal themselves and the simple people become angry and discontented, and one day angrily rebel against the sovereign. Many under the nobles become rebels, and then enemies from without will attack as well. The surrounding barbarians vie for supremacy in pillaging the kingdom, and finally the people will undergo the extremest suffering and the existence of the state and people falls into chaos.

" 'But if the sovereigns concentrate their thoughts on the lower levels, then the nobles live modestly, the officials rest faithful to their promises and do not forget the people. The farmers have abundant harvests, the women much clothing, and many of the wise in the country are attracted to the service of the sovereign. The nobles give respect to the sovereign, there is prosperity for the people, and the state becomes strong. So the people obey the law, and there are no enemies from the outside who attack the frontiers. The officials don't quarrel, and the people know nothing of weaponry in their midst. That is all a portrait of the human body.

" 'The perfect man always lets the heart-energy fill the lower body; when the heart-energy is fulfilled below, the seven evil powers will not become strong: joy, anger, fear, care (worry), musing, sorrow, and fright - and also, the four enemies from without will not attack: cold, heat, moisture and wind. Breathing and circulation of the blood remain strong, and heart and spirit are healthy. Mouth does not know the sweet and acid of medicine, and body need not suffer the pains of acupuncture needles and cautery by moxibustion. But foolish men always let the spirit rule above; and when it thus rises as it likes, the heart will injure the lungs, the inner organs shrivel, and the Six Relatives (senses) suffer and become inharmonious. Therefore, the old Chinese wise man Shitsuyen, says: "The breathing of the true man is breathing from the heels. The breathing of the simple man is breathing from the throat." The Korean doctor Kyoshun says: "If the Ki-spirit is situated just over the bladder, (in the Tanden) breath becomes wide; but if the spirit is sitting above - just under - the heart, then the breath becomes narrow and short."

" 'The Chinese, Joyoshi, says: Only one true spirit is in man. If this is taken down to the Tanden, then a yang power comes to life again. If you begin to know the kindling of this yang power, you will feel warmth. Generally, to care for life, you must keep cool the upper body, and keep warm the lower body.

" 'Then the twelve pulses and the twelve networks of connections between the inner organs will be in harmony with the twelve signs of the zodiac, the twelve months, and the twelve hours of the day, just as the possibilities of the six yang and yin powers fill a whole year after having fulfilled a round. There is a symbol from the book of divinations (I Ching): Above, five negative (yin) forces and below, one positive (yang) force.

— —
— —
— —
— —
— —
———

" 'That means: above is earth, below, thunder, or *thunder in the earth returning*; that is the sign of the living point between winter and summer (the winter solstice), and that means that the breath of the true man is the breathing through the heels. The sign showing above three negative (yin) and below three positive (yang) is the sign of January, or *Earth and Heaven in Harmony*; the seasons when all is imbued with live-giving energy for germination, and a thousand flowers smell of Spring.

```
            — —
            — —
            — —
            ———
            ———
            ———
```

" 'This signifies that the true man gives the fullness of power to the lower body. If you accomplish this, the breath and the blood become strong and powerful. But when below are five negative (yin) and above is one positive (yang), it signifies deprivation, or *Mountain and Earth stripped*; it is the season of September.

```
            ———
            — —
            — —
            — —
            — —
            — —
```

" 'Now mountains and forest lose their colors and the thousand flowers fade. That is the condition of many men who breathe through the throat. In this condition the whole body and the face become dry, the teeth will totter and decay. Therefore, the book *Enjinsho* says: "If all the six yang powers are absent, then men only consist of yin powers, and die easily." That is why you must know that you should always fill the lower part with spirit and power, and this only is the secret of the right care of life.

" 'Once upon a time Go Keisho purified himself and visited the master Sekidai, asking him very politely for the secret technique of distilling the elixir of Tan. The master answered him, 'I know well the holy secret of True Tan. But if one is not of the highest integrity, one must not teach another the secret.' Once Koseki taught it to the Yellow Emperor, Kotei; but for this the emperor cleansed his body during a period of twenty one days and then began respectfully to learn. Beside the Great Way there is no True Tan, and beside the True Tan there is no Great Way.

" 'Now, there is the Method of the Five Laws of ridding oneself of all desires; when you drop all desires and the five senses forget to function, then the whole-in-one power will subtly become manifest. That is why Taikakudoji, the Great White Hermit (or Man of the Way) said: "What I do with my own divine nature, with the spirit of myself, that becomes one with the primal divine nature of sky and earth." And if one concentrates the Great Spirit power in Tanden in the spirit spoken of by Mencius and holds it concentrated and cares for it throughout the months and years, and if one day he will turn out his Tanden, so one will see that inside and outside, the middle and the eight directions of wind, and the four places are a single great One; the one Tanden, oneself, yes, are the great true eternal Holy, which was before heaven and earth and will be after heaven and earth, beyond life and death. With that the Tan-exercise is finished. One becomes not a saint who rides on the winds and mists, flies over the earth great distances and goes easily over water, nor an acrobat, but a saint who stirs the great ocean to milk and changes the earth into gold. But as it has been revealed by the ancient sages, 'The elixir lies below the navel, the secret alchemical fluid is that of the lungs, which is to be taken to the Tanden and transformed into the elixir.' Thus, the teaching is, the liquid of the lungs (metal) is that which circulates in the Tan.'

"And then I said (said Hakuin): 'Reverently have I listened to you. So I shall put away my Zen meditation and endeavor to heal my illnesses. I am afraid only of letting down the heart's fire too far by cooling, as Rishishai says. If one concentrates too much his heart's fire in one place, would not the blood and breath perhaps stagnate?'

" And then Hakuyushi smiled and said, 'No. Did not Rishisai say that the character of the heart's fire (breath) is to mount up? Therefore it must go down, and the water (blood) that goes down by nature, should be permitted to rise. If the water goes up and the fire down, it is called the 'right to-and-fro' (exchange), and if the blending of the two happens in this manner it means: it is extinguished, it has been fulfilled, and if not: unfulfilled. Exchange is the sign of life. No exchange is the sign of death. If the teaching of Rishisai warns of going too far in letting down the heart's fire, he really just means to admonish in the going too far of the letting-down of the heart's fire, which was the error made by the method of Tanken, which cultivated only the water, or yin aspect.

" 'One of these ancients once said: If the minister fire goes up easily, the body will suffer. If the fire is given water, it is regulated. There is a Lord fire and a Minister fire. The Lord fire rules above and reigns over tranquillity (stillness aspect). The Minister fire rules below and reigns over activity (dynamic aspect). The Lord fire is ruler of the heart, the Minister fires are the servants thereof. The functions of the minister fires are of two kinds: that of the kidneys and that of the liver. The liver is compared to the thunder, the kidneys to the dragon. Therefore it is said: If you let the dragon descend into the depths of the ocean, no outbreak of thunder is possible. And if we harbor the thunder in the depths of the ocean, then we will have no suddenly upflying dragon. Sea and lake are both of water-nature; the content of this image reveals the secret of preventing the minister fire from erupting upward. Even once again let it be said: if one suffers exhaustion of heart and has pains, then the heart-fire arises in the vacuum thereof. Therefore, if the heart becomes hot one should let it down and submerge it into the water of the kidneys. This is called the balancing of the heart's fire; that is a way of extinguishing, restoration and true fulfillment (completed perfection).

" 'You, Hakuin, have let the heart's fire up, and therefore you suffer much illness. If you do not let down the heart-fire, you can never become healthy, even though you may know all the human and divine secrets of the world and master them.

" 'Do you imagine that I am a great distance from the Buddha because I look like a Taoist? No, for this is true Zen. If you break through and come to understand this one day, you will break out into a great laughing ("satori": to come to a great laughing).

" 'What can be said of the looking within is this; the not-looking is the right looking. 'Much looking' is the wrong looking. It is by too much looking that you came to such grave illness. Now you must go contrary to the path you have taken to illness by going the way of no-looking. Is it not so? If you now take your heart's fire and your mind's fire together and put them into the Tanden and the middle of the feet, then your breast and diaphragm will become cool by themselves; you will never have any more a shade of speculation or thought, nor a drop of thought's wave or passion's torrent. Don't say: You want to take away Zen! Buddha himself said bringing the heart into the middle of the soles of the feet will heal a hundred and one illnesses. Further, in the Agama Sutra you will find the technique of using the *So* cream for curing exhaustion of the spirit. It helps wonderfully to save one from weariness of heart. In the classic Tendai book 'Maka Shikwan' (Ch'i k'ai's Scripture on Meditation, *Stilling and Contemplating*), not only are the causes of illnesses discussed in great detail, but the methods by which to heal them are very exactly described. It offers twelve methods of breathing by which one can heal illnesses. And it also teaches that this be accomplished by taking certain ideas in mind. So comes the idea of 'child-of-the-navel'; that means to imagine a bean in the middle of the navel. Of greatest importance in the imagination is that the heart's fire descend; that means it is let down into the Tanden and to the center of the soles. This allows one not only to heal illness, but to further the unfolding of the Zen spirit, also.

" 'In the last analysis, there are two kinds of 'Stilling' and 'Meditation' exercises: Keien-Shikan and Taishin-Shikan, the former being the relative method of controlling mental associations, and the latter the absolute method of full awareness of reality. The latter is the perfect looking of truth, the first is concentrating the heart-force in the Kikai Tanden. If the pupil practices the latter, he gains much. Once master Dogen, founder of the temple Eiheiji, went to China during the Sung dynasty and saw the Zen master Nyoyo on the mountain of Tendozan. One day, in the 'Hall of Mysteries', Dogen begged to his master to give him the core of his teaching. The master said to him: "If you are sitting in za-zen put your heart in the palm of your left hand." That's the Keien Shikan (stilling) in one sentence, as taught by Chisha-Daishi in the book 'Sho Shikan' in which he tells how his brother was healed with this method, having been dangerously ill. Chisha-Daishi was the first to teach the secret of 'stilling' and 'meditation' in the context of looking within. By this method he saved Cheshen - one of his students - from the jaws of death. (This is recounted in detail in the Sho-Shi-kwan).

" 'Another one, the great priest Huku-un (1043-1121), taught: "I let fill my soul in the belly; that's my way to do right to other people, to rule them in the right manner, and to receive my guests. In this way I can rule inexhaustibly in both little and large congregations, for which I am the guest. Now, in my old age, the virtue of this practice is clear." Wonderful, wonderful!

" 'Here, in summary, is the teaching from the medical book Somon: "If all one's inner being becomes empty, the true force comes into fullness by itself.' If force and soul would protect the inside, so one must fill the body with them, the three hundred and sixty joints and the eighty-four thousand pores, until not even the tiniest hair lacks. One should know that this is the secret of nurturing life."

" 'Hoso, a saint who became eight hundred years old, said: "To make the spirit harmonious and to bring the force to its full power, one should close oneself in one's room, quietly arrange one's bed, level and warm, compose the pillow, which is to be ten centimeters high in order to lay the body down in the right way, close their eyes, concentrate the heart and the whole of one's spiritual forces in the middle, and place a tiny hair before the nostrils, and see that it is not disturbed by the breath. Already, after three hundred inspirations one comes to the state wherein the ears do not hear and the eyes do not see. In this condition neither cold nor heat will penetrate the body. Also, the sting of bee and scorpion can do no harm to one. This exercise brings one to a great age of three hundred sixty years, and so one comes near to being a saint."

" 'The poet Sonaikian Sotoba, of the College of Literature in China, says: "You only must eat if you are hungry, but before being satisfied, cease eating. Then take a walk until the activity makes the stomach empty. After this has been done, go into your quiet room, sit down in the right manner, and count your breathing mentally, to ten, to a hundred, and then to a thousand. Then the body becomes immovably strong, the soul is silent and remains quiet like an empty sky. If you stay in this condition for a longer time, then the breathing gradually stops; and if there is no more breathing out and breathing in, the breath comes in like clouds and goes out like mist through the eighty-four thousand pores. Then you come clear in such a way that all the illnesses which have existed since begilingless eternity must disappear, and many infirmities and weaknesses dissolve by themselves. It is as if a blind man suddenly can see, and no longer has need to ask another whither to find his way; but must only care for his force without speaking. Therefore you can comprehend this: Who wishes really to nurture the power of the eyes, will close them, and who wishes to nurture the capacity of his ears, is never anxious to hear; who nurtures his soul and the True Force, remains ever in silence."

" After this I interrupted him: 'May I ask you for the method of using the *So*, cream?' Master Hakuyushi replied: 'During the exercise, if you become conscious of a disharmony of the four elements within you, and of a weariness of body and soul, you should focus yourself and imagine the following: A form, as of the egg of a duck, made from *So*, - this fragrant, milk-colored liquid of wonderful clarity - is sitting upon the crown of your head; and then this liquid with the wonderful fragrance and flavor begins to make luminous the whole head, and to run down slowly over the shoulders, the elbows, over the two breasts, over the lungs, liver, stomach, intestines, into the body through the end of the vertebral column and down the entire back, as well. And likewise do the pains and griefs run down. All is cleared away by this liquid, all is eliminated as if having been washed out by flowing water. Really, you can hear this water slowly streaming down, flowing through the body, down to the legs, ending in the soles of the feet.

" 'The pupil shall perform this imagination several times further. If the downflowing *So* accumulates within the body and yields a rich warmth and humidness, then you feel as if an excellent doctor had composed rare, wonderful medicines and herbs and filled a bath in which you warm the lower body up to the navel, simmering in the *So* elixir. Because all depends upon soul and spirit, you smell in your nose a wondrously indescribable fragrance, and the body feels exquisitely soft, surpassing its state of being even in the prime of youth. A great joy courses within yourself because body and heart are in harmony. You feel much better than one of twenty or thirty years of age. At this time all maladies and griefs will dissolve, having so long accumulated, stomach and inner organs are harmonized, and the skin shines. If you continue practicing it further, there is not a single malady that may not be healed. What manner of virtue may not be collected? What manner of practice may not be mastered? You even enter upon the way ofperfection. How rapidly one obtains success depends upon the diligence of the pupil.

" 'When I was young, I was often ill, ten times more than you; all doctors had abandoned me, and not one of hundreds of methods which they tried succeeded. Therefore I had begged all the gods and Buddhas, all divinities, all the saints of heaven and earth for secret help, and by their grace, what fortune to come unexpectedly upon the method of *So*. An incredible joy arose in me; I practiced diligently, and in a month most of my illnesses disappeared. Since then I have felt light and tranquil in body and soul. As I practiced ceaselessly, like a stupid man, unmindful of the rising and setting of the moon or the passing of the years, thoughts of the world became fainter and fainter. Desires I once possessed, and such as men have today are forgotten. How old I am I do not know. In the middle of my life I was in the mountains of the province of Wasakas for about thirty years, unseen and forgotten by the world; and if I look back on this period it seems like a the dream of Koryan, in which one had dreamed a whole lifetime in just half an hour, arising and returning. And now I sit in these unpeopled mountains and I have cast free this withered vessel of a body. Though covered by but a few rough clothes, and even with the strong cold of winter penetrating these clothes, it cannot chill these wizened insides. For food, often there is nothing to eat for some months when the grain comes to an end, yet I never feel cold or hunger. What is this but the power of Naikan - the fruit of this practice of looking within? Now I have told you the secret, whose mysterious essence you shall never exhaust, ever and ever, all your life. Apart from this, what more can I say?'

"Now Hakuyushi closed his eyes and lapsed into silence. Tears in my eyes, I bowed. Then I began the backward journey, descending from the mouth of the cave, and down the mountain. Beyond the peaks shone the evening sun. Suddenly I heard the echo of a scuffling noise of sandalled footsteps. Very astonished, I looked back and in the distance I saw Hakuyushi, who had left his cave to see me home. Then he called to me, 'This mountain is seldom used. You can barely distinguish east and west. The guest will easily lose his way, so I myself will guide you in the right direction.'

"He went on his big, high clogs, and on a thin stick, over steep ledges and dangerous paths, as easily as he would go in a public street. He spoke and laughed and went before me, until we reached a distance of two kilometers, above a brook which I would thence ford, and there Hakuyushi said: 'If you follow this flowing stream, you will surely come to the White River valley of the village of Shirakawa.'

"Sorrow in my heart, I parted from him. I stood for some time, like a lone tree, and watched Hakuyushi going back. The old man slipped over the earth like a saint who receives wings and flies through the sky, leaving the human world behind. At the same time, I felt a longing and an awe within me, and to the end of my days I would regret not being able to spend my life following such a man.

"But then I slowly returned and practiced Naikan - inward-looking - in secret. After three years, my old illnesses were as if extinguished, without acupuncture, moxibustion or medicine. And not only were the illnesses healed, but so also were many incredible, impenetrable, indissoluble and inaccessible things made to become transparent - which I never achieved with various other approaches. Now, following the root and penetrating to the bottom, I had many experiences of great joy, and uncounted experiences of little joys. As says Master Mayoki: 'I had a grand satori eighteen times, and had innumerable small satoris.'

"Finally, for my part, I know that this revelation from Myoki does not deceive. It is true. In earlier times I dressed in two or three pairs of socks, but always my feet felt like ice; and now I wear no socks, even in the strongest winter I need no stove. I'm beyond seventy years of age and never ill. This is the success of this holy-divine method.

"Don't say, a half dead old geezer of Shoinji, has, in his final delirium, writen such nonsense and now seduces reputable people with it. What I wrote down was not written for the gifted who have won satori in one masterful attempt. It is done for the doubtful ones who are stupid, as I was, and who have already created both illnesses and cures, as I had. If such people read this and practice carefully, they will without doubt be helped. My only misgiving is that this will come into the hands of scoffing outsiders; then there will come a great laughing, and a noisy clapping of hands. When the horse munches the dried straw, it disturbs the midday siesta, and that is annoying if one wants to sleep at midday."

Recorded in the Horeki era (1757) the year of the Ox of the Hi-no-to in-signia, on the twenty-fifth day.
(The day entitled Hei, Shepherd's Purse) (14th March, 1757)

Reference:
From the Japanese by Karlfried Graf von Durckheim, from the German by Nikki Hanus, 1970. Revised by Joseph Marcello, 1999.

References

Chan, Luke, *101 Miracles of Natural Healing*, Benefactor Press, 1996. *Chi-Lel™ News*, various issues, 1996 - 1999.

Jin, Xiaoguang, *Personal Letter*, 1998.

Jung, Carl G., (Commentary by), *The Secret of the Golden Flower*, Harcourt Brace & Co., NY, 1962.

Montgomery, Ruth, *Born To Heal*, Coward, McCann & Geoghegan, NY, 1973.

Pang, Ming, *Introduction to Zhineng Qigong Science*, International Culture Publishing Company, August, 1994. (in Chinese)

Pang, Ming, *Fundamentals of Zhineng Qigong Science -The Hunyuan Entirety Theory*, International Culture Publishing Company, August, 1994. (in Chinese)

Pang, Ming, *Essences of Zhineng Qigong Science*, International Culture Publishing Company, August, 1994. (in Chinese)

Pang, Ming, *Practice Methodology of Zhineng Qigong Science*, International Culture Publishing Company, August, 1994. (in Chinese)

Pang, Ming, Technology *of Zhineng Qigong Science - Superintelligence*, International Culture Publishing Company, August, 1994. (in Chinese)

Weisenburger, Debra, *Chi-Lel™ News*, Vol. 1, Issue 3, October, 1996.

For further information about Chi-Lel™, including books, audio and videotapes, seminars and workshops, contact:

Benefactor Press
9676 Cinti-Columbus Road
Cincinnati, OH 45241
Telephone: 513-777-0588
Fax: 513-755-5722
Toll free: 1-800-484-6814

For further information about Zhineng Qigong contact:

Office of International Training
Huaxia Zhineng Qigong Recuperating Center
Zicaowu, Fengren County, Tangshan City
Hebei Province, P.R. China
Postcode: 064000
Telephone: 86-315-5115735
Fax: 86-315-5115733

Or

General Office
Beijing Shunyi Qigong Intelligence Science Center
Long Wan Tun, Ding Jia Zhuang, Shunyi County
Beijing, The People's Republic of China
Postcode: 101300
Telephone: 86-10-60462482

Glossary

Chigong: An ancient and contemporary practice for the improvement and enhancement of physical and spiritual health.

Chigongology: A body of knowledge explaining the theory and practice methods of chigong.

Soaring Crane Form: The former first-level practice of Zhineng Qigong.

Hunyuan: To form a new oneness by blending and transmuting two or more pre-existing substances.

jing: The essence, the body.

jingluo: The main and collateral chi channels, the networks of chi channels.

Lao Shi: Teacher.

Neiqiu: Inner perception.

Qi **(chi):** The most basic and vital, formless and invisible source matter in the universe.

shen: Spirit, consciousness, mind.

Superintelligence: Extraordinary or special abilities, supersensory perceptions.

xing: Body.

Yuanjing: The vital essence.

Yuanqi: The vital chi.

Yuanshen: The vital spirit.

Zishi Gong: International practice, twice a month (the fifteenth and last nights by Chinese Lunar Calendar), from 10:30 PM-12:00 Midnight (Beijing Time).

Zuchang Fa: A method for establishing and building up a chi field for group teaching and healing

Index

Authors' Biographies

MING PANG

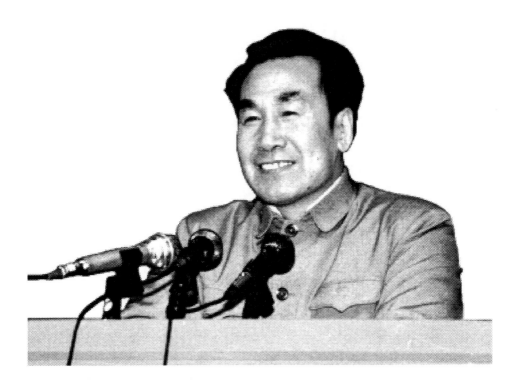

Birth and Childhood

Pang Ming (Pang Heming) was born in 1940. His ancestral home is in Dingxing County, Hebei Province. The originator and founder of Qigong Science, Ming Pang's development was nurtured and influenced by Traditional Chinese Medicine, especially acupuncture, as well as qigong and the martial arts, the practice of which he commenced in early childhood, and which subsequently continued under the tutelage of 19 Grandmasters.

Training and Development

After several years of study he received a diploma from Beijing Medical Training School, working at a clinic in a factory in Beijing. While not holding the degree of a medical doctor (M.D.), he has had some training in Traditional Chinese Medicine and also in Western medical practice (as it is taught in China). He possesses an extraordinary capacity for self-training and self-instruction. Due to his profound aptitude in the cultivation of qigong he learned extremely rapidly, reading books not word by word, but page by page, absorbing dozens of books a week.

Trials and Achievements

During the Great Cultural Revolution he came under scrutiny and was eventually dismissed from the clinic and sent for "physical reformation"- a political persecution that was undergone by all intellectuals in China in the 1960's. In the 1970's, he became a well-known expert in Beijing in both Traditional Chinese Medicine and Western medicinal practice. As an acupuncturist, he treated both ordinary workers and various high-ranking officials.

Commitment and Transformation

In June 1976, the decision was made to give up his medical career and to devote himself fully to qigong, as well as to the formulation of the Hunyuan Theory, but for many reasons this did not become a reality at the time. At the Day University of Beijing Haidian District, The Department of the Orient Qigong for Health, he was employed as an Associate Professor teaching qigong. In June 1981, he was wrongfully persecuted a second time, at which point he left the realm of qigong teaching and research and over the next three years devoted himself to self-cultivation at the Tanjue Temple in the Fragrant Mountain. After these three years of solitary practice he achieved remarkable ability. When he returned to the world of qigong again, he did so as a Grandmaster, and the founder of a new school of thought and science. Without this isolated three-year period of extremely painstaking self-cultivation (much like the six-year cultivation of the Buddha before his awakening), it is certain that he would not have founded what is now known by the name of Zhineng Qigong Science. The former initial practice level of Zhineng Qigong - the Soaring Crane Form - in some ways constituted a premature practice, due to the incidence of spontaneous and uncontrolled reactions on the part of its practitioners. But the later practice disciplines are much safer due to the fact that, after his three-year period of cultivation, Ming Pang had reached an extraordi-